THE MURDERER AND
HIS VICTIM

THE MURDERER AND HIS VICTIM

SECOND EDITION

By

JOHN M. MACDONALD, M.D.

Professor of Psychiatry
and
Director of Forensic Psychiatry
University of Colorado Health Sciences Center
Denver, Colorado

With a Chapter by

Stuart Boyd, Ph.D.

Tutor
St. Johns College
Santa Fe, New Mexico

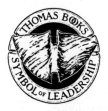

CHARLES   C   THOMAS   •   PUBLISHER
Springfield   •   Illinois   •   U.S.A.

Published and Distributed Throughout the World by

CHARLES C THOMAS • PUBLISHER

2600 South First Street

Springfield, Illinois 62717

© *1986 and l961 by* CHARLES C THOMAS • PUBLISHER

ISBN 0-398-05205-0 (cloth)

ISBN 0-398-06254-4 (paper)

Library of Congress Catalog Card Number: 85-24686

First Edition 1961

Second Edition 1986

Printed in the United States of America

Q-R-3

Library of Congress Cataloging in Publication Data

Macdonald, John M. (John Marshall), 1920-
   The murderer and his victim.

   Includes bibliographies and index.
   1. Murder. 2. Criminal psychology. I. Boyd,
Stuart, II. Title. [DNLM: 1. Criminal Psychology.
2. Homicide. .II. ....]
HV6515.M2 1986   364.1'523   85-24686
ISBN 0-398-05205-0. — ISBN 0-398-06254-4 (pbk.)

PREFACE

MURDER COMPELS attention and seldom a month passes without publication of a book on some sensational case of murder or mass murder. Books which provide a comprehensive report on this crime are less often encountered. The aims of this book are to review the origins and circumstances of murder; to explore the mind of the murderer, his repeated return to the scene of his crime, and his strange compulsion to confess. The victims, criminal investigation, punishment, and prevention of murder are also considered.

Psychiatric examination of over 400 murderers forms the basis of my personal experience. These murderers ranged from eleven to eighty years of age, and over thirty had committed more than one murder. One man alone had killed forty-four persons. These men, women and children provided numerous illustrative case histories that are used in this book. Attendance at over fifty homicide scenes immediately following the homicide in the company of homicide detectives provided additional insights into the ultimate crime.

This second edition has undergone extensive revision. New topics include research of the Behavioral Science Unit of the FBI Academy on crime scene and profile characteristics of organized and disorganized murderers, fantasy role playing games and homicide, the multiple personality, recent serial murderers, and a new chapter on the criminal investigation of murder. References additional to those articles or books quoted in the text are given in some chapters. These references have been selected because they contain original contributions or comprehensive reviews.

In preparing this book I have kept in mind the warning of Doctor Samuel Johnson that what is written without effort is in general read without pleasure. The enigma of murder will, I hope, compensate for any deficiencies in style.

ACKNOWLEDGMENTS

I WISH TO THANK many physicians, law enforcement officers, lawyers and criminal offenders who have helped me in one way or another. Doctors George I. Ogura, George E. Thomas, Seymour Z. Sundell, and Kathy A. Morall as well as Craig L. Truman, Attorney at Law, were most helpful. Dr. Doris Gilbert provided information on Jack Chester.

Police Chief Thomas E. Coogan of the Denver Police Department has continued to provide the generous cooperation and assistance which I received for many years from his predecessor, Arthur G. Dill. Division Chief, Investigative Division, Donald B. Mulnix, Commander Crimes Against Persons, Bureau, Captain Douglas A. White as well as Lieutenants James J. Fitzpatrick and Gary K. Walter were all most helpful.

I am particularly indebted to those detectives who served in the homicide detail during the last three years. It was a valuable learning experience to stand alongside them at homicide scenes and at the morgue; to watch their interviews and to listen to their discussions. Thank you Lieutenant David L. Michaud, Sergeant Thomas P. Haney, and Detectives Steven L. Antuna, Russel Brooks, James Burkhalter, Peter Diaz, Raymond P. Estrada, Donald A. Gabel, F. Gene Guigli, Ervin L. Haynes, Kirk Hon, George B. Kennedy, Richard E. Pennington, James A. Rock and, last but not least, John D. Wyckoff who has served longer in the homicide detail than any of his colleagues.

FBI Special Agents Donald A. Gunnarson, Neal W. Fore, Brian Jovic, Donald W. Lyon Jr. and William H. Matens have extended many courtesies over the years. I attended an excellent four day seminar on psychological profiling of criminal offenders taught by Special Agents William Hagmaier and Ronald P. Walker of the Behavioral Science Unit of the FBI Academy. The responsibility for any statements regarding the work of the FBI is solely mine, except for direct quotations from articles by special agents published in the *FBI Law Enforcement Bulletin*.

My thanks are due to many authors and publishers who have permitted reproduction of material. Permission to quote at length is greatly appreciated. For copyright purposes, the source of quotation has been listed, unless otherwise requested, under author, title and publisher in the references. Permission of the Controller of Her Britannic Majesty's Stationery Office has been obtained to quote from official reports.

This is the fourth book that Mrs. Carolyn Zwibecker has typed for me and, as always, she has been most skillful and remarkably tolerant of unreasonable requests. She has also made many useful suggestions.

CONTENTS

THE MURDERER AND
HIS VICTIM

CHAPTER 1

THE PROBLEM OF MURDER

"For I must talk of murders, rapes and massacres
Acts of black night, abdominable deeds."

Shakespeare, *Titus Andronicus*

EATH as the Psalmist saith is certain to all. Life itself is but the shadow of death, and death has so many doors to let out life. Murder, as a cause of death, attracts attention out of all proportion to its statistical significance. The tragedy of death from criminal homicide arouses, in all of us, hate and fear. These emotions are inflamed by exposure to a constant procession of murderers and their victims across the pages of our newspapers. Reports of murder repel and yet fascinate the reader. Fascination with this morbid subject remains yet unsatisfied and murder, as a literary theme, competes in popularity with its frequent companion — sexual deviation.

The problem of criminal homicide may be approached from several viewpoints. The policeman is concerned with the detection of the murderer, the discovery of clues and the subtleties of criminal interrogation. The District Attorney seeks the execution of justice, and perhaps the defendant as well, with one eye on the voter if election time is approaching. The defense attorney searches for some legal technicality which will save his client from the gallows. The psychiatrist explores the mind of the murderer and the motives behind the deed. The author's experience includes interviews with over 400 murderers.

The sociologist does not confine himself to the individual offender, but analyzes homicide statistics and considers tensions within society that contribute to this crime. Wolfgang, for example, studied 588 criminal homicides involving 621 offenders in Philadelphia. He noted

3

the locations and times of these crimes, the weapons used, the characteristics of the offenders and the victims, the relationships of the antago-
nists to one another, the circumstances of the crimes, the motives
involved, and what happened later to the offenders.

Wolfgang has suggested that from the subculture of violence in
densely populated areas of cities in the United States come most violent
crimes. A subculture of violence does not define personal assaults as
wrong or antisocial, and quick resort to physical aggression is socially
approved. When a blow of the fist is casually accepted as normal response to certain stimuli, when knives are commonly carried for personal defense, and a homicidal stabbing is as frequent as Saturday
night, then social control against violence is weak (22).

HOMICIDE DEFINED

Homicide is a general term used to describe the killing of one person
by another. Not all homicide is criminal. Lawful homicide includes justifiable and excusable homicide. The executioner who electrocutes the
condemned criminal on the order of a court, and the policeman who
shoots a felon in the lawful course of his duties commit justifiable homicide. Excusable homicide generally includes killing in self-defense and
accidental killings during the commission of lawful acts.

Criminal homicide includes murder and manslaughter. Murder is
defined as the unlawful killing of one human being by another with malice aforethought, express or implied. The meaning of "malice afore-
thought" requires consideration as "the 'malice' may have in it nothing
really malicious; and need never be really 'aforethought,' except in the
sense that every desire must necessarily come before—though perhaps
only an instant before—the act which is desired" (14).

Express malice refers to the actual intent to kill. It matters not if the
actual victim was not the intended victim. Malice is usually implied if
there was intent to inflict great bodily harm; if the act or its omission
was likely to cause great bodily harm; and if the killing occurred during
resistance to lawful arrest or commission of certain felonies.

Many states have divided murder into two degrees according to the
intent, premeditation or deliberation of the offender. The verdict of
murder in the first degree is usually mandatory when the murder occurred during the commission, or attempted commission, of certain
felonies such as rape, arson and robbery.

Manslaughter differs from murder in that there is no malice afore-thought, either express or implied. Voluntary manslaughter refers to an intentional homicide done under conditions of extreme provocation or mutual combat, in which there are mitigating circumstances. Adequate provocation occurs when a husband sees his wife in adultery.

Involuntary manslaughter is the killing of another human being without any intent to do so, by the commission of an unlawful act (e.g., an illegal abortion operation), or the commission of a lawful act in an unlawful manner (e.g, reckless driving). A building contractor is guilty of involuntary manslaughter if, by using defective materials, he constructs a building which later collapses because of his negligence, with fatal outcome.

Whether a person who kills another is found by the jury to have committed murder, manslaughter or excusable homicide sometimes depends as much upon the skill of his attorney as upon the circumstances of the killing. Dean Swift was uncharitable when he wrote in **Gulliver's Travels** that lawyers are "a society of men bred up from their youth in the art of proving, by words multiplied for the purpose, that, white is black and black is white, according as they are paid." Nevertheless, there is some point in Bierce's facetious comment that it makes no great difference to the person slain whether he fell by one kind of homicide or another — the classification is for advantage of the lawyers.

HOMICIDE RATES

The annual homicide rate in the United States increased between 1900 and 1930 when there was a peak of 9.8 homicides per 100,000 population, then the rate declined slowly in the 1940's and 1950's. There was a sharp decline during World War II when millions of young men were serving overseas in the armed services. Between the 1960's and the 1980's the homicide rate increased. There were 5.1 victims of murder and nonnegligent manslaughter per 100,000 population in 1960, 7.8 victims in 1970 and 9.7 victims in 1980 when there were 23,044 homicides.

Southern states have higher homicide rates (13 victims per 100,000 population) than other regions, and metropolitan areas (12 victims) have higher rates than rural areas (7 victims). Metropolitan areas with high rates in 1980 included Miami (32.7 victims), Houston (27.6), Los Angeles (23.3), New Orleans (22.3) and New York (21). In contrast

Boston (5.2), Lincoln, Nebraska (4.7) and Madison, Wisconsin (1.6) had low homicide rates according to **Uniform Crime Reports** of the FBI.

Many foreign countries, such as England, Ireland, France, Germany, and Switzerland to name a few, have much lower homicide rates than the United States. In these countries the rates range from 0.4 to less than two homicides, compared with nine homicides in the United States, per 100,000 population each year. Among the theories advanced to explain the high rates in the United States are the ready availability of handguns, great material wealth in the midst of poverty, the declining influence of the church and religious beliefs, the slow administration of justice compared with the swiftness and certainty of judgment in some other countries, the frontier spirit and a traditional opposition to any legal restriction on individual behavior.

Family disorganization resulting from a high divorce rate and great social mobility may adversely affect personality development of children, but it is difficult to measure its significance with relation to the homicide rate. Certainly many murderers come from broken homes and family discord is a prominent feature in the life history of criminal offenders. Much has been written about the relationship between crime and religion. Miner many years ago found that states with large proportions of church members had on the average lower homicide rates than states with small proportions. Other factors which influence the homicide rate were not taken into consideration. Any study of religion and crime which is based upon statistics of claimed church affiliation is suspect. Church affiliation may bear little relation to church attendance and even the latter is not a reliable measure of religious belief.

William Palmer, the English physician who murdered fourteen persons, was an unremitting church goer and never failed to be in his place on Sundays — and even used to be observed taking notes of the sermon upon the margin of his Bible. "Faith has a heavenly influence" he wrote upon one of these occasions. The human heart is a mystery even to itself, and who shall say whether Palmer was so profoundly and coldly hypocritical that these private notes made in his Bible were all part of his relentless scheme, or whether in that distorted egoism of the true criminal he did not perhaps hope that by certain concessions of his mind to the Deity he might not keep his immortal accounts squared? (12).

The community influences exerted by movies and television, have been held responsible for the increasing incidence of juvenile delinquency and adult criminality through disproportionate attention to morbid sexuality, sadism and crime. The quantity of violence on the television screen is staggering. In one week, mostly in children's viewing time, one station showed 334 completed or attempted killings. The different channels in one large city showed in one week 7,887 acts of violence and 1,087 threats of violence such as "I'll break your legs" (20). It has been estimated that the average American child by the age of fourteen has seen 12,000 killings on television.

Wertham is convinced that the moving visual image on movie or TV screen, complete with sound has a much greater impact on most children than the images they conceive in their own mind's eye from reading a story or having one read to them. When reading a violent story in book form, a child is protected by the limits of his own imagination, to which, in even the grisliest fairy story, something is left. On the screen violence and horror are spelled out. They are so much "realer," as a seven year old told Wertham.

Although some criminals state that they committed their crime after seeing a similar crime on a television show, it is possible that these crimes would have been committed in the absence of such a stimulus. "The devil made me do it" has long been proffered as an excuse for criminal behavior, and the devil may take many forms. Imitative violence captures national attention.

> In October 1973, six youths in Boston set upon a young woman carrying a can of gasoline to her car, forced her to douse herself with the gasoline and then set her afire, burning her to death. This happened two days after the nationwide showing of a movie, **Fuzz**, a police drama set in Boston, which contained a scene portraying teenagers burning a derelict to death "for kicks" (8).

There is much that is to be deplored in television programs and movies, but the extent of their influence on criminal behavior is not clear.

Two public groups, the National Coalition on Television Violence (NCTV) and Bothered About D & D (BADD) have claimed that the popular fantasy role-playing game **Dungeons and Dragons** has been a major factor in causing a number of suicides and homicides. Other critics claim that the game fosters not only violence but also an interest in occult beliefs. Some young persons spend twenty or more hours a week on this hobby. Games continue for many hours but can be interrupted at any time. Some campaigns have continued at regular group meetings for several years.

Each player, but not the Dungeon Master, creates a character by rolling dice to determine the relative strength or weakness of such abilities as intelligence, dexterity, strength and charisma. After each player has decided whether his character will be a fighter, thief, assassin, magic user, cleric or whatever the Dungeon Master assigns the players a task such as rescuing the king's kidnapped daughter from a heavily guarded fortress.

There is no playing board as in chess and **Monopoly,** but each player keeps a character sheet in which he lists his character's skills such as the ability to use special weapons, wear armor, administer poison, cast spells or become invisible. He will also record any increase in power resulting from combat experience. The Dungeon Master usually draws a map of the dungeons for his own information but he does not show it to the players. However he does give the players information from time to time about their present location. He also keeps a list of the monsters, demons, wild animals and mercenaries as well as a record of their skills.

The Dungeon Master's role is to test the skills of his players taking care to avoid making their task either too difficult or too easy. The players through their characters have to cope with the Dungeon Master's fantasy world of missiles, trap doors, monsters and diseases. A character can be struck by insanity due to a mental attack, curse or whatever. The twenty types of insanity include schizophrenia, catatonia, manic-depressive, sadomasochism, homicidal mania and paranoia.

The person with homicidal mania appears completely normal but occasionally he becomes interested in weapons, poisons and other lethal devices. At one to four day intervals he becomes obsessed with the desire to kill. If prevented from killing he will become uncontrollably maniacal and will attack the first person he encounters, but then he falls into melancholia for one to six days before becoming homicidal again (9). Gygax states that the Dungeon Master will have to assume the role of the insane character whenever the madness strikes, for most players will not be willing to go so far.

The outcome of any encounter between a character and a demon, dragon or other opponent is determined by rolling four, six, ten, twelve and twenty sided dice. The Dungeon Master acts as an impartial referee and knows well **The Advanced Dungeons and Dragon Masters Guide,** a book of over 200 pages in small type that contains complex combat tables and much intriguing information. For example, Lizard men who are non-human troops, tend to devour wounded men of either side if not strictly officered at all times. A vampire in gaseous form cannot be harmed by holy water (9). Characters can be killed, but they can be resurrected so the campaigns can continue for years.

In **Villains and Vigilantes,** another role-playing game the character used by the player is himself, with the addition of super-powers to fight crime and protect society. He may have to cope with "Big Bill" Buckford, one of several villains in the Crusher Crimewave Team. "Big Bill" bit the head off his pet dog at the age of six and his personality has not mellowed much since then. After a few years in and out of criminal and mental institutions he nearly murdered his entire family.

After being found unfit to stand trial he escaped from a medium security mental hospital. Bill, who weighs 540 pounds, once threw an elephant at police officers. He attacks any moving red object he sees. Supposedly he hates the color red because he was hit by a red sports car when he was small. Bill was not injured but his ice cream cone and the car that struck him were both demolished. The doctors tried to reattach the driver's lungs, but to no avail (5).

John Holmes, a professor of neurology and practicing Dungeon Master, reports: "The level of violence in this make-believe world runs high. There is hardly a game in which the players do not indulge in murder, arson, torture, rape, or highway robbery." The descriptions of violent persons and monsters in role-playing games have a whimsical quality which softens the violence. Play enables children to master situations and most children play these games without apparent ill effect. Avid players who kill themselves or others may well have psychological problems but these problems may not be the consequence of their game playing.

Homicide or suicide by a teenager is an especially tragic event. In the search for a cause of the tragedy it is easy for parents, family friends and others with a personal relationship to seize upon some untoward event (his best friend moved elsewhere or braces were put on his teeth that day) or time consuming involvement in some questionable activity (going out with the "wrong crowd," taking LSD, or playing fantasy games).

Such simple explanations deflect search for deeper causes of social isolation, lack of confidence, uncertainty about choice of occupation, or conflicts over sexual impulses. All too often the origins of an adolescent's despair are locked within his heart and he may not himself be aware of all the sources of his anguish.

HOMICIDE AND ALCOHOL

Homicide is frequently committed by persons who have taken alcohol prior to the crime. The role of alcohol as a cause of homicide is, however, difficult to evaluate. Although it is often stated that alcohol is a frequent cause of homicide, it should be noted that many offenses are assumed to be due to alcohol on insufficient grounds. It would be more accurate, in the light of available information, to say that homicide is commonly associated with indulgence in alcohol. Indulgence in alcohol does not, however, commonly lead to homicide. Excessive consumption of alcohol and homicidal behavior may have the same root cause in psychological conflict.

Wolfgang found that either or both the victim and the offender had been drinking immediately prior to the slaying in nearly two thirds of 588 homicides in Philadelphia. Offenders had been drinking in 54 percent and victims in 52 percent of the homicides. Alcohol was a factor strongly related to the violence with which an offender kills his victim. He noted that alcoholic indulgence by either the victim, the offender, or both, was much higher in weekend murders, than in those occurring during other days in the week. He also found a significantly higher proportion of murders occurred at weekends and suggested a possible association between alcohol, weekend slayings and the payment of wages on Friday.

The percentage of murderers taking alcohol prior to the crime in various cities is as follows: Memphis 86 percent, Columbus 83 percent, Chicago 55 percent, Helsinki 66 percent and Glasgow, Scotland 55 percent (10). Shupe reported the urine alcohol concentrations of thirty murderers who were arrested immediately after the crime. He found that 83 percent had been drinking at the time of the murder.

HOMICIDE AND DRUGS

In a study of 110 men charged with first degree murder in Missouri, Holcomb and Anderson found that 36 percent had abused drugs prior to the crime. Those who took drugs, alcohol, or both, had a greater likelihood of overkilling the victim. Kozel and DuPont checked the urinalysis data on over 9,000 persons arrested in Washington, D.C. Almost 25 percent of these persons had drug positive urines for heroin or for methadone. Those whose urine tested positive for heroin accounted for 9.7 percent of all homicides. In Philadelphia homicide was the leading cause of death among drug users, higher even than deaths due to the adverse effects of drugs (23).

Major drug abusers are not usually singled out for their scrupulous observance of the ten commandments, but even among major drug abusers there is some recognition that speed freaks (amphetamine abusers) in their behavior are likely to go over the edge. Their tendency to become extremely paranoid makes them dangerous associates. Ellinwood has described the histories of thirteen persons who committed homicide while intoxicated with amphetamines. Murders have been committed by persons under the influence of other drugs, especially LSD (acid) and PCP (angel dust). Paranoid beliefs, wild excitement and loss of pain perception are a dangerous combination in persons who have taken PCP.

Drug dealers and drug abusers contribute to the incidence of criminal homicide not only through acts of violence while under the influence of illicit drugs. Millions of dollars in profits are made from the sale of drugs and those who interfere with this trade do so at some risk. The dealer who sells poor quality drugs, the addict who fails to pay for his drugs, the snitch who provides information to the police, the person suspected of being an informant, and drug enforcement officers, especially in Sicily and Colombia can all become victims of homicide.

In large cities competition between gangs for control of sales and "copping corners" has been associated with a significant number of homicides, including many execution style slayings. In 1984 the Peruvian government temporarily halted a program financed by the United States to destroy coca leaves after nineteen men working on an erradication program were massacred.

THE CIRCUMSTANCES OF MURDER

In the United States about 40 percent of homicides involve disagreements between acquaintances, friends and neighbors. About 20 percent of homicides involve killings within the family. One half of these family killings are spouse killing spouse. About 10 percent of homicides occur during a robbery and another 10 percent occur during other felonies such as narcotics offenses, sex offenses, arson and other crimes.

THE SCENE OF THE CRIME

"The very air rests thick and heavily
Where murder has been done."

Joanna Baillie, *Orra*

More slayings occur in the home than outside the home. Men kill and are killed most frequently in the street, while women kill most often in the kitchen, but are killed most often in the bedroom (22). In both Philadelphia and Baltimore the most dangerous single place is on the highway — public street, public alley or field (28 to 30 percent of homicides). The most dangerous room in the house is the bedroom (19 to 20 percent), followed by the kitchen and living room which are equally dangerous (8 to 12 percent). Taverns are also a frequent place for homicides (8 to 9 percent).

Murder is more likely to occur in poor, densely populated, deteriorating city neighborhoods. Of 2,389 homicides in Chicago, 495 (21 percent) occurred in an area of 375 blocks. Thus, two percent of the blocks of Chicago accounted for 21 percent of the homicides. The blocks where these homicides occurred are among the most economically depressed areas of the city (3).

MURDER ON WEEKENDS AND HOLIDAYS

Weekends and public holidays are the main times for murder. For the most part homicide occurs during leisure time and is frequently associated with recreational activities. Drinking is often a factor in crimes of personal violence and Saturday night is the traditional time of the drinking spree. Homicide is generally committed against persons with whom one has personal feelings — friends, family members, lovers, acquaintances — and opportunities for personal contacts are much greater during leisure time.

Several studies have shown that homicide reaches a peak on Friday and Saturday nights. Almost two thirds of 588 criminal homicides in Philadelphia occurred between 8 PM Friday and midnight Sunday. In Baltimore 27 percent of 578 homicides occurred on Saturday nights. Throughout the week the most dangerous hours are between 8 PM and 2 AM accounting for almost 50 percent of homicides in Philadelphia. The least dangerous period of the day is between 8 AM and 2 PM. Only nine percent of homicides in Philadelphia occurred during these hours.

Depressed murderers have a noticeable tendency to murder between 6 AM and 8 AM. If one excludes such obvious exceptions as a burglar who meets a policeman on his way home from a night's work, or a man who has been drunk and quarrelling all night, one can say that murder at breakfast time is nearly always the act of the insane, or by a man so weighed down by circumstances that he is seriously ill mentally (7).

SEASONAL VARIATIONS IN HOMICIDE

In the United States homicides tend to be more frequent in the summer than in the winter, but there are usually more murders in December than in any other month of the year. The occurrence in Seattle many years ago of more homicides in winter than in summer was attributed to the distress and disorder among the large numbers of migratory seasonal workers who made the city their headquarters during cold weather (18).

If the seasons do affect the distribution of homicide, they probably do so indirectly, through their effect upon the social behavior of people. Thus, climatic conditions may be important, but for their social rather than their biological significance. As Howard Jones points out "The dark nights of winter in the northern hemisphere are very convenient aids to the thief or the burglar. Winter is also a time when nature is niggardly. Then, if at all, there will be high prices and material privation. The economic privation is likely to be at its strongest during the darkest months of the year. The light and (at least relatively) warm months of the summer, on the other hand, facilitate social intercourse. It is easier to meet people — and to fall out with them. The location of the main annual holiday during the summer tends to the same end."

COMMUNITY ATTITUDES TOWARD MURDER

Criminal homicide usually arouses an immediate aggressive response in society, especially if the victim is a child, a woman or a crippled person; if there are several victims or if the circumstances of the deed show great cruelty. Absence of remorse on the part of the slayer adds to the public indignation. On the other hand if the victim has a bad reputation, for example, as a criminal or as a brutal alcoholic husband the community may show considerable sympathy for the slayer. Many years ago in a Western state the dismembered body of a wealthy but extremely unpopular landlord was found in his own home. Although the trunk of the body was found in one room and the severed head in another room, the coroner's jury returned a verdict of death from natural causes.

An active newspaper campaign in support of the accused person may lead to substitution of manslaughter for murder charges by a vote conscious district attorney or may influence a jury to return a verdict of not guilty in spite of overwhelming evidence to the contrary. Newspapers in the United States also publish information which may prejudice the defendant in his later trial. Trial, or rather pretrial, by newspaper, which is so common in the United States, is not permitted in England. In 1949 an English newspaper published lurid stories of a man awaiting trial for murder but did not mention his name; nevertheless the identity of this man was obvious and it was possible that the newspaper reports might have prejudiced his defense. Three weeks later the company owning the newspaper was fined $28,000 and the editor was sent to prison for three months. The Lord Chief Justice ordered the directors of the newspaper into court and warned them — "In the opinion of the court what had been done was not the result of an error of judgment, but was done as a matter of policy in pandering to sensationalism for the purpose of increasing the circulation of the newspaper. Let the directors beware; they know now the conduct of which their employees are capable, and the view which the court takes of the matter. If for the purposes of increasing the circulation of their paper they should again venture to publish such matter as this, the directors themselves may find that the arm of this court is long enough to reach them and to deal with them individually."

Rebecca West has commented that if a gentleman were arrested carrying a lady's severed head in his hands and wearing her large intestine as a garland round his neck and crying aloud that he and he alone, had been responsible for her reduction from a whole to parts, it would still be an offense for any newspaper to suggest that he might have had any connection with her demise until he had been convicted of this offense by a jury and sentenced by a judge.

COMMUNITY REACTIONS TO AN UNUSUAL CASE OF MURDER

The following report by Arndt of community reactions to an unusual case of murder is of particular interest.

During late November, 1957, in a small Wisconsin farming community, Mrs. Bernice Worden disappeared from her general store. Blood stains were found on the floor. The last entry in her sales book was for antifreeze. Police investigations and inquiry as to her last customers led the sheriff to the farm of the 51 year old bachelor recluse, Ed Gein (the name rhymes with "wean"). The sheriff's visit to the Gein farm exposed bizarre activities which drew a horrified but fascinated press to document the news to the country.

Mrs. Worden was shot by Gein with a .22 rifle, was decapitated, eviscerated, and hung by the heels from a rafter in his "summer kitchen." During the questioning, Gein confessed to the 1955 murder of Mary Hogan, a tavern keeper in a nearby town, and to robbing fresh graves (only female bodies) in the local cemetery over a period of several years. One of the corpses was removed from a grave adjacent to his mother's burial plot.

Portions of viscera, sections of human skin, a box of noses and remains of extremities were found in the trash-littered, dingy rooms of his home. Ten human skulls neatly arranged in a row, books on anatomy, embalming equipment, pulp magazines, furniture upholstered with skin, and dirty kerosene lamps completed the macabre scene. Gein also stated he made belts and purses from skin sections. The largest piece of skin found, neatly rolled, was from an anterior chest, including the mammaries.

An immaculate portion of the house, his mother's bedroom and sitting room, had been sealed off by nailed doors and windows after her death in 1945.

Ed Gein was described as a relatively quiet, lazy, friendly, good-natured handyman and neighbor who earned his living doing odd jobs. Few people visited him as he was considered "peculiar," "dull-witted" and prone to discuss crimes, especially murders — the mistakes of criminals that exposed them to detection — and women. He did no courting as a youth and had few female friends during the years. Evidently he was accepted as a "town fool."

Although he often gave obvious clues to his bizarre activities — in a local group discussing the disappearance of Mary Hogan he joked, "She's up at the house now" — these were passed off as crude witticisms. When the final crime was uncovered, the body found hanging and dressed as if it were a deer, neighbors recalled that he had frequently given them portions of "venison," although he remarked, while under psychiatric observation, "I've never shot a deer."

Grim jokes about Gein were told throughout Wisconsin. All ages participated in the humor, and before the Christmas holidays, the children were chanting:

"Twas the night before Christmas
And all through the school
Not a creature was stirring
Not even a mule.
The teachers were hung

From the ceiling with care
In hope that Ed Gein
Soon would be there."

Their favorite carol was paraphrased: "Deck the walls with limbs of Mollie."

The humor can be roughly divided into three categories: (1) cannibalism, (2) sexual perversion, and (3) combination of the first two categories.

Cannibalism. Examples of this type of humor are the following:

As he said to some late arriving guests, "Sorry you weren't a little earlier—everybody's eaten."

His telephone number was "O-I-C-U-8-1-2."

Someone asked him how his folks were—he replied "Delicious."

He couldn't operate his farm—all he had left was a skeleton crew.

He used the cremated ashes of his victims to make "Instant People."

One of the favorites in the taverns was to order "Gein Beer"—"That's lots of body but no head."

Sexual Perversion. The following are some examples of this category:

They let him out of the hospital on New Year's Eve—so he could dig up a fresh date.

They say he was real popular with girls—there were always a lot of women hanging around his place.

His girl friend stopped going with him because he was such a cut-up.

As a hearse went by he said: "Dig you later, Baby."

All the women in the area are going to Plainfield for used parts.

They changed the population sign at Plainfield because it "gruesome."

Cannibalism and Sexual Perversion. Illustrations of this category are as follows:

They could never keep him in jail—he'd just draw a picture of a woman on the wall and eat his way out.

He's the author of that article: "I've Had My Fill of Women."

"There was a man named Ed
Who wouldn't take a woman to bed
When he wanted to diddle,
He cut out the middle
and hung the rest in a shed."

Arndt concludes his report by pointing out that the people of Wisconsin chose the mechanism of grim humor to allay the grief and horror aroused by the horrifying crimes of Ed Gein. It might be added that gallows humor serves a similar purpose.

REFERENCES

1. Arndt, G.W.: Community reactions to a horrifying event. *Bull Men Clin, 23*:106, 1959.
2. Bierce, Ambrose: *The Collected Writings of Ambrose Bierce.* New York, The Citadel Press, 1946.
3. Block, Richard: Homicide in Chicago: a nine year study. *J Crim Law, 66*:496, 1975.
4. Criminal Justice Commission. *Criminal Homicides in Baltimore, Maryland, 1960-1964.* Baltimore, 1967 (processed).
5. Dee, Jeff and Herman, Jack: *Crisis at Crusader Citadel.* New York, Fantasy Games Unlimited, 1982.
6. Ellinwood, E.H.: Assault and homicide associated with amphetamine abuse. *Amer J Psychiat, 127*:1170, 1971.
7. Gibbens, T.C.N.: Sane and insane homicide. *J Crim Law, 49*:110, 1958.
8. Group for the Advancement of Psychiatry. *The Child and Television Drama.* New York, Mental Health Materials Center, 1982.
9. Gygax, Gary: *Advanced Dungeons and Dragons; Dungeon Masters Guide.* Lake Geneva, Wisconsin, TSR Inc., 1979.
10. Holcomb, W.R. and Anderson, W.P.: Alcohol and multiple drug use in accused murderers. *Psychol Rep, 52*:159, 1983.
11. Holmes, J.E.: Confessions of a dungeon master. *Psychology Today, 14*(10):84, 1980.
12. Jesse, F.T.: *Murder and Its Motives.* London, Harrap, 1952.
13. Jones, Howard: *Crime and the Penal System.* London, University Tutorial Press, 1956.
14. Kenny, C.S.: *Outlines of Criminal Law.* London, Cambridge University Press, 1947.
15. Kozel, N.J. and DuPont, R.L.: *Criminal Charges and Drug Use Patterns of Arrestees in the District of Columbia.* Rockville, Maryland, National Institute of Drug Abuse, 1977.
16. Macdonald, J.M. and Kennedy, Jerry: *Criminal Investigation of Drug Offenses.* Springfield, Charles C Thomas, 1983.
17. Miner, J.R.: Church membership and the homicide rate. *Human Biology, 1*:562, 1929.
18. Schmid, C.F.: Study of suicides in Seattle. *Social Forces, 4*:745, 1926.
19. Shupe, L.M.: Alcohol and crime. *J Crim Law, 44*:661, 1954.
20. Wertham, Fredric: *A Sign for Cain.* New York, Macmillan, 1966.
21. West, Rebecca: *A Train of Powder.* New York, Viking Press, 1946.

22. Wolfgang, M.E.: *Patterns in Criminal Homicide.* Philadelphia, University of Pennsylvania Press, 1958.

23. Zahn, M.A. and Bencivengo, Mark: Violent death, a comparison between drug users and nondrug users. *Addict Dis, 1*:283, 1974.

CHAPTER 2

THE MURDERER

"Carcasses bleed at the sight of the murderer."
John Burton, *Anatomy of Melancholy*

PHYSICAL APPEARANCE

LOMBROSO, the Italian criminologist, believed that there was a direct relationship between physique and crime. In this viewpoint he was preceded by many artists and authors. East draws attention to the immortal pictures of William Hogarth, the eighteenth-century satirist, illustrating the principles of good and evil in scenes from the lives of the Two Apprentices. The results of Industry and Idleness were forcibly presented by contrasting success and honor in the one with crime and ruin in the other, and the latter in all its ugliness must have impressed those who reflected upon the lessons which the twelve engravings taught. In the nineteenth century the inimitable illustrations of George Cruikshank depicting Fagin, Bill Sikes and other characters in the work of Charles Dickens also emphasized the association of crime and evil-doing with personal ugliness.

Ellis has given a number of examples from literature which relate criminal behavior to physical appearance. When Homer described Thersites as ugly and deformed, with harsh or scanty hair, and a pointed head like a pot that had collapsed to a peak in the baking, he furnished "evidence" as to a criminal type of man. According to the well known story, a Greek physiognomist who examined Socrates' face judged that the philosopher was brutal, sensuous, and inclined to drunkenness; and Socrates declared to his disciples that such, although he had overcome it, was his natural disposition. He was himself a physiognomist, he disliked a certain man who was of pale and dark complexion, such signs, he said, indicating envy and murder. Ellis mentioned the fact that long ago men referred to the organic peculiarities which they believed separated the criminal from the ordinary man and quoted in support among others the proverbs "salute from afar the beardless man and the bearded woman," and "Distrust the woman with a man's voice."

Lombroso described murderers as having cold, glassy eyes, long ears, strong jaws with strongly developed canines and thin lips with a menacing grin. He stated that assassins possess a peculiar face stamped by the seal of a brutal and impassable instinct. Lombroso's theory of the born criminal type with certain physical abnormalities was discredited by Charles Goring who compared 3,000 British criminals with a similar number of nonprisoners including Oxford and Cambridge university students.

Certainly Lombroso's description of the murderer is not supported by the appearance of many persons charged with criminal homicide. Hentig quotes a description of a vicious murderer, "He was about 35 years old, a handsome and upstanding figure of a man, who looked at the world with reposed and pleasant eyes. He was a good looking fellow and one, moreover, whose pale, spiritual face suggested anything but the killer or libertine."

Abrahamsen in his classification of types of murderer, includes murder due to physical inferiority. No less than twenty of 120 sane homicides studied by Gibbens suffered from a fairly marked physical defect, such as heart disease, diabetes, epilepsy, cancer and severe head injury. Another curiosity was that eight were recorded as being 5'1" in height, or less. Quite a number of murderers are timid, resentful and embittered men turning upon their tormentors and killing stronger men — a feature which hardly accords with Hooton's description of the average homicide as being taller and stronger than other offenders. Hill found that thirteen of 105 English murderers sent for electroencephalographic (brain wave) examination had physical deformities, such as deafness, lameness, and paralysis of face and arms. The murderer is much more often the underdog than is usually believed.

AGE

In general those who kill are younger than those who are killed. Wolfgang's analysis of persons involved in the Philadelphia homicides was made by five-year age classifications, according to the mean annual rate per 100,000 for specified age groups. Offenders had their highest rate (12.6) between ages 20 and 24, and their second highest rate (11.9) between ages 25 and 29. As men and women grow older they become less homicidal but more suicidal. Persons 50 years of age and older account for seven percent of those arrested for murder in the United States (8). Women are likely to be offenders at later ages than men.

FEMALE MURDERERS

"Rarely is a woman wicked, but when
she is she surpasses the man."
Italian Proverb

In the United States male criminal homicide offenders outnumber female offenders in the ratio of approximately six to one. The low homicide rate among women as compared with men has been attributed to biological differences. Social factors have also been implicated. Hacker has shown that the male-female crime ratio varies widely in different countries. The female share of the total amount of crime is greatest in those countries where women are most emancipated. It reaches vanishing point in those countries of the East and Middle East, where their social experience is rigorously circumscribed.

Elwin in his study of a primitive Asiatic Indian society reports a low incidence of homicide among Maria women. "The reason . . . is possibly connected with the strong aboriginal belief that it is supernaturally dangerous for a woman to take life. This is the ultimate reason why there are no woman priests for the priest has to offer sacrifice. Maria women are not supposed to kill goats or even chickens. They are not permitted to join in hunting. The only pursuit of the kind which is not taboo to them is fishing — but fish are cold blooded creatures."

Female offenders usually kill their husbands, lovers (heterosexual and lesbian) or children. Infanticide is almost always performed by the infant's mother, usually an unwed girl who wishes to conceal her pregnancy. It is of interest that the number of women arrested for criminal homicide in the United States declined during the war years, possibly because of the absence of husbands or lovers in the armed services.

CRIMINAL RECORDS

"Taking murderers as a class," said one witness to the Royal Commission on Capital Punishment "there are a considerable number who are first offenders and who are not people of criminal tendencies. The murder is in many cases their first offense against the law. Previous to that they were law abiding citizens and their general tenor of life is still to be law abiding." Many other witnesses said the same thing and similar opinions have been widely expressed in other countries.

This viewpoint is not supported by studies in the United States. The Philadelphia data on 621 criminal homicide offenders have shown that 64 percent of offenders have a previous arrest record, that of these 66 percent have a record of offenses against the person, and that of these 73 percent have a record of aggravated assault. Many of the persons previously arrested were convicted, but given relatively light sentences and probably little constructive attention. The facts suggest that homicide is the apex crime — a crescendo built upon previous assault crimes.

MOTIVES FOR MURDER

Thomas Griffiths Wainewright, the journalist critic and wit, whose circle of literary friends included Charles Lamb, Coleridge and De Quincey, was asked why he killed such an innocent and trustful creature as Helen Abercrombie. After a moment's reflection he replied, "Upon my soul I don't know, unless it was because she had such thick legs."

Wolfgang found that among 621 criminal homicide offenders the most frequent motive was an altercation of relatively trivial origin such as an insult, curse or jostling (36.6 percent). Domestic quarrel (13.4 percent), jealousy (11.1 percent) and altercation over money (10.3 percent) together accounted for over a third of the cases and were followed by robbery (7.9 percent), revenge (4.8 percent), accidental (4.5 percent), self-defense (1.3 percent), other (7.1 percent) and unknown (3.1 percent).

Thus, in eight of every ten cases the police recorded motives were a vaguely defined altercation, domestic quarrel, jealousy, argument over money and robbery. As Wolfgang noted, underlying causes and unconscious motives usually lie beyond the realm of police investigations. Psychological factors in homicide will be reviewed in Chapter 5, madness in Chapter 9, character disorder in Chapter 10 and mental retardation below.

MENTALLY RETARDED MURDERERS

"Him have the gods given wisdom,
Neither as a digger nor as a ploughman,
Neither in aught whatsoever."

Homer

Mentally retarded persons seldom commit murder, however when the mental retardation is coupled with defects in temperament and character, control over homicidal impulses is weakened. Parental rejection, erratic discipline, lack of understanding and physical handicaps such as obesity or poor vision aggravate feelings of inferiority and may lead to explosive outbursts of rage. Crude sexual offenses or murder may be committed as lightly as some minor deception (15). Aggression may be directed toward more talented brothers and sisters or toward some chance acquaintance as in the following tragedy.

When the bodies of two small boys were found at the foot of a perpendicular 175 foot cliff on the south side of Castle Rock near Golden, Colorado, it was assumed that they were the victims of an accidental fall from the mountain top. The coroner decided that no inquest was necessary as the deaths were clearly accidental. Later police investigation, however, revealed that they had been hurled off the cliff top to their deaths by a sixteen year old mentally retarded youth. He had been placed on probation a year earlier for auto theft, was unemployed and tended to associate with much younger children. His general social adjustment was poor.

He had met the two boys, aged eight and eleven, while climbing the mountain on a Saturday afternoon. On the mountain top he decided that the older boy's shoes would fit his younger brother, whose shoes had gaping holes in the soles. He made the older boy take off his shoes and stockings and he took the boy's cheap wristwatch which he wanted for himself. According to the sheriff, "The accused seized the older boy by both wrists, pulled him to the edge of the cliff, then put both hands on the boy's shoulders and shoved him into space. The boy screamed for help while hurtling to the rock ledge below. The other boy meanwhile watched, petrified. He, too, was seized, dragged to the edge and pushed off."

The slayer told the sheriff he killed the boys so that they wouldn't be able to tell that he had robbed them of a pair of shoes, stockings and a watch. Seemingly insensitive to the situation, he displayed no remorse.

He demonstrated with his heel against the jail floor how his victims dug
their heels into the unyielding rock as they tried to resist being pushed to
the edge. Psychological tests confirmed that he was mentally retarded
with an IQ of 62. He was sentenced to life imprisonment.

James T. Straffen at the age of eleven was committed by a Juvenile
Court to a residential school for mentally retarded children. He was discharged from the school at the age of sixteen but was arrested a year later for burglary. It was disclosed at the trial, that in order to spite a girl
friend with whom he was displeased, he had wrung the necks of five
chickens belonging to her parents. He had also assaulted a thirteen year
old girl, and told her "What would you do if I killed you? I've done it before." The girl escaped injury. Once again he was committed to an institution where he remained for four years.

Within six months of his release at the age of twenty-one he strangled
a five year old girl, who was gathering flowers in a meadow. He also
bashed her head against a stone "because she did not scream." Less than
a month later he strangled a nine year old girl. Statements he made to
the police suggested that his motive was to spite the police. Neither girl
had been sexually assaulted.

A psychiatrist reported that Straffen was mentally retarded (IQ 64)
with little or no moral sense. Straffen felt no more emotion in killing
girls than a normal person would in killing a fly. He showed no regret or
remorse, but rather took pleasure and pride in speaking of his delinquent actions. At trial on a charge of murder he was found insane and
committed to Broadmoor Security Hospital. Within six months he escaped and it was four hours before he was recaptured.

During his short period of liberty he murdered a five year old girl.
When the police asked him about his activities while outside the institution, he replied that he did not kill the little girl on the bicycle. A highly
incriminating statement, as no one had told him about the crime. Although Straffen had been found insane by reason of mental defect at his
first trial for murder he was found sane at this trial and was sentenced to
death. The sentence was later commuted to one of imprisonment.

SADISTIC MURDERERS

The sadist delights in cruelty and may gain sexual excitement from
inflicting pain and humiliation on others. The sadistic murderer is
almost invariably a man but the female offender is no slouch in her

exercise of cold, pitiless cruelty. These persons who seem driven to maim or kill over and over again figure prominently in the ranks of serial murderers. Their indifference to the suffering of others enables them to take part in acts of mass murder. Long periods in a penitentiary or a mental hospital do not seem to turn them away from their homicidal inclinations. While in custody their behavior is without reproach and their custodians are too often deceived by this unreliable predictor of dangerousness.

Sadism is not confined to any single psychiatric disorder and may occur in antisocial, schizoid and obsessive personalities, in schizophrenia and indeed in persons who do not seem to have any psychological abnormality apart from their sadistic behavior. Sadistic murderers do not come from a single mold nor do they always behave alike apart from their cruelty and their need to show their power over others. Nevertheless it is useful to review some of the features that may be encountered.

There is no consistent pattern of parental behavior but there may be a stern, overly punitive father and a promiscuous, seductive or domineering mother. Parental rejection, if present, may extend to giving up for adoption all the children, or perhaps just one child is discarded. At every step in the description of the sadist and his background it should be emphasized that other persons with similar life experiences may lead lives of Christian charity. The possible psychological effects of various child-parent relationships will be discussed in Chapter 5.

The sadist's childhood may include a history of bedwetting, repeated enemas for no clear reason, firesetting which extends beyond playing with matches or accidental fires to a fascination with fire and repeated acts of arson. Extreme cruelty to animals can include disembowelling a pet rabbit or pouring gasoline on a dog and setting it alight. Skillful questioning may be necessary to elicit this information which too often remains forever a family secret.

Abnormal sexual development shows itself in possession of quite remarkable collections of pornographic magazines and pictures, especially pictures showing a terrified woman, tied hand and foot, at the mercy of her assailant; pornographic paraphernalia; women's clothing especially panties which may have been slashed with a knife, wigs and even sanitary napkins. One offender had a garden shed stuffed from floor to ceiling with pornographic magazines and a large suitcase full of women's panties which had been stolen from clotheslines and from burglaries of homes. Another man had hundreds of pairs of women's shoes in an outhouse.

There may be repeated acts of, but not always arrests for, indecent exposure, window peeping, obscene telephone calls, arson, burglary and theft. Petty sexual offenses may progress to sexual assault but the first arrest may be for a brutal rape murder.

Brittain notes that the sadistic offender often considers himself to be underendowed as regards his sexual organs even when they are normal as they commonly, though not invariably, are. This feeling of sexual inferiority as compared with other men may partly explain why many persons find it difficult to urinate or undress when others are present, and so earn themselves a reputation for excessive modesty (3). Some are family men, others have difficulty relating to women and some are homosexual.

Their occupation may provide an opportunity to come in close contact with death and dying. Paradoxically these men work as doctors, nurses, operating room technicians and paramedics whose objectives are to preserve life. The connection to death is closer in meat cutters, packing company employees who slaughter animals, morticians and mortuary attendants. Others choose occupations which give them power, for example they apply for positions as security guards or police officers.

These men may have collections of Nazi medals, insignia, uniforms or other memorabilia. A less usual, but not rare, finding is an inordinate interest in, or even practice of black magic (3). Other bizarre findings reported by Brittain include offenses in churches; desecration of graves; an interest in monsters such as dinosaurs, werewolfs and vampires; possession of anesthetics, dolls, or life-sized models of women, and equipment to make a room resemble an execution chamber; as well as an interest in underwater swimming or practice of seeing how long the breath can be held underwater.

Curiously the sadistic murderer may profess strong religious convictions, quote from the scriptures, refrain from the use of tobacco, alcohol and illicit drugs, yet show no remorse for repeated sadistic murders.

Fascination with firearms is common and these men often have a collection of handguns as well as handcuffs and other police equipment. Yet often death is inflicted with a knife or ligature. Death comes too quickly from a shotgun blast or a bullet in the chest, but it can be prolonged through intermittent slow strangulation. Preliminary knife wounds need not be lethal and blows with a blunt instrument can be rationed.

Tying up the victim permits both demonstration of power over the victim and slow torture. Bite marks are usually found on the breasts and around the genitals. Sadism in sex murderers is reviewed in Chapter 8. Methods of attack and other features of sadistic murderers are further considered in the profiles of organized and disorganized murderers in Chapter 13.

MAFIA HIT MEN

A question has been raised about the mental make-up of hit men or executioners for the Mafia and other organized crime groups. These men are seldom seen by psychiatrists as they would not dream of entering a plea of not guilty by reason of insanity when charged with a crime. They avoid punishment by hiring the most adroit attorneys, by killing or intimidating vital witnesses, and by bribing judges or other officials in the criminal justice system.

John Shanley, formerly head of the Central Investigation Bureau of the New York City Police Department has stated that when an organized crime family member has violated the rules or has refused to abide by a superior's decision and the punishment is death, the killing is kept within the family. This eliminates the development of vendettas, makes it easy to perform the task and paves the way for the disappearance. If a dispute between members of this subsociety threatens gangland peace, the heads of the families may talk it out because "the only winners are the cops" when open violence occurs.

If murder is the only solution to the problem discussed, the homicide is assigned to the mob to which the victim belongs. Within a short time the man disappears. In five instances within three years, a member and usually his car have vanished without a trace. These obliterations were carried out by **Judases,** "friends" — possibly actual blood relatives — completely trusted by the victim. The victim showed no fear, no change from routine, prior to his disappearance.

This technique has great advantages. There is no apparent violence, no sprawled body in a bullet-punctured car, no gruesome pictures, no inflamed press and public. Usually, sometime after the victim was last seen, he is reported as a missing person in the jurisdiction in which he resides. Frequently, this is a small town adjacent to the city but, regardless, there is no body and no complaint of homicide. The case is carried as a missing person, a disappearance (19).

Some gangland slayings are not concealed because they are intended to warn others who might be tempted to break the rules. Louie Mileto was paid $5,000 a month to cut (dilute) heroin for sale. He made the mistake of keeping some of the heroin to sell himself. There are those who say that Louie's hands were chopped off at the wrist as a warning to others that he was trying to take what he shouldn't have been taking. Louie was beaten rather severely, probably in Manhattan, New York, and then placed in a meat locker, where he froze to death. His body was chopped with an axe, and his remains were placed in the trunk of a car, which was driven to upstate New York and set on fire.

A hit man for a Chicago organized crime syndicate was introduced to me by a police intelligence unit detective. Dressed in expensive but not flashy clothing, polite and courteous but businesslike, he had the appearance of a very successful company director. Although he denied ever having killed anyone, he admitted that he had been offered contracts to kill persons both in the United States and in Europe. He described the steps that had been taken to facilitate matters. Photographs were provided of the intended victims and their homes together with information on their work activities.

In his opinion men become professional killers because of "the money, the prestige, being accepted, it takes little skill, after the first one or two it's not that great a thing anymore. You have to maintain the respect of others, you have to have power, that means money. The families get together, a society all to itself. There's a lot of social life. You have to be known, trusted, tested, accepted." His coment that killing takes little skill and is not that great a thing after one or two, he attributed to another member of the crime syndicate.

Despite his genteel appearance he was clearly a man of violence and he admitted having stabbed a prison guard. He went on to describe fights in a Federal Penitentiary, usually a killing with a knife. "If I walk up to hit somebody, I have to worry about him walking up behind me and stabbing me tomorrow." It seemed clear that he had no intention of allowing another inmate to survive a knife fight.

Dietz has provided the viewpoint of a Mafia "leg buster" who had to rationalize his assaultive behavior as being reasonable under the circumstances: "When I have to go out and hurt some guy who hasn't paid up I might even like the guy. Then I think to myself, if this guy did what he was supposed to do, I wouldn't have to go out there. Now I have to take a chance on getting hurt or getting arrested and it's all his fault. He knows the rules. And he's gonna beg and cry and make me feel like a rat. The dirty fuck. Why is he doing this to me. I've always been straight with him. I ought to break his head. Anyhow, by the time I have to go I'm so mad at the sucker for putting me in this position that I walk up to him and knock him across the room" (4).

A victim of organized crime described a brutal assault by two members of a Chicago syndicate who came to Denver in search of her husband. The two men appeared to be totally without any feelings of anger or resentment toward her. They were just doing their job, like soldiers in wartime they were obeying orders. They were doing what they had been trained to do.

"I never open my door to strangers. I don't know why I did it. They had the all American look, sweaters, Joe College. They just pushed their way in. They wanted to know where my husband was. They said they were going to look around. They went upstairs and quickly came down. I knew right away they were just interested in finding him, they weren't interested in anything in the house." She was taken by the men that evening to a deserted construction site outside the city limits where she was questioned again about her husband.

"I kept saying I didn't know where he was, that I hadn't seen him for a week. While one man was talking to me, the other man would hit me from behind. The first man put a sock in my mouth, I couldn't breathe, it seemed like I was going to suffocate. I said I wouldn't scream. They just pushed it back in. They beat me on the legs and knees. It seemed a long time. They'd stop and ask questions.

"I knew they'd fractured my arm, I didn't hear anything break but it just hung down. I couldn't pick it up anymore. They said they didn't want to hurt me, they just wanted to know where my husband was. I never lost consciousness. I could see stars, I was in shock, my teeth were chattering. I kept falling over, they'd make me get up. They began to believe I didn't know where my husband was, or they didn't believe I'd tell them. It's strange, there wasn't anything obvious in their actions. I just knew they weren't going to do anything more to me. One man got a table leg out of the car. He said he was going to break my arms and my legs. He told me 'You're not going to walk for help, you're going to crawl.' "

Both her arms and one leg were broken. She thought he had also broken a knee cap but no fractures were visible on x-rays. She also had a laceration on the side of her head as well as many bruises and abrasions on her face, arms, legs and knees.

AGENTS OF GENOCIDE

"All men are merciful, and all men are murderers.
Doting on dogs, they build their Dachaus."

Aldous Huxley, *Ape and Essence*

Genocide refers to the deliberate, systematic extermination of a racial, political or cultural group. An early example of genocide was Pharoah's order (**Exodus** 2.22) that all male Hebrew infants should be cast into the river. In World War II Hitler gave orders for the "final solution" of the Jewish problem in Europe. The Nazi objective was the complete extermination of all Jews in Europe and it has been estimated that six million Jews were massacred.

Rudolf Hoess, an SS officer who served at Dachau and Sachsenhausen before being appointed commandant at Auschwitz Concentration Camp, acknowledged that he personally arranged the gassing of two million persons between 1941 and 1943. At the Nuremburg trial of war criminals he testified concerning his duties.

"I visited Treblinka to find out how they carried out their exterminations. The camp commandant at Treblinka told me that he had liquidated 80,000 in the course of one-half year. He was principally concerned with liquidating all the Jews from the Warsaw Ghetto. He used monoxide gas, and I did not think that his methods were very efficient. So when I set up the extermination building at Auschwitz, I used Cyklon B, which was a crystallized prussic acid which we dropped into the death chamber from a small opening. It took from three to fifteen minutes to kill the people in the death chamber, depending upon climatic conditions. We knew when the people were dead because their screaming stopped. We usually waited about one-half hour before we opened the doors and removed the bodies. After the bodies were removed our special Kommandos took off the rings and extracted the gold from the teeth of the corpses.

"Another improvement we made over Treblinka was that we built our gas chamber to accommodate 2,000 people at one time whereas at Treblinka their ten gas chambers only accommodated 200 people each. The way we selected our victims was as follows: We had two SS doctors on duty at Auschwitz to examine the incoming transports of prisoners. The prisoners would be marched by one of the doctors who would make spot decisions as they walked by. Those who were fit for work were sent into the camp. Others were sent immediately to the extermination plants. Children of tender years were invariably exterminated, since by reason of their youth they were unable to work.

"Still another improvement we made over Treblinka was that at Treblinka the victims almost always knew that they were to be exterminated and at Auschwitz we endeavored to fool the victims into thinking that they were to go through a delousing process. Of course, frequently they realized our true intentions and we sometimes had riots and difficulties due to that fact. Very frequently women would hide their children under the clothes, but of course when we found them we would send the children in to be exterminated. We were required to carry out these exterminations in secrecy but of course the foul and nauseating stench from the continuous burning of bodies permeated the entire area and all of the people living in the surrounding communities knew that exterminations were going on at Auschwitz."

Adolph Eichmann, the former SS officer, was kidnapped in 1961 from outside his home in Argentina and flown to Israel to face charges of causing the killing of millions of Jews. Arendt in her book on Eichmann's trial and execution referred to the banality of evil and stated that Eichmann, except for an extraordinary diligence in looking out for his personal advancement, had no motives at all. The terrifying thing about the executives of the "final solution", about Eichmann for example, is not that they were cruel men but that they were conscientious functionaries who in different circumstances would have retired with presentation gold watches after fifty years with respectable firms (12).

THE CANNIBAL

*"A gastronome of the old school who preserves
the simple tastes and adheres to the natural
diet of the pre-pork period."*

Ambrose Bierce, *The Devil's Dictionary*

Americans are unfit for human consumption: they contain more DDT in their body fat than is permitted in meat by our own pure food laws. Many years ago a King of Fiji stated that human flesh, or "long pig" as it was called tasted like pork but he complained that white men spoilt their flesh by eating too much salt.

Schneider considers that the flesh of an adult Western human, with its tissues built up over the years on an intake based largely on meat would require fairly lengthy marination to render it fit for the table. In his opinion Charles Lamb's well known suggestion of dressing only milk-fed infants for the pot was perhaps wiser from the epicurean stand-point than he knew (18).

In former times primitive tribes would eat the flesh and drink the blood of brave enemy warriors to acquire their valor. Lombroso mentions the Australian aborigine, who in reply to an inquiry as to the absence of old women in his country said, "We eat them all!" and on being remonstrated with for such treatment of his wives, answered, "For one whom we lose, a thousand remain."

A small portion of the body of a murdered man may be eaten in order that his ghost may not trouble the murderer. This practice is also said to have the effect of causing the relatives of the murdered man to lose heart, or to prevent them from exercising the right of revenge.

Cannibalism is occasionally reported in civilized society. Men cast adrift at sea or otherwise deprived of food may kill their companions in order to survive. The famous American hunter, John Johnson, escaped from Blackfoot captivity and his only food during his 200 mile trek to safety was the leg of a Blackfoot captor he had killed. In 1847, Crow Indians killed and scalped his pregnant wife. In revenge Johnson killed, scalped and ate the raw livers of any available Crow Indians, thereby acquiring the nickname "Liver-Eating" Johnson (21).

In Lake City, Colorado, Alfred Packer was found guilty of murdering and consuming five companions. The judge, a Democrat, pronounced sentence: "There were seven democrats in Hinsdale County and you, Alfred Packer, you ate five of them. I sentence you to be hanged by the neck until you are dead, dead, dead . . ." The facts are true, except for the judge's sentencing speech. Mr. Packer did commit the crime but he did not, as is often stated, wipe out the democratic majority in sparsely populated Hinsdale County.

In 1874 Packer acted as a guide for five men who set out from Ouray in winter through the San Juan mountains for Los Pinos. The trip should have taken one week but fifty-five days later Packer arrived alone. He told a tale of becoming lame, of being deserted by his companions, and of surviving on dry berries and boiled mocassins. Packer looked suspiciously well fed and fit after his ordeal; indeed, instead of asking for food, his first request was for whiskey (20). Furthermore he had too much money on him.

Bodies of the five missing men were later found with strips of their flesh cut away. Packer admitted that he had lived on human flesh but claimed that he had killed only one man in self-defense. He was granted a new trial on a legal technicality and in 1886 he was sentenced to forty years imprisonment. Paroled in 1901 he lived near Denver until his death in 1907.

In 1884, ten years after Packer had killed and eaten his five companions, the yacht **Mignonette** sank in a storm on a voyage from England to Australia. The crew of four, at sea in a small open boat in the South Atlantic nearly 2,000 miles from land, had only two tins of turnips to eat and a turtle which was caught on the fourth day. On the nineteenth day Captain Tom Dudley killed the seventeen year old cabin boy, and to use his word, the men "feasted" off the youth's body until they were rescued by a passing vessel on the twenty-fourth day.

On their return to England the crew were surprised to find themselves under arrest. After all it was an established custom of the sea to eat cabin boys in such circumstances. Some people thought that they should have drawn lots to select the next item on the menu rather than kill the weakest member. Five English judges, however, ruled that one must not kill one's shipmates in order to eat them, however hungry one might be (20). A seaman who became a prosecution witness escaped punishment but the captain and ship's mate were sentenced to death. This sentence was commuted to six months in prison.

Cannibalism due to a taste for human flesh in the absence of any lack of food is not common. Twentieth century cannibals include Albert Fish (see below) and Edmund Kemper, the "Co-ed" killer of Santa Cruz County, California (Chapter 8).

Albert Fish in 1928 persuaded the parents of a ten year old girl to let him take their daughter to a children's party. The young girl was never seen again and all efforts to trace her abductor failed. In 1934 the mother received the following letter in the mail.
My dear Mrs. Budd:

In 1894 a friend of mine shipped as a deck-hand on the steamer Tacoma, Captain Davis. They sailed from San Francisco for Hong Kong, China. On arriving there he and two others went ashore and got drunk. When they returned the boat was gone. At that time there was a famine in China. **Meat of any kind** was from one dollar to three dollars a pound. So great was the suffering among the very poor that all children under twelve years were sold to the butchers to be cut up and sold for food in order to keep others from starving. A boy or girl under fourteen was not safe in the street. You could go in any shop and ask for steak, chops or stew meat. Part of the naked body of a boy or girl would be brought out and just what you wanted cut from it. A boy or girl's behind, which is the sweetest part of the body and sold as veal cutlet, brought the highest price.

John stayed there so long he acquired a taste for human flesh. On his return to New York he stole two boys, one seven, one eleven, took them to his home, stripped them naked, tied them in a closet, then burned everything they had on. Several times every day and night he spanked them, tortured them, to make their meat good and tender. First he killed the eleven year old boy because he had the fattest ass and of course the most meat on it. Every part of his body was cooked and eaten, except head, bones and guts. He was roasted in the oven. All of his ass boiled, broiled, fried, stewed. The little boy was next, went the same way.

At this time I was living at 409 East 100th Street, rear right side. He told me so often how good flesh was, I made up my mind to taste it. On Sunday, June 3, 1928, I called on you at 406 West 15th Street, brought you pot cheese — strawberries. We had lunch. Grace sat on my lap and kissed me. I made up my mind to eat her, on the pretext of taking her to a party. You said yes she could go.

I took her to an empty house in Westchester I had already picked out. When we got there I told her to remain outside. She picked wild flowers. I went upstairs and stripped all of my clothes off. I knew if I did not I would get her blood on them. When all was ready I went to the window and called her. Then I hid in a closet until she was in the room. When she saw me all naked she began to cry and tried to run downstairs. I grabbed her, and she said she would tell her mamma. First I stripped her naked. How she did kick and bite and scratch. I choked her to death, then cut her in small pieces so I could take the meat to my rooms, cook it and eat it. Her sweet and tender little ass was roasted in the oven. It took me nine days to eat her entire body. I did not have (intercourse) with her although I could have had I wished. She died a virgin.

Although the letter was unsigned, the police succeeded in finding the writer, Albert Fish, a 65 year old housepainter and father of six children. He confessed that he had strangled the girl and dismembered her body.

"He took parts of her body home with him, cooked them in various ways with carrots and onions and strips of bacon, and ate of them over a period of nine days. During all this time he was in a state of sexual excitement. He ate the flesh during the day and thought about it during the nights. His state of mind while he described these things in minute detail was a peculiar mixture. He spoke in a matter of fact way, like a housewife describing her favorite methods of cooking. You had to remind yourself that this was a little girl he was talking about. But at times his tone of voice and facial expression indicated a kind of satisfaction and ecstatic thrill" (23).

His previous criminal record included arrests for grand larceny, false checks and for sending obscene letters through the mail. He had been admitted to several mental hospitals only to be released within a short time on each occasion. Nevertheless he was clearly suffering from a paranoid psychosis. His children reported that they had seen him stand alone on a hill with his hands raised shouting "I am Christ!" He would hit his nude body with a nail-studded paddle until he was covered with blood.

He admitted to Frederick Wertham, M.D. that for years he had been sticking needles into his body near his genitals and had not been able to pull them all out. X-rays showed twenty-nine needles in his body. He told Wertham that he felt driven to torment and kill children. Sometimes he would gag them, tie them up, and beat them, although he preferred not to gag them for he liked to hear them crying.

Estimates of the number of children he murdered varied from five to eighteen. At his trial for the murder of Grace Budd his plea of insanity was rejected and he was sentenced to death by electrocution. Ironically when he took his little ten year old victim by train to Westchester she noticed that he had left behind the package containing his knife on the train. She hurried back and brought it to him. With these tools she was dismembered.

PUNISHMENT OF MURDERERS

> *"Blood though it sleeps a time, yet never dies*
> *The Gods on murderers fix revengeful eyes."*
>
> Dryden, *The Cock and the Fox*

The story is told in Greek mythology of the madness of Hercules during which he slew his wife and six children. When his sanity returned he became aware of his awful deed and had to be restrained from killing himself. Overcome with guilt he was unable to accept the assurance of Theseus that he could not be held responsible as he had not known what he was doing. On consulting the oracle at Delphi he was informed that the stain of the crime could be removed only by great acts of penance. For twelve years he labored under the orders of Eurystheus, performing the almost impossible tasks known as the twelve labors of Hercules.

The modern-day murderer is not required to perform superhuman tasks of endurance, and the duration of his penance may be much shorter than that demanded of Hercules. In 1982 about half of the convicted murderers released from state prisons in the United States had served **less than six years**. More than half of all state prisoners released from prison in 1982 after serving time for manslaughter had served less than 2.3 years. A life sentence is seldom a life sentence. In 1981, 840 prisoners serving life sentences for murder or other crimes were released from state prisons. Half of such offenders had served fifty-one months or less, two-thirds were found to have served seven years or less (22). Capital punishment is reviewed in Chapter 14.

REFERENCES

1. Abrahamsen, David: *Crime and the Human Mind.* New York, Columbia University Press, 1944.
2. Arendt, Hannah: *Eichmann in Jerusalem: A Report on the Banality of Evil.* New York, Viking Press, 1973.
3. Brittain, R.P.: The sadistic murderer. *Med Sci Law, 10*:198, 1970.
4. Dietz, M.L.: *Killing for Profit: The Social Organization of Felony Homicide.* Chicago, Nelson Hall, 1983.
5. East, W.N.: *Society and the Criminal.* Springfield, Illinois, Charles C Thomas, 1950.
6. Ellis, Havelock: *The Criminal.* New York, Scribner and Welford, 1890.
7. Elwin, Verrier: *Maria, Murder and Suicide.* London, Oxford University Press, 1943.
8. Federal Bureau of Investigation: *Uniform Crime Report 1982.* Washington, D.C., Government Printing Office, 1983.
9. Gibbens, T.C.N.: Sane and insane homicide. *J Crim Law, 49*:110, 1958.
10. Harlan, Howard: Five hundred homicides. *J Crim Law, 40*:736, 1950.
11. Hentig, Hans von: *The Criminal and His Victim.* New Haven, Yale University Press, 1948.
12. Hewitt, Douglas: Freedom of expression. *Times Lit Suppl.*
13. Hill, D. and Pond, D.A.: Reflections on 100 capital cases submitted to EEG. *J Ment Sci, 98*:23, 1952.
14. Hooten, E.A.: *The American Criminal.* Cambridge, Harvard University Press, 1939.
15. Lewis, A.J.: Psychological medicine. In Price, F.W. (Ed.): *Textbook of the Practice of Medicine.* London, Oxford University Press, 1950.
16. Lombroso, C.: *Crime, Its Causes and Remedies.* Boston, Little Brown, 1918.

17. Royal Commission on Capital Punishment Report. London, H.M. Stationery Office, 1953.
18. Schneider, Edward: Cannibals. *Times Lit Suppl,* February 29, 1980.
19. Shanley, J.J.: Testimony on organized crime. In *Hearings Before Permanent Subcommittee on Investigation,* 88th Cong., 1st sess., 1963.
20. Simpson, A.W.: *Cannibalism in the Common Law.* Chicago, University of Chicago Press, 1984.
21. Thorp, R.W. and Bunker, R.: *Crow Killer.* Bloomington, Indiana University Press, 1958.
22. United States Department of Justice: *Prison Admissions and Releases,* 1981, 1982.
23. Wertham, Fredric: *The Show of Violence.* New York, Doubleday and Company, 1949.
24. Wolfgang, M.E.: *Patterns in Criminal Homicide.* Philadelphia, University of Pennsylvania, 1958.

CHAPTER 3

METHODS OF MURDER

"Better one safe way than a hundred
on which you cannot reckon."

Aesop, *Fables*

MURDER is usually brutal, direct and simple: a slash or stab with a knife, a shot from a pistol or shotgun, a crashing blow from a billiard cue or a rock (7). These methods of murder, together with the use of hands, fist or feet account for over 90 percent of criminal homicides in the United States. Poison, fire, explosives, narcotics, drowning and other less common methods account for less than 10 percent of criminal homicides.

FIREARMS

In the United States firearms are used in about 60 percent of homicides. Revolvers and semi-automatic pistols are the weapons of choice in about 50 percent of homicides. A semi-automatic pistol is easier to conceal beneath a sport coat or suit coat but is less reliable than a revolver and is apt to jam at an awkward moment, especially if it has not been kept clean and in good working condition.

In recent years Mafia hit men have used .22 caliber semi-automatic pistols. The bullets are of small caliber but several can be fired in quick succession. As the Mafia often use members who are acquainted with the intended victim ideal circumstances can be arranged for tidy termination. The use of a silencer or noise suppressor reduces the risk of interference by busybodies.

Wolfgang in his study noted that the use of a pistol or revolver was highest in the younger and older age groups. He suggests that these age groups (as do women who slay men) require some weapon to maintain distance between themselves and their victims, and to offset their limited physical power when involved in an episode of violence. In line with this probable explanation Wolfgang points out that fatal beatings with blunt instruments or with fists alone show the highest frequency for the ages twenty to twenty-nine when most males are in their physical prime.

Submachine guns, such as the Israeli Uzi which can fire 600 rounds a minute, and automatic machine pistols, such as the Mach 10 which can fire 1145 rounds a minute have been used for close range assassinations. As the Mach 10 can fire up to nine rounds in half a second little time is required for a kill. A Mach 10 was used in June 1984 to kill Alan Berg, a radio talk show host noted for his abrasive style, hostility toward extreme right-wing groups and outspoken support of gun control. He was shot at close range as he was stepping out of his car in the driveway of his apartment house and was found lying on his back with one foot still inside his car. A brown paper bag was still clutched in his right hand. Thirteen .45 caliber bullets caused 34 gunshot wounds several of which could have caused his death.

KNIVES

Knives or other cutting weapons are used in about 20 percent of homicides in the United States. In a stabbing, offenders under twenty years of age seem most often to select a pocket knife and those over forty to select a kitchen knife (18).

MURDER BY POISON

Pollak has suggested that murder by females may be less easily detected because female murderers resort to poison to a much higher degree than men. Medea, in the myth of Jason and the quest of the Golden Fleece, is the prototype of the female poisoner. Euripides has brilliantly portrayed the evil character of Medea who poisoned her rival and punished her faithless husband by murdering the children she bore him. Some of the most heartless murders have been committed by female poisoners.

The Marquise de Brinvilliers who poisoned countless hospital patients as well as her father and two brothers, gave as her reason for attempting to poison her daughter, the fact that she was growing too tall (11).

Sixty-six year old Mrs. M. E. Wilson of County Durham, England, remaried in November 1957, just over a year after the death of her first husband. When someone commented at the wedding reception that there would be a lot of sandwiches and cakes left over, she replied, "Just keep them for the funeral, although I might give this one a week's extension." This remark was recalled when her husband died two weeks later.

The bodies of her two husbands were exhumed and autopsies revealed that they had both died from phosphorus poisoning (phosphorus is a constituent of some rat poisons). It was clear that she had married her elderly victims for their money and had then murdered them. She was sentenced to death, but the sentence was later commuted to imprisonment. Had it not been for her unfortunate joke at the wedding reception, she might have escaped detection.

A particularly tragic case of poisoning occurred in Colorado in 1944. Charles F. Silliman purchased some rat poison at a drugstore. He asked for strychnine as he did not want commercial rat poison. After putting the poison in a bottle of brandy he offered his wife a drink. She poured herself a glass of the mixture and was holding it in her hand when their four year old daughter came running into the house. In the presence of her father the girl said, "Mama, I want a drink." The child took a sip and handed the glass back to her mother who also imbibed. Shortly afterwards first the daughter and then the mother died in convulsions. After the police found the poison bottle in the glove compartment of Silliman's car, he confessed the crime for which he was later executed.

One of the most infamous poisoners, an English physician, Dr. William Palmer, who earned the title "Prince of Poisoners," also employed strychnine. He was arrested after he had murdered at least fourteen of his friends and relatives. During his trial when the Lord Chief Justice Campbell rebuked his defense counsel, Palmer passed down a note from the dock: "I wish there were 2½ grains of strychnine in old Campbell's acidulated draught" (3).

Arsenic is more often employed in homicidal poisoning than strychnine. It is colorless, odorless and tasteless and therefore can be added to the victim's food or drink without arousing suspicion. The delay between ingestion and appearance of symptoms is an added advantage for the poisoner. Moreover, the principal symptoms, nausea and vomiting, occur in many disorders besides arsenic poisoning. Should murder be suspected, however, it is a simple matter to detect whether the victim was poisoned with arsenic, as the substance is stored in the hair and nails. Despite this drawback, arsenic continues to enjoy considerable popularity among poisoners.

Thallium, another substance used in rat poison, may also cause abdominal pain and vomiting. Sometimes there is diarrhea but it is followed by severe constipation. When small doses are administered gastrointestinal symptoms can pass nearly unnoticed. Violent unbearable pain in the legs and feet, especially in the big toes, is followed by loss of hair so that the victim may become completely bald.

Graham Young, a fourteen year old schoolboy, was convicted in 1962 of administering poison to his father, sister, and a school friend. Evidence was presented that made it reasonably certain that he had poisoned his stepmother with thallium, but her death had been attributed to natural causes and her body had been cremated (ten years later he boasted that he had killed her). He was committed to the Broadmoor Security Hospital with a recommendation that he should not be released within fifteen years. While in the hospital he was suspected of attempting to poison other patients by putting cleaning substances in their tea (9).

Within nine years he was released from the hospital after his psychiatrist reported that it was extremely unlikely that he would poison again. Within a month of his obtaining a job in the storeroom of a photography plant, his supervisor, Bob Egle, became ill with severe diarrhea. The supervisor went on vacation but the day after he returned to work he complained that his fingers were numb, he staggered as if he was drunk and he could not sleep that night because of severe backache. Following his admission to a hospital paralysis spread through his body and his condition grew steadily worse.

Egle died eight days later. After an autopsy his death was attributed to a rare form of peripheral neuritis, the Guillian-Barre syndrome, and his body was cremated. Young was chosen to replace Egle as storeroom supervisor and to represent the employees at the funeral. He was curiously knowledgeable about the rare disorder which caused Egle's death. Other employees became sick, two lost all their hair and another man died. At a meeting of employees to discuss the mysterious epidemic a doctor ruled out radiation poisoning and poisoning with a heavy metal such as thallium. He stated that medical experts were searching for an unusual virus that might be causing the sickness among employees.

Young drew attention to himself by asking rather indignantly why heavy metal poisoning had been ruled out. He showed detailed knowledge of metal poisoning, asked the doctor whether the symptoms of those with illness differed from those of the two men who had died, and he insisted on knowing whether the doctor was suggesting that loss of hair was psychosomatic (9). The manager called the police who noted that the epidemic began after Young's employment at the plant. Police inquiries revealed Young's prior convictions for poisoning.

Thallium was found in the body of the second employee to die. Egle's ashes contained nine milligrams of thallium. It was the first time in criminal history that a murder charge had followed the exhumation of ashes (9). In a search of Young's bedroom police found a vial containing more than twice the fatal dose of thallium in the pocket of one of his jackets. There were also bottles with traces of thallium and antimony. There were drawings of a bottle with the word poison on it, of gravestones, and of a man with hair on his head and another drawing of the same man with an astonished expression on his face and his head almost bald (19).

There was also a diary in his room in which his victims were listed by their initials. "F. is now seriously ill. He is unconscious and has developed paralysis and blindness. It is likely that he will decline in the next few days . . . The lastest news from the hospital is that F. is responding to treatment. He is being obstinately difficult. If he survives a third week he will live. That could be inconvenient. I am most annoyed. He is surviving far too long for my peace of mind." This victim died three days later.

In 1972 Young was convicted of murdering his two fellow employees and of administering poison to four others. He was sentenced to life imprisonment. His early life showed many of the features of the sadistic murderer (Chapter 2). He was cruel to mice, poisoning them and then performing autopsies. When his sister complained about this behavior he drew a tombstone with her name on it. He also drew coffins with his parents' names on them.

He was fascinated by the Nazi movement wearing a Nazi swastika and arm band. On the walls of his room were pictures of Hitler and Nazi leaders. He read books on Black Magic and stuck pins in wax images. His books included volumes on poisons and poisoners. He boasted that one day he would be as famous as Doctor William Palmer, who killed fourteen persons with poison. Repeatedly he made statements which should have aroused suspicion that he was a poisoner.

While poisoning his family in 1962 he talked frequently about medicine and toxicology. He told one of his victims at the photography plant that it was easy to poison somebody and that after an autopsy the doctor would say that death was due to natural causes. When this victim complained of a bitter taste in his coffee, Young replied, "What's the matter? Do you think I'm going to poison you or something?" The victim regarded this remark as a joke. Yet twenty minutes later he had to rush to the toilet because he felt he was about to throw up.

The next day he was in bed sick and the following day he saw a doctor because his legs felt numb. Yet for three days he continued to go to work and to have coffee with Young. His toes became painful, his hair began to fall out and eventually he was admitted to a hospital. Fortunately he survived. Young told police after his arrest that he had ceased to see his victims as people, they had become guinea pigs. His sister reported that in 1971 before his arrest he complained that he could not get close to people adding "There's a terrible coldness inside me" (19).

A disturbing aspect of the 1971 murders and poisonings, which caused such great suffering for the victims, was that not one of the forty-three doctors, including medical consultants as well as general practitioners, diagnosed poisoning.

Cyanide is occasionally used by murderers. In Chicago on September 29, 1982 a twelve year old schoolgirl took a capsule of Tylenol®, an analgesic, for her sore throat and fell lifeless to the floor. A few hours later a young post office employee, who had taken the day off to play with his children, took some Tylenol for chest pain, collapsed, had a convulsion and died. At the house that evening the grief stricken relatives assembled, neighbors brought coffee, donuts, and aspirin, but the family had their own extra-strength Tylenol, which they passed around. The deceased man's wife took a capsule, so did his brother, and both died within minutes (4).

That night two firemen discussing the deaths remembered that paramedics had reported that the young schoolgirl had taken Tylenol. The next morning tests showed that the capsules, all from lot 2880 contained potassium cyanide, and autopsies confirmed that the victims had died from cyanide poisoning. The same day a young woman suffering from headaches also died, as did a young mother who had just given birth to her third child. Despite official warnings not to take Tylenol, the next day an airline flight attendant was found dead in her apartment with poisoned capsules in her bathroom. She was the seventh and final victim.

In June 1984 James W. Lewis, age thirty-seven, was convicted of trying to extort $1,000,000 from the makers of Tylenol, and sentenced to ten years in prison. He admitted writing a letter to the makers demanding the million dollars to stop the killing. The US attorney contended that the extortion attempt was a motive for the murders and a confession of murder, but he added that Lewis was not charged with the murders because there was insufficient evidence.

MURDER BY INSULIN

It was perhaps unwise of Kenneth Barlow, an English male nurse, to inform a colleague "You could kill someone with insulin as it can't be found very easily, unless it is a very large dose." It was certainly unwise of him to tell a nursing orderly, that one could commit a perfect murder with insulin, as the drug could not be traced because it dissolved into the blood stream.

These remarks were recalled when Barlow was tried for the murder of his second wife. He claimed to have found his wife under the water in the bath and stated that as he was not strong enough to get her out, he applied artificial respiration. But the police officers noted that the sleeves of his pajamas appeared quite dry.

With the aid of a magnifying glass several puncture marks were found on his wife's buttocks and the presence of insulin was detected in her body. At first Barlow denied having given his wife any injections, but later he claimed that he had given her injections of ergometrine to induce an abortion. He was found guilty of murder and sentenced to life imprisonment. His first wife died the year prior to the murder of his second wife. At the inquest the doctors were unable to state the cause of death, but agreed that it was from natural causes (5).

MURDER BY RATTLESNAKES

On May 1, 1942, Robert S. James was hanged in San Quentin Penitentiary for a rather unusual murder committed seven years earlier. In order to dispose of his fifth wife he purchased some rattlesnakes which were tested on live chickens, but the chickens survived. Another snake was purchased and it was put in a cage with a rabbit. The rabbit lived and the snake died. Finally some snakes were obtained with enough venom to kill chickens and rabbits.

The unfortunate Mrs. James was told that a medical student had agreed to perform an operation for abortion and she allowed herself to be blindfolded and strapped to a table in her home for the operation. The box containing the rattlesnakes was placed over her left foot and the snakes bit her many times. James' accomplice then removed the rattlesnakes for resale to the snake dealer. The snake bites were not immediately effective and the impatient James drowned his wife in the bath, then placed her body in a lily pond in the yard of their Los Angeles home. The coroner returned a verdict of accidental drowning.

Some months later James unwisely confided to a girl friend information regarding the death of his wife. She wrote an anonymous letter to the police who obtained a confession from the accomplice. James was sentenced to death for the crime.

Almost certainly James also murdered his first wife at Manitou Springs, Colorado in October, 1932. She apparently drowned in a bathtub and the coroner termed the drowning an accidental death. Harry Galbraith, a Colorado Springs reporter, suspected murder at the time, but was unable to persuade the coroner to conduct an autopsy. James collected a $5,000 life insurance policy and departed for Los Angeles.

Galbraith suspected murder because of an unusual automobile accident in September, 1932, for which James gave two different explanations. The car ran off the Pikes Peak highway at an elevation of 13,000 feet. James was unhurt, but his wife suffered a skull fracture and remained unconscious in a hospital for several days. On recovery she could not recall details of the accident. Despite the suspicious circumstances there was insufficient evidence to enable criminal prosecution.

MURDER BY MOTOR VEHICLES

Motor vehicles have been used as guided missiles to commit murder. In Reno, Nevada, on Thanksgiving Day 1981, Priscilla Ford, age fifty-three, drove her car down a crowded sidewalk scattering mangled bodies for more than a block in front of the casinos. In court she claimed it was an accident caused by somebody tampering with the steering system of her car, but Reno police sergeant Duane Isenberg testified she told him after her arrest that she planned to kill as many people as she could. There was psychiatric testimony that she was a paranoid schizophrenic who had the delusion that she was the reincarnation of Christ but she was found guilty of six counts of first degree murder and twenty-three counts of attempted murder.

In Los Angeles in 1984, Daniel Lee Young, age twenty-one, was arrested after he drove his car into people on a crowded sidewalk killing one person and injuring fifty-four others. Police reported that the car jumped the curb at thirty-five miles per hour and continued down the sidewalk until it crashed into a bus kiosk. Young calmly left his car and tried to melt into the crowd. He told police "Somebody will have to grieve for these people, but I will get a lot of publicity as a result of the trial."

Two of the victims who survived suffered brain damage and a third was in critical condition after one leg was amputated below the knee. Young, who had a burglary conviction, had been treated briefly in a mental health clinic after he poured gasoline over himself and threatened to light a match. Convicted on one count of first degree murder and forty-eight counts of attempted murder, he was sentenced to 106 years in prison.

A woman drinking with her boy friend in a tavern was told that he was going with another girl. She became enraged, ran to the parking lot and with her car she rammed her boy friend's car three times. Then she caught sight of him on the sidewalk and tried to run him down. "I floorboarded the pedal and headed up the sidewalk after him. I hit a building and a tree. I fully intended to run him down." She did not reveal this information to the police as she feared she would be charged with attempted murder. Her boy friend, fearing publicity was equally reticent and she was fined $100 for careless driving (13).

The suicidal person may aim his car at an oncoming vehicle thereby endangering the lives of other persons on the highway. A woman, following an argument with her husband, jumped into her car and drove it into a truck at the nearest intersection. "All of a sudden it came on me to ram into the truck and get it over with. I didn't think about it till I saw the truck coming along the highway. I put on the gas and headed for the truck." The suicidal driver may attempt to kill himself and his passenger on an impulse by driving off a mountain road, at a bridge abutment or into a cliff as in the following example where the driver was seriously injured:

A man who was driving his wife home reported, "I was just driving along. She said 'Now what have you started drinking for?' Right after that I did it. I felt no good, might as well end it all. I had the urge, I turned and ran right into a rock, a big rock cliff 75 feet high, all solid rock. I hadn't thought about it before. At the time it didn't enter my head I might have killed her."

The influence of auditory hallucinations was seen in a thirty-two year old schizophrenic woman who, while driving with her husband and five children, deliberately crashed into the rear of another car at eighty miles per hour. She did this because voices told her to do so in order that the family could all be born again. Both cars overturned but fortunately no one was seriously injured and she was fined $10 for careless driving. Although her husband neglected to advise the police or court of her abnormal mental condition, he brought her to the hospital for treatment three days later (13).

HOMICIDE AND SUICIDE BY AIRCRAFT

In 1977, three months after he was fired from his job as a pilot for an airline company at Alice Springs, Australia, the thirty-three year old man stole a Beechcraft Baron aircraft from an airport almost 700 miles away. He was overheard singing hymns on the aircraft radio and saying "It is better to die with honor than live with dishonor." The plane approached the Alice Springs airport, without its landing gear down, crossed over the runway at an acute angle and levelled out at a height of sixteen feet before crashing into the offices of the airline company.

In addition to the pilot, three employees of the airline, including the owner's son, died instantly and a further employee died later. Police found a "shrine" in the dead pilot's apartment with pictures of his graduation day, a flying trophy, his log book, and a plan of his fatal flight (6).

Samuel Byck, a forty-four year old tire salesman, planned to kill President Nixon and members of his administration by crashing a commercial jetliner into the White House. He described his plan in a tape recording, copies of which were sent to several well-known persons. "I hope to force the pilot to buzz the White House—I mean, sort of dive towards the White House. When the plane is in this position, I will shoot the pilot and then in the last few minutes try to steer the plane into the target, which is the White House . . . Whoever dies in Project Pandora Box will be directly attributable to the Watergate scandals."

Byck was upset over the failure of his marriage, his financial problems and the refusal of the Small Business Administration to grant him a
loan. He complained that there was corruption in the SBA, the Federal
Government and the Nixon administration. In 1972 it was reported that
he had suggested that someone ought to kill President Nixon and he was
questioned by the Secret Service. A psychiatrist who had treated him for
emotional problems told the investigators that he did not consider Byck
a threat to himself or others. He described Byck as "a big talker who
makes verbal threats and never acts on them." In 1973 he was arrested
for picketing without a permit in front of the White House. His signs
called for Nixon's impeachment (2).

On February 22, 1974, Byck acted on his threat to skyjack a jet plane
and crash it into the White House. At Dulles International Airport near
Washington, D.C. he joined the passengers waiting at Gate C to board
Delta Flight 523 for Atlanta. He killed the security guard with two shots
from a .22 caliber pistol, ran down the ramp, boarded the plane, fired a
warning shot and told the pilots to take off. When it was explained that
the wheel blocks would have to be removed he shot the co-pilot in the
stomach.

On hearing shots from inside the plane Byck shot the co-pilot in the
head and the pilot in the shoulder. Before losing consciousness, the pilot
notified ground control, "Emergency, emergency, we're all shot . . ."
Byck reloaded his pistol, seized a passenger as a hostage, and once again
shot the pilot and dying co-pilot. A shot through a window in the door of
the plane was followed by two more shots which wounded Byck in the
chest and stomach. He then shot himself in the head with his own pistol.
Authorities later found a briefcase gasoline bomb under his body (2).

HOMICIDE BY FIRE AND BOMB

Fires and explosions are used to conceal murder. Many cases of arson
and bombing are not recognized as being due to criminal acts, especially
when the fire or explosion destroys evidence pointing to the origins of
the destruction. Thus a case of arson may be dismissed as being caused
by faulty electrical wiring or a carelessly discarded cigarette. An explosion due to a bomb is attributed to a leaking natural gas pipe. Arson for
revenge, to obtain money from an insurance company or from other
motives may cause loss of life, whether or not this was intended, as in
the following example:

Three teenage youths in Aurora, Colorado decided to drive to a wealthy neighborhood to siphon some premium quality gasoline from a parked Cadillac for use in their own car. On the way they were cut off by a truck driver with whom they became involved in a heated argument. One of them later recalled that a passenger in the truck attended a local high school and they obtained his address from the high school yearbook.

The group spent some time that evening deciding on appropriate revenge. Their first plan was to leave an obscene note in the truck but one of them put some gasoline in a bottle with the intention of fire bombing the truck. When they came back to the getaway car, they informed the driver that they "did the house." The driver later recalled, "I really freaked out, it was a drag because everybody would be asleep." Over the radio they heard the truck driver and four members of his family died in the fire.

In Los Angeles Humberto de la Torre, age twenty-two set fire to a residential hotel in 1982 to spite his uncle who managed the hotel. Supposedly the uncle had embarrassed the young man by berating him in front of friends for alleged gang involvement. Twenty-five persons died in the fire. The defense attorney, requesting a lenient sentence, said that de la Torre was not motivated at the time by the intent to hurt anyone. The judge imposed twenty-five consecutive life sentences. To be eligible for parole de la Torre would have to serve half the 625 year sentence.

A young man in Ash Flat, Arkansas, upset over his wife leaving him for another man, went to her lover's home and placed a stick of dynamite between the mattress and the bed springs. He attached a fuse which ran from under the bed out through the window, which had been partially boarded over because the lovers were fearful of attack. The husband waited two days after placing the bomb before returning to light the fuse after the lovers had retired to bed.

At the time of the explosion, the man was lying on top of his girl friend, and her body took the full force of the explosion. His hands were burned, but he was not seriously injured; he drove her to the hospital, where she was pronounced dead on arrival. Three months before the bombing, the lovers had moved out of their trailer home following a mysterious explosion which originated in the stove. A month later, someone fired a shot at the lover from some trees near their isolated home. Following the tragedy, the woman's husband was found guilty of second degree murder and sentenced to twenty-one years in prison.

Eric Brown, a nineteen year old English soldier, was upset over his father's tyrannical temper which persisted after his father was injured in an accident that left him paralyzed below the waist. One day his father was blown to pieces in his wheelchair. Eric had placed a land mine in the upholstery of the wheelchair. A single bomb may cause the loss of many lives as for example John Gilbert Graham's bombing of a United Airlines plane which killed forty-four persons including his mother (Chapter 7).

PSYCHIC HOMICIDE

In Meerloos' opinion those persons who push others into suicide, commit psychic murder. He gives the example of an engineer who gave his harsh, domineering alcoholic father a bottle of barbiturates to "cure" his alcoholism. He was very well aware what he expected his father to do, and two days later he received a telegram announcing the suicidal death of his father. Another example was a doctor who denied his wife psychiatric treatment for her depression. He was having an affair with his secretary and he took a vacation with her and his young daughter, leaving his wife at home alone. After two days she committed suicide on his unconscious demand.

VOODOO MURDER

Sorcerers and witches use black magic and other diabolical practices to secure the death of a person who has been a cause of offense. Voodoo death has been reported from the Island of Haiti, Africa, Australia and other countries. It has been suggested that poisons have been used surreptitiously to kill the victims. This may be true in some cases, but there are numerous cases on record of death occurring as a direct result of voodoo. The intended victim must know what is being done against him and he must fear it.

The Australian witch doctor may cause the death of a fellow aborigine by pointing a bone at him. Basedow has described the efficacy of this procedure. "The man who discovers that he is being boned by an enemy is, indeed, a pitiable sight. He stands aghast, with his eyes staring at the treacherous pointer, and with his hands lifted as though to ward off the lethal medium, which he imagines is pouring into his body. His cheeks blanch and his eyes become glassy and the expression of his face becomes horribly distorted . . . He attempts to shriek but usually the sound chokes in his throat, and all that one might see is froth at his mouth. His body begins to tremble and the muscles twist involuntarily. He sways backwards and falls to the ground, and after a short time appears to be in a swoon; but soon after he writhes as if in mortal agony, and covering his face with his hands, begins to moan. After a while he becomes very composed and crawls to his wurley. From this time onwards he sickens and frets, refusing to eat and keeping aloof from the daily affairs of the tribe. Unless help is forthcoming in the shape of a countercharm administered by the hands of the Nangarri, or medicine-man, his death is only a matter of a comparatively short time. If the coming of the medicine-man is opportune he might be saved."

In a review of murder by witchcraft, Christina Hole describes the making of a figure, resembling the intended victim, out of wax, clay, wood or metal. Something connected with the victim, such as a strand of his hair, nail clippings or shreds of his clothing was usually included in the image. This figure was baptized in the victim's name and then stabbed with pins, thorns or nails, and either melted slowly before a fire or left to decay in earth or running water.

The victim suffered whatever was done to the image, because this was now the same as himself. He felt with agonizing pain the thorns or pins thrust into limbs or back, wasted away mysteriously as the image melted or decayed, went mad when it was stabbed through the head, and died suddenly when the heart was pierced (10).

OTHER METHODS OF MURDER

Relatives of brain damaged or terminally ill patients sometimes unplug respirators, nurses have been convicted of administering medicines such as muscle relaxants and anesthetics in fatal doses, and spouses have dropped electrical hair dryers into their mate's bath water. In Germany a paranoid schizophrenic built himself a flame thrower and an iron lance with which he attacked a primary school. Eight children and two female teachers died, mostly of severe burns, while twenty-two more victims were injured.

DISPOSAL OF THE VICTIM'S BODY

"How long will a man lie i' the earth ere he rot?"

Shakespeare, *Hamlet*

How often must Hamlet's leading question to the grave digger have passed through the tortured minds of the world's murderers in the still hours when darkness hems them in and the small voice of conscience whispers to them. For to every shedder of blood there comes inevitably the dread moment when, his revenge or hatred satisfied, he finds himself alone with the cold clay of his enemy, and knows that his victim has suddenly become an enemy indeed, a far greater peril to him in death than ever he had been in life (17).

In 1935 a 14-foot shark was captured by two Australian fishermen and placed on exhibition in an aquarium. Some days later the shark vomited up, among other things, a well preserved human arm. Tattoo marks on the arm and fingerprints revealed that the former owner of the arm was James Smith, a forty year old man who had left his home, never to return, some nine days before the capture of the shark.

It was suggested that on leaving home he had gone to a seaside cottage with another man. It was reported that a tin trunk and a mattress had disappeared from the cottage and a rope and three mats from the owner's boat. The distinguished forensic pathologist, Sir Sydney Smith has reviewed this most unusual case. "My tentative reconstruction of the case was that Smith and his companion had quarreled over something or other, and it had ended with Smith being killed. His body was probably cut up in the cottage on the mattress and the mats taken from the boat. The parts of the body were placed in the tin trunk, which was completely filled without the arm. Unable to get this in, the murderer cut it off and attached it to the outside of the trunk with the rope from the boat, tying one end of it around the wrist. The trunk and its contents and the blood soaked mattress and mats were then taken out to sea and dumped. The arm worked loose and was swallowed by the shark.

"What a queer series of coincidences it was that brought the crime to light! The trunk was a little too small to take all the remains, and the only part of the body with a distinguishing mark was the part left out. This part worked loose and was swallowed whole by a shark — and, out of the thousands of sharks that infest the beaches of Australia, that particular shark had to be caught alive and exhibited in the aquarium.

Further, out of all the sharks put in aquaria, that one had to become sick and vomit up the contents of its stomach, including the arm which led to the identification. It is a trite saying, but true, that fact is stranger than fiction" (16).

The suspect who was charged with the murder of Smith, was acquitted. A man who was expected to be one of the most important witnesses was murdered before the trial.

When F.B. Deeming rented a house for six months on behalf of a fictitious Colonel Brook, he insisted that the agreement to rent should include a clause permitting him to cover the kitchen and scullery floor with cement. He explained that Colonel Brook had an extreme prejudice against uneven floors. Douthwaite has commented that no more conclusive proof of premeditated murder has ever been furnished than Deeming's insistence upon this extraordinary provision. In the light of later events he could not more definitely have proclaimed his intentions, if instead of cement, he had ordered tombstones.

Disposal by burial presents certain difficulties. Disappearance of the victim raises a hue and cry which may extend to inspection of cellars and basements. Animals may uncover the shallow grave and new tenants may remodel the house. In 1950 Timothy Evans was tried and hanged for murder after the dead bodies of his wife and child were found hidden in the house in which he had rented rooms. In 1953, later tenants of rooms in the same house in London discovered human remains hidden behind a wall. Four bodies were discovered in the house and two in the garden. All the victims were women, two of whom had been dead for over eight years. A former tenant Reginald Christie confessed, before his execution, that he had murdered the six women. It has been suggested that he also murdered Evan's wife and child.

Many murderers have attempted to dispose of bodies by burning them. Professor Webster of Harvard University placed the body of his fellow physician, Dr. George Parkman, in a laboratory furnace. A suspicious college porter found a set of charred false teeth in the furnace, with fatal consequences for Webster. The French murderers, Lamarre and Petiot, were betrayed by vast columns of smoke from the chimneys of their homes.

The poisoner in his anxiety to ensure rapid cremation of his victims, may arouse suspicion. Nurse Dorathea Waddingham would probably have escaped the gallows if she had not forged a letter in her victim's handwriting requesting cremation after death. The physician had issued a certificate of death from cerebral hemorrhage, but discovery of the forgery led to an autopsy.

Dismemberment facilitates disposal of bodily remains but despite all precautions, blood may soak through crevices to leave tell-tale stains. The celebrated French murderer, Voirbo, filled the head of his victim with molten lead and threw it into the river Seine. Other parts of the body were cut into minute pieces and scattered abroad. The legs were dumped into a well which was used by a local restaurant. The diners complained about the taste of the water and the limbs were discovered.

Another murderer took more care over his task. William Sheward of Norwich, England, spent three evenings cutting up his wife, and he took infinite pains in strewing the portions over a wide area. Although some of the remains were discovered, it was not possible to establish the victim's identity. Eighteen years later he walked into a police station and confessed the crime for which he was later executed.

A young university student, who cut up his father so that he would fit into suitcases, disarmed the suspicions of a taxi driver, who had noticed blood seeping from one of the suitcases, by remarking that it contained venison. The student was detected after he tried to dispose of his father from the deck of a passenger ship. Vere Gould was less successful in disarming suspicion. When the stationmaster complained that blood was oozing from Gould's trunk, Gould blandly replied that it contained poultry.

The English murderer, Wainright, was foolish enough to leave the parcels containing his victim in the care of a youth while he summoned a cab. Donald Hume hired an interior decorator to varnish the kitchen floor on which he had dismembered Stanley Setty, a used car dealer. The interior decorator helped him carry the parcel containing Setty's torso to his car. Hume dropped the remains from an airplane into the English Channel, but the torso was washed ashore onto the Essex mudflats where it was discovered.

Roger Moore, who was confined to a wheelchair, faced a difficult problem disposing of the body of his roommate. Some years earlier, while serving a sentence for burglary in the Colorado State Penitentiary, Moore was stabbed in the back and paralyzed below the waist. He rented an electric saw, cut the body into pieces, borrowed a child's red wagon, pulled it behind his wheelchair and left body parts in plastic garbage bags outside other homes in the low income housing project.

A young girl leaving for school the next morning found one of the bags on the doorstep. Another girl felt the bag and thought it contained a human arm. It did, and police who searched the housing project found other bags containing a leg, another leg, a foot, and the trunk of the body. Notes in Spanish on the bags stated, "Death to the murderers of the barrios" and were signed "The Vigilantes." Moore was arrested on a jet plane about to leave from Denver for California. Two hands were found in his suitcase and the head, an arm and a foot were found in the refrigerator in his apartment.

Edmund Kemper, the serial murderer (Chapter 8), after decapitating his mother cut out her larynx and put it down the garbage disposal. "This seemed appropriate," he said, "As much as she'd bitched and screamed and yelled at me over the years" (12). A Roto-Rooter service-man found that the cause of a blocked toilet in the home of Dr. Harvey Lothringer was a mass of sludge in the main house trap leading to the sewer. Small fragments of human tissue and bone had apparently been passed through the disposal, or flushed directly down the toilet (8). Dr. Lothringer, who pleaded guilty to second degree manslaughter, said that a nineteen year old girl had died during an illegal abortion operation in his home.

Denke, the German mass murderer, profitably disposed of the bodies of his victims through his business as a butcher on the black market. The names, weights and dates of slaughter of his victims were entered in his ledger. He pickled their flesh in tubs of brine and stored the salted joints in a backyard shed. Bones were stacked tidily in a kitchen cupboard, and fat rendered down (3).

Georges Serrat was the first offender to dissolve the bodies of his vic-tims in corrosive acid. He died on the guillotine in 1933. John George Haigh, the English acid bath murderer, claimed to have killed nine per-sons, but this may have been an exaggeration as the police have credited him with only six deaths.

When questioned by the police regarding the disappearance of his last victim, Haigh stated, "I will tell you all about it. Mrs. Durand Deacon no longer exists. She has disappeared completely and no trace can ever be found again. I have destroyed her with acid. You will find the sludge which remains at Leopold Road. Every trace has gone. How can you prove murder if there is no body?"

Haigh inveigled his elderly victim to accompany him to his store-house where he shot her in the back of the head. After removing her coat and jewelry he put her body in a 45-gallon tank. After a cup of tea at a nearby restaurant, he filled the tank with sulphuric acid. The following day he called in to see how "the reaction in the tank had gone."

Two days later he returned to find the reaction almost complete, but a piece of fat and bone was still floating in the sludge. He emptied off the sludge with a bucket and tipped it onto the ground outside the storehouse. More acid was added to the tank. Four days after the murder he completely emptied the tank.

Examination of the sludge revealed gall stones, an intact set of dentures, part of a left foot and fragments of human bone. Haigh, who was nicknamed "old corpus delicti" by his fellow prisoners, claimed that the foot was from an earlier victim. He was executed.

REFERENCES

 1. Basedow, Herbert: *The Australian Aboriginal.* Adelaide, Preece, 1925.
 2. Clarke, J.W.: *American Assassins: The Darker Side of Politics.* Princeton, Princeton University Press, 1982.
 3. Dickson, Grierson: *Murder by Numbers.* London, Robert Hale, 1958.
 4. Dunea, George: Death over the counter. *Brit Med J, 286*:211, 1983.
 5. Furneaux, Rupert: *Famous Criminal Cases,* 5. New York, Roy Publishers, 1958.
 6. Goldney, R.D.: Homicide and suicide by aircraft. *Foren Sci Int, 21*:161, 1983.
 7. Harlan, Howard: Five hundred homicides. *J Crim Law, 40*:736, 1950.
 8. Helpern, M. and Knight, B.: *Autopsy.* New York, St. Martins Press, 1977.
 9. Holden, Antony: *The St. Albans Poisoner: The Life and Crimes of Graham Young.* London, Hodder and Stoughton, 1974.
10. Hole, Christina: *A Mirror of Witchcraft.* London, Chatto and Windus, 1957.
11. Jesse, F.T.: *Murder and Its Motives.* London, Harrap, 1952.
12. Lundee, D.T.: *Murder and Madness.* New York, Norton, 1975.
13. Macdonald, J.M.: Suicide and homicide by automobile. *Amer J Psychiat, 124*:475, 1967.
14. Meerloo, J.A.: Suicide, menticide and psychic homicide. *Arch Neurol Psychiat, 81*:360, 1959.
15. Pollack, Otto: *The Criminality of Women.* Philadelphia, University of Pennsylvania Press, 1950.
16. Smith, Sir Sydney: *Mostly Murder.* London, George C. Harrap, 1959.
17. Whitelaw, David: *Corpus Delicti.* London, Geoffrey Bles, 1936.
18. Wolfgang, M.E.: *Patterns in Criminal Homicide.* Philadelphia, University of Pennsylvania Press, 1958.
19. Young, Winifred: *Obsessive Poisoner: The Strange Story of Graham Young.* London, Robert Hale, 1973.

CHAPTER 4

VICTIMS OF HOMICIDE

"In a sense the victim shapes
and moulds the criminal."

Hans Von Hentig,
The Criminal and His Victim

IT IS PERHAPS distressing that, statistically, one stands a much greater risk of being murdered by a member of one's own family than by a stranger. The homicide offender rarely selects as his victim a stranger. More often his victim is someone with whom he has been familiar for a prolonged period of time.

Svalastoga, in a study of 172 Danish murderers, found that in nine cases out of every ten, murderers chose their victims within their circle of relatives or acquaintances. Six selected victims from among the members of their own family, three selected victims from among acquaintances and one selected a victim whom he did not know personally before the event. In this sample the fifty-two female killers only rarely went outside the family circle and none of them killed strangers.

In England, Norwood East found that only 6.6 percent of 300 insane murderers and only 16.5 percent of 200 sane offenders killed strangers. In the United States, too, the victim is more often than not a relative or close friend of the offender. In Wolfgang's study 63 percent of 550 victims were relatives, close friends, paramours or homosexual partners of the principal offender. Only 12 percent of the victims were strangers. Recent FBI figures for the United States show that each year between 15 and 17 percent of homicide victims are strangers.

THE CRIME PROVOCATIVE FUNCTION
OF THE VICTIM

"The murdered is not unaccountable for his own murder,
And the robbed is not blameless in being robbed . . .
Yea, the guilty is often times the victim of the injured
And still more often the condemned is the burden
bearer for the guiltless and unblamed."

Kahlil Gibran, *The Prophet**

The innocent bystander who is fatally wounded in the course of a shootout between police and bandits is a chance victim of circumstances beyond his control. Not infrequently, however, the victim may be in large measure responsible for his own fate. The contributory role of the victim to the criminal act finds dramatic portrayal in poetry, literature and folklore. Franz Werfel's novel, **Not the Assassin, but the Victim is Guilty,** has been summarized by Ellenberger:

"The hero of the novel recounts how he saw one day in an amusement park a good looking boy working with his father in a shooting gallery. He was engaged in picking up the hats of the wooden heads at which people threw balls, as well as the balls themselves, and seemed to be enjoying it. Thirteen years later, this young man killed his father. The crime seemed all the more inexplicable in that the father had literally adored his son.

"In contrast with the young murderer, the hero of the novel had been strictly reared by his father, a tyrannical, ambitious officer who showed no affection. For this reason, the hero hated his father bitterly. Affiliation with a nihilistic group brought him almost to the point of slapping his father's face. This is why the hero felt he understood the secret of this crime: By systematic cultivation, the father built such an immense accumulation of aggressive feelings in the son that these finally were turned toward their author, that is against the father himself. In ending his story, the hero declares, identifying himself with the young parricide, 'I, the assassin and he the victim are both guilty! But he is a little more guilty than I.' "

Study of the victim's role is hampered somewhat as "dead men tell no tales." Nevertheless there are many cases on record where there is clear

---

*Reprinted from **The Prophet** by Kahlil Gibran with permission of the publisher, Alfred A. Knopf, Inc. Copyright, 1923, by Kahlil Gibran; renewal Copyright, 1951, by administrators of Kahlil Gibran Estate and Mary C. Gibran.

evidence that the victim by continued brutality, alcoholic excesses, or other provocative behavior, contributed in large measure to his own demise.

Some persons, by reason of their unconscious needs, are destined to become victims. Just as there are accident prone persons, so also there are persons who are prone to become victims. Thus, there may be a symbiotic relationship between the criminal and his victim. Potential victims include the depressed sufferer, the masochistic character, the tormentor, the sexually provocative, the acquisitive person and persons who themselves have criminal or antisocial tendencies.

THE DEPRESSED VICTIM

The depressed person who seeks self-punishment is likely to have his needs met by the criminal to the satisfaction of both parties. Von Hentig has drawn attention to the most peculiar Peltzer murder case and the depressed victim who indifferently walked into the trap the murderer had set for him.

An elderly man went to a bar in a black ghetto neighborhood with a high crime rate. When he flashed six to eight fifty dollar bills in the bar a woman warned him, "Don't be flashing that money, it isn't safe, they'll get you here." He was seen leaving the bar with another man and later his body was found in an alley. He had been shot with his own gun and an informant reported that he had been killed during a robbery. A suspect claimed that, "I must have made him mad, he pulled out a gun, I was trying to grab it away from him and the gun went off.

A relative wondered whether the death was a "manipulated suicide." The victim had been depressed following the death of his mother. He was a quiet man who did not drink, gamble or carry a gun. He lived from paycheck to paycheck and did not carry large sums of money. It was completely out of character for him to go to a bar in a black neighborhood.

Neustatter has described the remarkable case of a depressed mental hospital patient who kept asking other patients to kill him. Eventually another patient agreed to strangle him for a few dollars and his victim was found unconscious with a belt around his throat on the verge of death. The assailant was charged with attempted murder, but the judge thought there was insufficient evidence, as so much of it came from mental hospital patients and the accused was found not guilty. Following his transfer to another hospital the assailant complained ruefully that this was the last time he would ever try to do anyone a favor.

Ellenberger adds that not only a great sorrow but also a great joy constitutes a danger. "To quote a German proverb, 'Nothing is harder to endure than a succession of happy days.' What the Germans call 'the drunkenness of good fortune' (Glücksrauch) has cost many people dear. It is thus for instance that one can explain the death of the archeologist, Winckelmann (1786). After completing his great masterpiece, the man became famous to the point of being invited by princes and even by the Empress, who conferred on him a gold medal. During his trip, he encountered at Trieste a stranger, struck up an acquaintance with him, and without the least investigation as to his identity, showed him the gold medals and threw himself blindly into the fatal trap which his assassin set for him."

THE MASOCHIST

In masochism, which is a sexual perversion, sexual gratification is obtained or enhanced by the suffering of pain. Masochists derive pleasure from being abused or dominated and they tend to place themselves repeatedly in self-defeating situations. The term is derived from the name of Leopold von Sacher-Masoch, an Austrian novelist. On the strength of a considerable number of his novels and stories, Krafft-Ebing took the scarcely warrantable liberty of identifying his name, while yet living, with a sexual perversion (9).

In his youth Sacher-Masoch liked to look at pictures of executions and dream of torture by a cruel woman. After his marriage he persuaded his wife to whip him nearly every day with whips that had nails attached to them. It is difficult to believe that a masochist in his wish for punishment would agree to his own murder, but many masochists willingly expose themselves to the risk of severe bodily injury or murder at the hands of brutal husbands or lovers.

A young woman who for ten months was a prostitute in London describes her love for a young man. She learns that he has just been released from jail after serving a long term for grievous bodily assault of a former girl friend. He broke her jaw in three places. When advised to leave him alone she replies to herself, "It's out of the question, I am committed physically and emotionally." Inevitably she herself suffers severe bodily assault a short time later. Even though she had warning of the assault, she returned with him in a taxi to her apartment. She made no attempt to escape and merely took half-hearted measures to protect herself, while he was paying the taxi-driver.

"Mechanically, I made provisions for the attack. I move all small things out of the way, hid all the knives, move chairs against the wall. Useless, really these little safeguards, but I must do something. My cheek stings and my arm aches. I sit on the edge of the bed after this is done, waiting for him. At least I shan't have far to fall.

"Pete comes back in; takes off his jacket with deliberation, hangs it up neatly and rolls up his sleeves. Then he drags me off the bed, hurling me into the far, empty corner of the room. He stands over me, menacingly. I bring up my arms to shield my face. He pulls me to my feet, pushes my useless defense out of the way, and holds me against the wall by my throat, constricting it so that I am choking . . . He brings his knee into my stomach and digs it in hard . . . Crash goes my head against the wall . . . He pushes me into an easy chair, standing behind me and holding my head back with an arm under my chin. Then he takes his nail file, with its cruel curved tip, out of his pocket, and holds it close to my cheek . . . tearing agony down my face. Dragging, zig-zagging pain from cheekbone to chin . . . With a frantic leap upwards, I push past him and rush to the door, lurching and missing it, then finding the handle locked, locked, locked and he has me again. Pounding of feet . . . Pete shouts, 'you're too bloody late' "*

The young woman was perhaps fortunate to be admitted to a hospital rather than a morgue.

Many women were attracted by the serial murderer Kurten (Chapter 8). "Kurten was clean and smart and well groomed; he looked about thirty, his voice was soft and persuasive; and his manners were perfect. But there was something else, something primeval and, to many women, regrettably attractive. 'Women were mad after Peter,' his wife said. When she had at first refused to marry him because he seemed to go about with so many women, he had said 'I shall kill you if you don't marry me,' and obviously meant it.

"In her book on the case Margaret Wagner compresses Kurten's secret into seven words, 'gentleness of manner and forcefulness of action.' He realized this himself. 'Brutality belongs to love,' he would murmur neatly as he kissed away blood forced from the mouth of a half strangled

---

*From **Streetwalker** published anonymously in 1959. Quoted by permission of The Bodley Head (London) and The Viking Press Inc. (New York), publishers.

victim. And police reports showed how often a girl thus attacked — and thus placated — would want to go with him again. A girl whom he had severely hurt by throttling her twice in one evening said in evidence, 'I said I would not see him for another month. But I could not sleep that night for thinking of him and hoping he would marry me . . . I know he is a scoundrel, but I am certain he is not the Dusseldorf murderer' " (5).

A thirty-one year old man asked his girl friend if she loved him. When she replied, "If you don't know now, you never will," he struck her on the back of the head, knocking her down, then he shot her in the head, in each hand, and in the right shoulder. He then dragged her into the bathroom and tried to drown her. She fought her way out of the bathroom and he pulled her into the bedroom where he tried to smother her. Charges of assault to murder were withdrawn after his girl friend married him and refused to testify against him. One month prior to the assault a brother of the assailant had murdererd his wife.

Ellenberger cites a case described by Locard which is of interest: A rich farmer of advanced years came one day to seek out Locard. He explained to him that he lived on an isolated farm with a young woman whom he had married, even though she was poor, because she was very beautiful and he loved her without being sure that it was reciprocated. For some time he had experienced symptoms, and he found a peculiar taste in his soup and in his coffee. The day before, while his wife believed that he slept, he had observed that she was manipulating a packet of powders. He had been able to fetch a little and he brought it to Locard. An analysis promptly showed that it was a case of poison. Locard set himself to direct a complaint to the magistrate, but the man protested: It was not that which he desired. "What I would like is an antidote to counteract the poison. I would like to last as long as possible, I love her very much!"

THE TORMENTOR

The tormentor usually dies by the hand of one of his family. The autocratic mother or wife who is constantly criticizing her son or husband may find that even a worm will turn. The sadist who threatens the lives of others may lose his own. Provoked beyond all measure, the long-suffering wife of the alcoholic tormentor may take her revenge in an impulsive act of violence; or a son may protect his mother from assault by stabbing or shooting his father.

A twenty-five year old alcoholic refinery worker brutally ill-treated his wife from the time of their marriage. He had frequent affairs with other women and on one occasion he brought a girl friend home. Before he closed the bedroom door his wife could see him starting to undress the girl. Although steadily employed and able to afford a late model car he allowed his wife insufficient money for housekeeping. At the end of the week she would have to beg neighbors for money or food to feed her children. There was a compartment in the refrigerator containing special food for her husband's exclusive use.

"He disciplined me and the children very sternly. We didn't go no place without his permission. In fact I was forbidden to call anybody unless they called me. I could talk to them if they called me. I was forbidden to use the phone. We asked permission to watch television. We didn't ever criticize or anything like that. I never asked questions. He stated to me quite frankly that what he told me I should know and what he didn't state to me was none of my business. We didn't disobey him.

"He beat me quite often, it could be over something like forgetting to put the ketchup on the table, or maybe I hadn't the coffee table just as he thought it should be, or the drapes were maybe pulled. They were little things. He threatened if I left him, he would come and get me with a gun. It seemed like every time we got into an argument, or I disagreed with him in any way, the gun came out of the drawer."

He would grab her by the hair, pull her off the couch, stand over her and beat her with his fists. Even when she was pregnant the physical assaults continued. On one occasion a physician had to use fifteen sutures to repair lacerations above and below her eyes. After particularly severe beatings she sought refuge in neighbors' homes.

One night he left home to buy some beer and did not return till 4 AM, the following morning. He boasted that he had been out with a married woman. When his wife remonstrated with him he ordered her out of the house. She protested that there was a snowstorm and she did not want to take the children out at that time in the morning. He told her to leave before he awakened or she would be unable to walk out of the house. Then he told her to do "her job," that is to perform fellatio on him. She complied, but not to his satisfaction, and he hit her on the back of her head and pulled her hair.

About six o'clock in the morning she obtained her husband's revolver and shot him in the right temple. She was found guilty of second-degree murder, but a mistrial was declared. At her second trial, she was found guilty of voluntary manslaughter and she was placed on three years' probation.

The tormentor is further considered below.

VICTIM PRECIPITATED HOMICIDE

The term victim precipitated homicide has been used by Wolfgang to describe those cases in which the victim was the first to show and to use a deadly weapon, to strike a blow—in short, the first to commence the interplay of resort to physical violence. He gives the following examples:

"A husband accused his wife of giving money to another man, and while she was making breakfast, he attacked her with a milk bottle, then a brick and finally a piece of concrete block. Having had a butcher knife in hand, she stabbed him during the fight.

"In an argument over a business transaction, the victim first fired several shots at his adversary, who in turn fatally returned the fire.

"A victim became incensed when his eventual slayer asked for money which the victim owed him. The victim grabbed a hatchet and started in the direction of his creditor, who pulled out a knife and stabbed him.

"During a lovers' quarrel, the male (victim) hit his mistress and threw a can of kerosene at her. She retaliated by throwing the liquid on him, and then tossed a lighted match in his direction. He died from the burns.

"A drunken victim with knife in hand approached his slayer during a quarrel. The slayer showed a gun, and the victim dared him to shoot. He did.

"During an argument in which a male called a female many vile names, she tried to telephone the police. He grabbed the phone from her hands, knocked her down, kicked her, and hit her with a tire gauge. She ran to the kitchen, grabbed a butcher knife, and stabbed him in the stomach."

This Philadelphia study showed that in 150 or 26 percent of the 588 homicides, the victim was the first to show and use a deadly weapon, or to strike a blow in an altercation. Furthermore, in these cases the victim

(62 percent) was more likely than the offender (54 percent) to have a previous arrest or police record. Almost one third of 578 homicides in Baltimore were victim-precipitated (2). As Wolfgang notes, in most cases of victim-precipitated homicide the roles and characteristics of the victim and offender are reversed:

"In many cases the victim has most of the major characteristics of an offender; in some cases two potential offenders came together in a homicide situation and it is probably only chance which results in one becoming a victim and the other an offender. At any rate, connotations of a victim as a weak and passive individual, seeking to withdraw from an assaultive situation, and of an offender as a brutal, strong and overly aggressive person seeking out his victim, are not always correct. Societal attitudes are generally positive toward the victim and negative toward the offender, who is often feared as a violent and dangerous threat to others. However, data in the present study — especially that of previous arrest record — mitigate, destroy or reverse these connotations of victim-offender roles in one out of every four criminal homicides" (24).

Wolfgang properly restricts victim precipitated homicides to those cases where the victim is the first to resort to physical violence. When an assailant makes a serious threat to kill, the victim by his response may tip the delicate balance between threat and homicide. Words and looks can wound as well as blows and bullets. Harsh criticism, belittling sarcasm, or a contemptuous glance by the recipient of a homicidal threat may have fatal consequences.

It is unwise for a wife to respond to her husband's display of a firearm during an argument with provocative comments, such as "What are you going to do, big man, kill me?" and "You haven't got the guts to kill me." A very vain girl friend did not say "Don't shoot me," but "Don't shoot me in the face." Her boy friend altered his aim and shot her in the chest. How different the response of a child when his severely depressed mother said she was going to kill him, "Oh no, momma, I know you wouldn't do that."

A man threatened by his homosexual partner, who held a knife at his throat, said, "I dare you, I think you're chicken." A daughter, overhearing father beating mother, came between her parents. Her mother said, "Never mind, honey, let him kill me." After she left the home to seek help, her father obtained his revolver from another room and killed his wife. One mother threatened by her daughter responded angrily, "We'll see who kills who first."

FEMALE VICTIMS

> *"It can perhaps never be sufficiently impressed upon*
> *the mind of a young girl that she should not have a*
> *lover; for if she does, and if she bears him children —*
> *or threatens to — he is quite likely to murder her before*
> *he marries the woman he has chosen as his wife."*
>
> Richard Baker, *The Fatal Caress*

Women are more often victims than offenders in criminal homicide and the great majority of female victims are slain by men. The relative danger to women increases when the homicide rate is low. Thus, the percentage of female victims in England (57 percent of 551 criminal homicides) is higher than in the United States (24 percent of 588 criminal homicides in Philadelphia). This is in accord with Verkko's Law. "In countries of high frequency of crimes against life the female proportion of those killed is small; and vice versa: in countries of low frequency of crimes against life the percentage of female victims is perceptibly greater than in countries of high frequency of crimes against life."

In Wolfgang's study there were 100 husband-wife homicides, 53 victims were wives and 47 were husbands. The number of wives killed by their husbands constituted 41 percent of all women killed, whereas husbands slain by their wives make up only 11 percent of all the men killed. Eighty-seven percent of all the females were slain by males.

Lonely middle-age spinsters and childless widows are ready victims for the serial murderer (Chapter 7). It is extremely rare for a person to be murdered before the eyes of another individual. This shows the protective value of company. Love making, which excludes such companionship, is one of the most adequate means of isolation (12).

Women stand in danger of assault and murder by rapists. This risk is not confined to young women as there are many cases in which unattractive elderly women have been raped and murdered. Some women by their provocative dress and behavior contribute to their selection as victims by sexual offenders. The young child who is sexually assaulted and murdered is properly regarded as the victim of the adult assailant. Nevertheless it is well known that small girls will sometimes act in a very seductive manner toward strangers and their behavior may be the first link in the chain which leads to their murder.

PROSTITUTES AND MURDER

Murder is an occupational hazard of prostitution. Detection of the murderer is difficult because of the clandestine nature of the profession. The clients, who come by night, are usually strangers who are invited with little question into the girl's apartment. The client may be overcome with guilt and rage following sexual relations with the prostitute or he may be a sadist whose intention is murder rather than intercourse. Dr. Neill Cream and "Jack the Ripper" come to mind, although the former did not restrict his murderous activities to prostitutes.

The prostitute may be murdered by her "pimp," the procurer who exploits her. According to Puybaraud when a crime takes place in the couple of pimp-prostitute, it is always the prostitute who is killed. He states that between 1870 and 1890, more than a hundred pimps were condemned to death or to penal servitude for life for murder, in the police district of Seine alone. He cites the case of a certain Drogmatchoff who, having murdered the woman who supported him for forty years, gave as an excuse: "I believed that she was showing ill will."

Söderman states that when a macquereau (pimp) gets his hooks into a prostitute there is almost no way she can escape from him except by death. Even so, he once came upon a case of a pimp who had cut the throat of this woman, and her last words were "I love you." A macquereau will beat and torture his woman if she fails to earn as much money as he expects. Often he will beat her for fun without any reason (22). In contrast, German authors describe the ferocious jealousy of the prostitute in connection with her pimp. Should there be a crime it is not she who is killed, but rather that she kills the pimp through jealousy (8).

MODELS

In August 1957, the parents of a young model reported that she was missing from her home in Los Angeles. She was last seen in the company of a man who wished to take photographs of her. Eight months later a young divorcee disappeared after going out with a man she met through a lonely hearts club. In July 1958, another model, a former striptease dancer, disappeared from her apartment in Los Angeles. Three months later thirty year old Harvey Glatman was arrested on a country road by a highway patrolman who caught him struggling with a girl for possession of a revolver.

The girl informed police that she was a model and that she had agreed to pose for some "cheesecake" photos for $20. Instead of driving her to a studio, Glatman drove away from Los Angeles, and he then attempted to tie her up. She resisted his efforts and in the struggle for the gun a shot was fired which caused a superficial wound on her leg.

In Glatman's apartment were found pictures of the missing divorcee and missing models. The pictures showed the girls, fully clothed, gagged and bound with rope. Other pictures showed the girls nude or partially clothed. There was a picture of each victim with a sash cord around her throat. Curiously one series of pictures included Glatman's driver's license. He explained that this was to identify himself. He confessed that he lured his victims to their death by posing as a photographer. His first victim agreed to being tied up when he said he was taking pictures for a crime magazine. The pictures were to portray a terrified girl at the mercy of a rapist. The pictures he took were very realistic. The girls were disrobed, photographed, sexually assaulted, then strangled.

On being charged with the murder of two of his victims, Glatman pleaded guilty and blocked all efforts of his attorney to enter a plea of not guilty by reason of insanity. When he was sentenced to die for each of the two murders, the defendant jokingly asked, "How can they carry out two death penalties?"

He was first arrested in Denver at the age of seventeen after he had tied up and robbed two Denver women. While awaiting trial he kidnapped a young girl from a street in Boulder, Colorado and drove her to a canyon near the town where he tied her up and sat beside her all night. He left her in the morning, but at nightfall he returned and released her unharmed. The girl did not press charges, but he was sentenced to one to five years for his first crime. In 1946, he was arrested in New York for stealing purses from women as they were walking home late at night from bus stops. A five to ten year sentence was imposed and he was released in 1951.

Some modeling agencies and free lance models in their newspaper advertisements welcome amateur as well as professional photographers, others go even further and offer to lend or rent cameras to those "photographers" who do not have their own equipment. Following the Glatman killings the Los Angeles City Council drafted an ordinance requiring models and photographers, specializing in nudes, to register with the police and show evidence of good moral character.

CHILDREN

The danger of murder begins at birth. "Early in the seventeenth century the practice of killing illegitimate children directly after they were born had become a very common occurrence. The unmarried woman of that time who became pregnant did not resort to illegal operations. Abortion then was rare, infanticide quite common. Just the converse obtains at the present time—illegal operations being very common, infanticide comparatively rare.

"So frequent had the crime of infanticide become that in the reign of James I an Act of Parliament was passed to deal with the matter. Briefly, the provisions of the Act were as follows. If a woman delivered of a child, which, being born alive, would be a bastard, endeavored by burying, drowning, or other means, by herself or by others, to conceal its birth so it would not be possible to determine whether it were born alive, it was murder unless she could prove by one witness at least it was born dead. The law was regarded as so unfair and severe that in practice it seems that judges, juries and even the prosecution entered into a conspiracy to defeat its harshness.

"Many fictions and judicial evasions were resorted to in order to evade the Act. For example it was held that if the mother had provided clothes for the expected child she had not concealed the birth; if she knocked on the wall during the actual birth she had called attention to the birth, and again was not guilty of concealment, and so on. The Act, however, remained in nominal force till the reign of George III, when in 1803 it was repealed" (20).

As DeGreeff has well emphasized, direct infanticide is much less frequent than indirect and disguised infanticide: It is no accident, he says, if in Belgium the mortality among the babies of unmarried mothers is double that of other babies of the same age.

The term baby farmer was applied to women who adopted babies, usually illegitimate, on payment of a fixed sum or on continuing payment of money and then murdered their charges. Mrs. Dyer, the infamous English baby farmer, disposed of one of her charges in the Thames River, but made the mistake of wrapping the body in a piece of brown paper bearing her own name and address! Jesse attributes this incredible piece of carelessness to the fact that she had pursued her trade for so long that continued immunity had stolen away her caution. It will never be known how many children met their death at her hands.

Infanticide is socially approved among Eskimos. "Infants are only potentially productive. If conditions permit, the Eskimos will always endeavor to raise their babies to adulthood. Too often, however, harsh circumstances do not permit. It is then up to each family to decide for itself; are its present resources (both human and material) sufficient to maintain the baby through its non-productive years? There will be no social blame or legal sanction if a negative decision is reached. Baby girls are the most frequent victims of homicide . . . one Netsilingmiut mother had borne twenty children — fifteen girls and five boys. Ten of the girls she had killed at birth" (13).

Children seldom own property or large sums of money. When their parents are wealthy, other relatives may seek to kill the child in order to inherit a fortune which they might not otherwise obtain. The danger of kidnapping and murder faces children of wealthy parents. The hostage may be killed whether or not the ransom is paid, as in the Bobbie Greenlease case. In September 1953, a woman called at the Notre Dame de Sion convent school in Kansas City and claimed that she was Bobbie Greenlease's aunt. She was allowed to take him away on the pretext that his mother had suffered a heart attack. Almost a week later the millionaire father paid $600,000 to the kidnappers but it was later discovered that the boy had been murdered soon after the kidnapping. Indeed his grave had been prepared before the abduction.

Subsequently, a man who had been spending heavily was investigated by the police and found to have over $250,000 in his luggage. He was Carl Austin Hall who had turned to crime after squandering over $200,000 which he had inherited on the death of his father, a well-known lawyer. An alcoholic and drug addict, he had once served fifteen months of a five year penitentiary sentence for robbery. His partner in crime was Bonnie Heady, widow of a bank robber who had been killed by law enforcement officers after escaping from jail. The couple were executed for their crime.

In earlier times the children of royalty were sometimes murdered by the person who was next in line of inheritance. The child may be in the murderer's way for other reasons. Von Hentig quotes the case of a woman whose husband had not been heard of for ten years and who wanted her lover to return to her. He had left because she had a twelve year old boy who was troublesome. The mother drowned the boy to win her lover back.

Elizabeth Downs was accused in Oregon of shooting her children in 1983 because they interfered with her relationship with a boy friend in

Arizona who did not want to be a father. She claimed that an unkempt man flagged her down on an isolated country road, then shot her and the children when she refused to give him the car keys. However her nine year old daughter whose wounds caused her to suffer a stroke that impaired her speech and her use of one arm testified that her mother shot her and her siblings. A seven year old daughter was killed and a four year old son was paralyzed from the waist down. She was convicted of murder and attempted murder.

Children have been killed by severely depressed or schizophrenic mothers (Chapter 9). Often these mentally disordered mothers then kill themselves or attempt to do so. Other children have been killed by fathers upset over divorce or threat of divorce. These fathers usually have an antisocial personality disorder rather than severe depression or schizophrenia. A man angered by his wife's desire for a divorce told her "If you want war you shall have it, but the children you shall not have." He killed his three children (11). Those children of battering parents increase the risk of homicidal assault when they cry too much or show open disobedience. The young child is sometimes menaced by jealous brothers or sisters.

THE ELDERLY

The elderly person, especially if he is believed to be in possession of a large sum of money, faces the risk of robbery-homicide. The tendency of some elderly persons to hoard their money in their home rather than place it in a bank adds to their danger. Von Hentig draws attention to the large number of deaths by fire, 15,000 each year in the United States, and points out that in all such fires babies and old people are the main sufferers. Too many people, in his opinion, are burned by exploding oil burners, or while burning weeds or leaves in the barnyard, or are said to have fallen asleep while smoking and thus ignited their bedding. He suspects that the possibility of murder is overlooked.

Older persons are excellent subjects for poisoning as sudden death in later life does not arouse the suspicion that would accompany death of a younger person. Many doctors are only too ready to attribute unexpected death in the aged to a heart attack.

Among Eskimos, elimination of elderly nonproductive members of the community is socially approved. "Although others may decide that the days of an aged one are done, the request for death usually comes from the old person. The actual killing should be performed by a relative to preclude the possibility of vengeance. Infanticide is casually accepted, but not so senilicide and invalicide. Emotional bonds are not easily severed that have built up through the years and not infrequently the aged one has to insist upon his demand-right to be killed; the kinsman is forced into performance of his duty.

"Weyer records a poignant example: A hunter living on the Diomede Islands related to the writer how he killed his own father, at the latter's request. The old Eskimo was failing, he could no longer contribute what he thought should be his share as a member of the group; so he asked his son, then a lad about twelve years old, to sharpen the big hunting knife. Then he indicated the vulnerable spot over his heart where his son should stab him. The boy plunged the knife, but the stroke failed to take effect. The old father suggested with dignity and resignation, 'Try it a little higher, my son.' The second stab was effective, and the patriarch passed into the realm of the ancestral shades.

"Stabbing is but one form of Eskimo senilicide. Hanging, strangulation, blocking up in a snow house to freeze to death, and abandonment in the open wastes by traveling groups are all used by various Eskimos" (13).

THE ACQUISITIVE

"One is never so close to being deceived
as when one wishes to deceive."

La Rochefaucauld

The confidence game criminal selects as his victim someone with larceny in his soul. In confidence games the aim is to show the victim how he can make money dishonestly and then beat him in his attempted dishonesty. The acquisitive victim usually loses his money rather than his life.

The mass murderer, Jean Baptiste Troppmann, succeeded in persuading Jean Kinck, who was worth 100,000 francs, to leave home and wife, in anticipation of quick profit from an illegal money-making scheme. "There was, he confided, in an old and apparently abandoned chateau at Herrenfluch, Alsace, a room in which good friends of his own had installed the last word in up-to-date machinery for the manufacture of spurious coin; machinery which turned out its products with such versimilitude that after a long term of operations the authorities were not even aware that base coin was in circulation. So successful had been the operations of the syndicate that now they were in a position to retire from business, leaving premises and plant for any reliable and trustworthy successors, who were prepared to pay a matter of 5,000 francs for the goodwill of the concern (6)."

Jean Kinck's cupidity resulted not only in his own death, but also in the murder of his wife and their six children.

OCCUPATIONAL RISKS

Certain persons by reason of their occupation face added risk of death from criminal homicide. Law enforcement officers, royalty, political leaders, physicians, lawyers, and prostitutes are exposed to special danger. Bank tellers, druggists, taxi drivers, and nighttime clerks in convenience stores may be killed by armed robbers. Although relatively few stickups end in murder, armed robberies account for 12 to 13 percent of deaths from criminal homicide. The Boston Police Department, in a survey of taxicab robberies in eighteen cities, found that there was an average of one murdered cab driver per 1,200 cabs each year (17).

PRESIDENTS

"A president has to expect those things."

Harry S. Truman

Four of the first thirty-eight presidents of the United States were assassinated and attempts were made on the lives of several others. Since the murder in 1865 by John Wilkes Booth of Abraham Lincoln, whose guard neglected his duties by leaving the president's presence, elaborate precautions have been taken to protect the lives of our presidents. All the modern secret service procedures could not save John F. -Kennedy in 1963 from the rifle bullets of his assassin, Lee Harvey Oswald. Lattimer has drawn attention to the extraordinary series of similarities between the assassinations, a century apart, of Lincoln and Kennedy.

"Both presidents were shot in the back of the head on a Friday before a public holiday, while seated beside their wives. Another couple was present in both instances, of which the man was also wounded by the assassin but not fatally. Both men had gross missile damage to one cerebral hemisphere: both were given closed-chest cardiac massage and artificial respiration. In each case only partial autopsies were allowed and insistent claims were made later that in each case the fatal shots must have come from a different direction. Both claims were later discredited: press photographs of the body were forbidden in each case.

"The wives concerned were both married at twenty-four, both had three children, and both lost a child while in the White House. Both held the wounded heads of their husbands and endured an agonizing period of waiting while doctors unsuccessfully tried to save the victims. Both presidents had a slight ocular abnormality with a 'wandering eye.' Both enjoyed rocking chairs. Each man was over six feet and had previously been a boat captain. Both were immediately succeeded by vice-presidents called Johnson" (15).

Knight in his review of Lattimer's book further notes that both assassins were Southerners in their twenties, both learned of their victim's movements from the newspapers, using this knowledge to choose their assassination sites. Both were trapped by officers named Baker—though Oswald was released when Baker found he worked in the book depository. Both were psychologically the same type, deprived of a father figure and overshadowed by elder brothers. Both had the habit of writing down their thoughts and plans and in each case, these journals were not made available to the investigating commissions.

PHYSICIANS

The physician is exposed not only to the risk of contagious disease in the exercise of his profession, but also to the risk of being murdered by one of his patients. D'Heucqueville reports that each year in France three to seven physicians are mortally or gravely wounded by patients. For the most part these patients have been known to be mentally ill for a long time prior to the assault. They fall into three groups.

In the first group are paranoid patients who kill mental hospital doctors or doctors who have been responsible for their commitment to mental hospitals. Paranoid persons who have failed in their applications for workmen's compensation or military pension for alleged physical illness or disability may kill doctors who have given unfavorable testimony or have denied their application.

The second group includes the hypochondriac who blames the physician for having created or aggravated their illness. A surgeon may be held responsible for the failure or complications of a surgical operation. The hypochondriac is preoccupied with his symptoms and his entire life may be focused around his illness. As complaints are often related to the anus, genitals or lower abdomen; surgeons, gynecologists and urologists are particularly exposed to these patients. Impotence may be blamed on an operation for hemorrhoids. Delusions of contamination or innoculation with syphilis lead to feelings of resentment and anger.

The physician often loses sight of the patient but in the shadow, plans for vengeance ripen. A claim for damages in a court of law is accompanied by virulent defamation of the physician.

The third group consists of female patients with "erotomania" who are convinced that their doctor is madly in love with them. The patient seeks help for a multitude of complaints and will not leave the consulting room before obtaining "the wages of the love object." She besieges the doctor with telephone calls and begs him to visit her in the intimacy of her home. Harmless acts on the part of the doctor are interpreted as evidence of his love for her. Although every doctor is exposed to this problem, psychiatrists and psychoanalysts are in a particularly vulnerable position. When these patients fail in their quest they resort to anonymous letters, open accusations of scandal and in extreme cases to use of a revolver.

Yet another group of patients might be added to D'Heucqueville's list. Each year there are reports of threats to kill or the murder of plastic surgeons by dissatisfied clients. The following case illustrates the occupational hazards of plastic surgery.

JS, a tailor with a saddle nose, consulted a physician because of earache. He was persuaded to undergo an operation to correct the deformity of his nose. Unfortunately the operation was a failure and disfigured him more so than before. Following the operation JS developed paranoid delusions regarding the physician. Five years later, following an unsuccessful attempt to kill the physician, he was placed in an institution, but he was released after a relatively short period. Twenty-seven years later he succeeded in killing the physician (10).

INFORMERS

*"The business I'm in right now
you can't get life insurance."*

confidential informant

The confidential informant who betrays his criminal associates to the police, whether for money or to escape punishment for his own illegal acts, places his life in jeopardy. In order to discourage betrayal, the Mafia and other organized crime groups place great emphasis on the code of secrecy and punish severely those who transgress this code. New recruits are taught the code of **omertá,** manliness, and honor: a man does not betray his comrades.

Informers shot to death in an ambush are fortunate indeed compared with those who are kidnapped, tortured and then murdered. These torture-killings serve as a grim warning to others. An untidy method of disposal is to blow up the informant. The bomb is placed under the hood of the victim's car near the dashboard, and when the driver turns on the ignition to start the car he ends his own life. There is the risk that the intended victim may lend his car to a friend, but the mafiosi probably console themselves with the thought that only persons of doubtful character would associate with informants.

AGE

In general those who are killed are older than those who kill. The majority of victims are between twenty-five and thirty-five years of age, whereas the majority of offenders are between twenty and thirty years of age.

CRIMINAL RECORDS OF VICTIMS

Almost 50 percent of the 588 victims of criminal homicide in Wolfgang's study had a previous police or arrest record. In the cases of victim precipitated homicide it was found that the victim (62 percent) was more likely than the offender (54 percent) to have a previous arrest or police record.

FAILURE TO HEED WARNING OF MURDER

There are numerous cases on record where the victims were given more than adequate warning of their fate yet failed to heed the warning signs. The victims of Palmer, the English poisoner, feared and distrusted him. His mother-in-law declared it would be the end of her if she went to stay in his house. Yet she went to live with him uttering these words, "I know I shall not live a fortnight." She was right; the fortnight saw her buried from Palmer's house, and he became the possessor of nine houses (14).

Arthur Major, an English truck driver threw away his luncheon sandwiches remarking, "I'm sure that woman is trying to kill me." A flock of starlings settled down on the abandoned sandwiches and Major's companion was horrified to see one of the birds topple over dead. It was astonishing that Major was not warned by this sinister event, particularly as he already suspected his wife, but he did nothing and eventually met his death as a victim who had been forewarned (19). Mrs. Major was hanged for poisoning her husband with strychnine.

A thirty-three year old man thought that he was chosen to be the savior of the world and accused his wife of being the devil. At night he would sit up with a loaded gun as he thought people were spying on him. Four months after brief treatment in a psychiatric ward he returned home one evening with some wooden stakes which were used on animal carcasses at the packing house where he was employed. He announced that he was going to obtain a hammer from a relative.

His wife became alarmed when she noted that there was one wooden stake for each member of the family she was convinced that he was going to kill her and the children. She told him "I know you're going to kill me. That's OK if you want to kill me and it makes you happy. When I lay down tonight you're going to pound that in my heart and kill me. But you do it, if that's what you want to do. Before you do it, buy me a six-pack of beer because I don't want to know about it." He denied that he was going to kill her, bought her a six-pack of beer and later burned the stakes. He did not kill her but the next day he killed one of his employers by driving a wooden stick in his victim's chest. Later he explained that the employer was the devil and the only way to kill the devil was with a wooden stick through the heart.

WHOSE FINGER ON THE TRIGGER?

At Siderno, Italy in 1952 two young Italian brothers, Frank and Gene Archina, married two American sisters, Rose and Mary Macri in civil ceremonies. The couples did not live as men and wives as the girls' father, Frank Macri, Sr., had insisted that the marriages should not be consummated until solemnized in the Roman Catholic Church at Denver, Colorado. The purpose of the civil marriages was presumably to enable the brothers to enter the United States as husbands of American citizens.

The young couples lived, but not together, in Frank Macri's Denver home. The husbands kept requesting church wedding services but their father-in-law refused to agree until the Archinas' saved enough money to pay for an elaborate wedding service and receptions, furniture, home and so on. This situation gave rise to frequent arguments and much ill feeling.

On Sunday afternoon, on January 24, 1954, following the noon meal, Frank Archina again approached his father-in-law on the subject and a fight developed. According to Frank Archina's wife, Rose, her husband kicked his father-in-law in the leg and then dashed upstairs to his room. Frank Macri thereupon took his wife and daughters to a back bedroom on the first floor and hid his wife and daughter, Mary, in a closet. Rose called her brother from the backyard where he was washing his car. As she joined her mother and sister in the closet her father was leaving the bedroom with a double barreled shotgun in his hand. She described the ensuing events as follows:

"I heard several shots and I heard a scream. Someone screaming, then I saw Frank Archina opening the closet door. He had a gun, a double barrel. He shot my mother twice. She was kneeling. She said, 'Please don't shoot me.' He shot her in the mouth twice. He reloaded the gun and shot my sister in the arm and side twice. He opened the gun and put in a new shell. He put the muzzle at my neck and pulled the trigger. I heard a click, it didn't go off. (A 20 gauge shell was later found in the 16 gauge shotgun.) He looked under the bed and then jumped out the window."

When the police arrived they found Frank Macri, his wife and son dead. Mary was still alive despite serious wounds but she died later in a hospital. Archina was picked up in a tavern. He stated that at the peak of the argument his father-in-law threatened to kill him and attempted to slash him with a knife. He claimed that he blacked out when his father-in-law pointed a shotgun at him and that he could remember nothing more of the tragedy. At his trial he was found guilty of first degree murder and sentenced to death. The Supreme Court of Colorado reversed the conviction and ordered a new trial.

Three years later during his re-trial, Robert Koch, a schoolteacher and former neighbor of the Macris', informed the defense attorneys that he entered the home before the police and spoke to mortally wounded Mary Macri. On the afternoon of the shooting he heard a booming noise and then heard someone shout for help. In the home he found twenty-six year old Frank Macri, Jr., lying on his back dead with a wound in his left shoulder. He next saw Frank Macri, Sr., lying in the hallway on top of his shotgun. He removed the gun and placed it in the kitchen. "Good housekeeping, I guess," he explained.

Hearing moans from the bedroom he went there and found Mrs. Macri and her daughter in the closet. Mary was still alive and seemed to be more worried about her mother than herself. She told him, "Don't let them hurt him (Frank Archina). We made him do it." In these dramatic words, "We made him do it," one of the victims of the quadruple slaying placed the blame not on the homicide offender but on his victims.

Frank Archina was found not guilty by reason of insanity at his second trial. In explanation of the verdict one of the jurors remarked, "The evidence showed that Archina emptied double barrel blasts into both his mother-in-law and sister-in-law while they cringed in a bedroom closet. A sane man would not have to pull a trigger twice at that range to kill somebody."

Archina was given a probationary release from the State Hospital in 1958 to be deported to Italy. On arrival in Italy he was promptly jailed. Italian law provides that Italian citizens who commit crimes abroad which carry penalties greater than three years in prison must be tried in Italian courts when the citizen returns to that country.

REFERENCES

1. Anonymous: *Streetwalker.* London, The Bodley Head, 1959.
2. Criminal Justice Commission: Criminal homicides in Baltimore, Maryland 1960-1964. Baltimore, 1967 (processed).
3. DeGreeff, E.: *Introduction à la Criminologie,* Vol. 1. Bruxelles, Vandenplass, 1946.
4. D'Heucqueville, G.: Les assassins de medecines. *Presse Medicale, 1*:1053, 1933.
5. Dickson, Grierson: *Murder by Numbers.* London, Robert Hale Ltd., 1958.
6. Douthwaite, L.C.: *Mass Murder.* New York, Henry Holt and Company, 1929.
7. East, W.N.: *Society and the Criminal.* Springfield, Charles C Thomas, 1950.
8. Ellenberger, Henri: Psychological relationships between criminal and victim. *Arch Crim Psychodyn, 1*:257, 1955.
9. Ellis, Havelock: *Studies in the Psychology of Sex.* Philadelphia, F.A. Davis Company, 1927.

10. Gross, Hans: *Criminal Psychology.* Boston, Little Brown and Company, 1915.
11. Harder, Thoger: The psychopathology of infanticide. *Acta Psychiatr Scand, 43*:196, 1967.
12. Hentig, Hans Von: *The Criminal and His Victim.* New Haven, Yale Univ. Press, 1948.
13. Hoebel, E.A.: *The Law of Primitive Man.* Cambridge, Harvard Univ. Press, 1954.
14. Jesse, F.T.: *Murder and its Motives.* London, Harrap, 1952.
15. Knight, Bernard: Murder of two presidents. *Brit Med J., 282*:1864, 1981.
16. Lattimer, J.K.: *Kennedy and Lincoln: Medical and Ballistic Comparisons of Their Assassinations.* New York, Harcourt Brace Jovanovich, 1980.
17. Macdonald, J.M.: *Armed Robbery: Offenders and Their Victims.* Springfield, Charles C Thomas, 1975.
18. Neustatter, W.L.: *The Mind of the Murderer.* London, Christopher Johnson, 1957.
19. O'Donnell, B.: *Should Women Hang?* London, W.H. Allen, 1956.
20. Parry, L.A.: A dissertation by William Hunter on the uncertainty of the signs of murder in the case of bastard children. *Brit Med J, 2*:1143, 1931.
21. Puybaraud: *Les Malfaiteurs de Profession,* 1893.
22. Sodermann, H.: *Policemen's Lot.* New York, Funk and Wagnalls Company, 1956.
23. Svalastoga, K.: Homicide and social contact in Denmark. *Amer J Sociology, 62*:37, 1956.
24. Wolfgang, M.E.: *Patterns in Criminal Homicide.* Philadelphia, Univ. of Pennsylvania, 1958.

CHAPTER 5

THE PSYCHOLOGY OF MURDER

"Thus speaks the red judge, 'Why did this criminal
murder? He wanted to rob.' But I say unto you: his
soul wanted blood, not robbery; he thirsted after the
bliss of the knife. His poor reason, however, did not
comprehend this madness and persuaded him: 'What
matters blood?' it asked; 'don't you want at least to
commit a robbery with it? To take revenge?' And he
listened to his poor reason: its speech lay upon him
like lead; so he robbed when he murdered. He did
not want to be ashamed of his madness."

Nietzsche, *Thus Spake Zarathustra*

THE PSYCHOLOGICAL basis of homicide has long fascinated not
only psychiatrists and psychologists, but also philosophers and
writers. Indeed there can be few persons who are not interested in the
mind and motives of the murderer. Newspaper headlines and the popularity of murder mysteries testify to the ever present public concern over
the problem of human aggression. Profound intuitive understanding of
the murderer is revealed in the writings of Shakespeare **(Richard II,
Hamlet, Macbeth)**, Simenon **(The Murderer)**, Dostoyevsky **(The
Brothers Karamazov, Crime and Punishment)** and other authors.

The explanation of murder is usually sought in such obvious conscious motivations as lust, greed, envy, revenge and anger. Often indeed
there is clear evidence of such factors, but even when they are present
they seldom provide an adequate explanation for the crime. The murderer himself may seek to explain his conduct in like manner. Yet the
mainsprings of human conduct are so complex as to cast doubt on such
simple solutions.

The conscious confessions of criminals and a statement of the circumstances of the crime be it ever so complete, will never sufficiently explain why the individual in the given circumstances had to commit just that act. External circumstances very often do not motivate the deed at all, and the doer, did he wish to be frank, would mostly have to acknowledge that he really did not himself exactly know what impelled him to do it, most often however, he is not so frank, not even to himself, but subsequently looks for and finds explanation of his conduct, which was in many ways incomprehensible, and psychically only imperfectly motivated, that is to say he rationalizes something irrational (11).

For example a young man who was arrested after he had made several homicidal assaults on women was quick to agree with the district attorney that his assaults were for the purpose of sexual gratification. At first sight this explanation appears satisfactory. After rendering his victims unconscious he would proceed to rape them. But surely sexual intercourse can be achieved at less cost. The man was of pleasing appearance and experienced little difficulty in establishing social relations with members of the opposite sex. He lived in a large city where it was relatively easy to make the acquaintance of prostitutes. Furthermore intercourse with an unconscious woman in a dark alley with the ever present risk of detection can scarcely be pleasurable.

Not all his victims were rendered unconscious. He would pick up a young girl at a drive-in or on the city streets and drive to a lover's lane. On arrival without any attempt at seduction he would tell the girl to remove her underclothing. Removing a large hunting knife from the glove compartment he would ostentatiously clean his fingernails while commenting on the dangers of physical resistance. In these circumstances one would not expect to find a loving embrace. On psychiatric examination I pointed out to the young man that he must harbour considerable feelings of hostility toward the opposite sex.

When he rejected this suggestion, I reminded him that he had fractured the skulls of two women, attacked others with a hatchet and in other ways physically assaulted a number of women. Grudgingly he agreed that perhaps he had acted in a hostile manner toward a number of women. He acknowledged that the fleeting tense moments with his victims were not the most appropriate circumstances for sexual union. I then asked if any woman had made sexual advances to him. There was indeed one such instance, an attractive young woman who, while on a date made it clear that she was willing to have sexual relations with him.

He added rather primly that this suggestion upset him and he drove her straight back to her home.

After further discussion he began to realize that sexual gratification was not the explanation for his assaults on women. He requested psychiatric treatment for which he was eligible under a sexual psychopath law. I pointed out that treatment would mean exploration of the source of his hostility to women, and that this hostility probably originated in his childhood. As the only significant members of the opposite sex in his early life were his mother and his grandmother attention would be focused upon them. At this he became extremely angry and flexing his biceps, shouted out that he would bust the teeth out of any blankety blank psychiatrist who suggested that his mother had anything to do with his problem.

As this was precisely what I was doing I thought it wise to change the subject. His extreme reaction brought to mind Shakespeare's comment, "The lady doth protest too much, me thinks." When his anger subsided he became very anxious and volunteered that he had committed a number of assaults which the police did not know about; stating "I'm cutting my throat by doing this" he gave time, place and circumstance of these earlier crimes. He knew that I would report this information to the court as I had previously told him that the examination was not confidential.

Although he claimed that his relationship with his mother was a good one and that she disapproved of his wayward behavior, it was significant from his account that she had in the past shielded him from the police and hence from detection and that she gave tacit approval for his delinquent behavior. When she visited him on the ward she would sit close to him in a conspiratory manner and the pair would stop talking whenever a nurse approached within earshot. On one occasion, however, the two were overheard reviewing with obvious pleasure one of his earlier offenses. His mother in her childhood had been placed in a home for delinquents, and had later been acquitted on the charge of murdering her husband.

This youth was committed to the state hospital for treatment. One time his mother was driving him away from the hospital on leave and the sun was in her eyes, so she pulled down the sun visor. When she did this a packet of contraceptives fell in her lap. She commented what a fool her other son was to use contraceptives as they took a lot of pleasure out of sex. Surely an inappropriate comment in the circumstances. The son later revealed that he used to bring a stripper home in the hope that his mother would tell him not to do this, but she never did.

At the age of thirty-two after a period of confinement in the state penitentiary he was released. Within two months he decided to ask me to treat him and, unknown to me, he was within ten feet of me outside the University Hospital when he realized it was too late, for he had already killed a woman. Within a year of his release from the penitentiary, he raped a number of women and stabbed four of them. He was suspected of killing two women and he pleaded guilty to one murder. Alongside the body of the victim outside a church, the words, "I hate women" were written in the snow.

Originally he did not reveal his great feelings of anger at his grandmother, who was given responsibility for his care after the birth of a younger brother when he was thirteen months of age. "I was given away by my mother and shunned by my grandmother, a cold blonde bitch on wheels, a cold unloving monster. My feelings about my mother are just as screwed up. I had this sense of worthlessness, of being not loved, of being a little monster. Every time I suffer, I'm made to suffer, it's a woman that does it, and I suffer without the possibility of forgiveness. Somewhere in the back of my mind I've got the impression even this institution is a woman." He was referring to the state penitentiary where he was serving a life sentence.

Another example comes to mind in which an attempt to explain the circumstances of murder led to rationalization which took no heed of unconscious motivations. A young man after shooting a drinking companion of a few days acquaintance, stuffed the body of his victim in the trunk of his car. He then drove from Colorado in the direction of Arizona. He was arrested before reaching that state, where he had previously been employed as a miner.

At the trial the district attorney claimed that he was driving to Arizona to hide the body of his victim in an abandoned mine. Again this might appear to have been a reasonable explanation. But was it? The accused was a man of very superior intelligence. Indeed, with an IQ of 138 he was in the top 3 percent of the population from the viewpoint of intelligence. If his aim had been to hide the body of his victim, the State of Colorado offered admirable opportunities. In this age few persons walk more than 200 yards from their parked car, and the Rocky Mountains afford excellent hiding places.

Furthermore, instead of driving straight to Arizona he proceeded in a leisurely fashion. In the heat of summer the body soon began to decompose. A girl friend whom he picked up in his travel inquired about the smell coming from the back of his victim's car, and he replied with considerable aplomb that it was a crate of limburger cheese. Eventually, the smell became sufficient to attract so many flies that the curiosity of the police was aroused when he left his car overnight outside a hotel. It would appear that while ostensibly fleeing to avoid arrest he was unconsciously behaving in a manner which would result in his detection.

It is clear that to understand murder we must look for deeper, less obvious explanations of the criminal's conduct than is usually provided by the clues available in newspaper reports or in the deliberations of men who must, perforce, deal mostly with conscious things. Lust, greed, envy, revenge and anger are the motives commonly held responsible for murder. As these motivating forces are so common and murder so rare, further inquiry is required into the causes and control of the urge to kill.

THE URGE TO KILL

The urge to kill another human being, the ultimate form of aggression, will be reviewed in general terms. Freud regarded aggression as an instinct and he thought, therefore, that a certain amount of aggressive behavior by human beings was inevitable.

The psychoanalytic concept of the mind in terms of id, ego and superego has been aptly described by Rado as personifications of passion, common sense and conscience; reflecting satanic temptations, the adaptive task and divine commandments. The id is the source of the instincts and throughout life it constantly seeks expression of asocial drives. The viewpoint that we are all potential criminals is not peculiar to psychoanalysis. It is in conformity with the Christian belief that we are all sinners. Thus St. Paul writes "for the good that I would I do not: but the evil which I would not that I do," and "The flesh lusteth against the Spirit and the Spirit against the flesh" is but another way of describing the struggle of the id with the superego.

Goethe spoke in similar vein when he said, "There is no crime of which I do not deem myself capable." Dostoyevsky in **The Brothers Karamazov** gives dramatic expression to the same theme. "Nobody in the world can be the judge of the criminal before he has realized that he himself is as much a criminal as the one who confronts him," and again, "Everyone pretends to hate evil, but deep down they all like it, all of them."

Dollard considers that aggression is always a consequence of frustration. He cites the case of a man who asked for psychiatric care because he was afraid that he would murder his wife, After some examination it turned out that the couple did not wish to have any more children and were achieving this end by strict continence. He felt frustrated, but because of his early training could not pick a fight with his wife and indeed felt that he should love her instead of hating her. The aggression eventually came out as a strong fear of doing murder, and he could not control or understand this fear.

In support of his viewpoint Dollard quoted figures to show the influence of poverty, illiteracy, mental retardation, smaller than average stature, ugliness, deformity, ill health, membership of a minority group, illegitimacy, unwholesome home conditions, demoralized neighborhoods and other frustrating factors on the crime rate. It should be noted that aggression is but one of many possible responses to frustration. The suggestion that frustration is the only cause of aggression is not supported by experiments with animals. For example, Scott found that the best way to train a mouse to be highly aggressive is not to frustrate him but to give him success in fighting. Scott's experiments suggest that frustration leads to aggression only in a situation where the individual has a habit of being aggressive.

Early childhood experiences play an important role. Prolonged separation of a child from his mother (or mother figure) in the early years may affect the development of aggressive behavior. Parental rejection may have the same effect. If one has suffered great deprivation oneself, one will feel inclined to inflict equal suffering on someone else (2). The total child-parent relationship will foster or discourage aggressive responses. The child who finds that angry outbursts produce the results which he desires will tend to repeat this form of behavior. Extreme indulgence or domination will adversely affect personality development and either may stimulate aggressiveness. Excessive punishment and frustration arising from undue restriction of the child's behavior are especially likely to generate aggression. However the former may also inhibit expression of hostility, particularly within the home.

An important source of aggression in family life is rivalry among the children for parental approval. The Biblical account of the murder of Abel by his brother Cain suggests that the motive was jealousy. The first child receives much care and attention from his parents. Following the birth of the second child both parents may neglect the firstborn, who bitterly resents the sibling who has usurped his position in the family. The resulting hostility, which may be repressed, may not be recognized by the parents. For example, an older sister may ostensibly pat the baby, saying how much she loves it, while actually beating it on the back as hard as she dares (26). There are many cases on record, including the example described in Chapter 11, where a jealous brother or sister has been responsible for the death of the envied infant.

There are many unconscious motivations for the aggressive criminal act, one for example being that it is a protest against passivity and enforced submission. Enforced passivity in childhood may result from a long period of illness. Schilder's studies on aggressive criminals, including murderers, have shown that the aggressive reaction is often merely a reaction to a passive role which the individual feels has been enforced upon him.

"Too much caressing may increase the child's sense of passivity. Passivity and dependence may appear as femininity. Acts of aggression, especially with a gun, help to restore the threatened masculinity. Mouth and especially anus may be linked up with the idea of passivity and femininity of which the violent criminal action is the negation. The criminal action also counteracts the fear of castration. The deeds of violence are psychologically often a self-defense. In many of the cases, there was a special animosity against homosexuals and a tendency to beat them up" (25). A need to demonstrate masculinity may contribute to the motives of persons who take part in duels or Russian roulette.

Individual differences in aggressive behavior may result from brain disease or brain injury. Although the effect of heredity is disputed, Scott's research on dogs suggests that there are hereditary differences in aggressiveness.

PARENTAL BRUTALITY

Parental brutality not only generates aggression in the child but also provides a model for future behavior. The father is usually the brutal parent, but the mother often does little to protect her children and sometimes encourages her husband to punish them. She may also be a victim of her husband's cruelty. I was requested to examine a youth who had been charged with the murder of his father, and his sister who had been charged with aiding, abetting and conspiracy to commit this murder. Both had long been victims of physical and verbal abuse in the home.

The sixteen year old youth recalled his father beating his mother, his sister and himself as far back as he could remember. Between the age of four and twelve seldom a day went by without physical punishment by his father. The worst beating at the age of nine was so severe that he had trouble walking and breathing because of his injuries. Between seven and twelve his father frequently injured his son's gums while forcibly brushing his teeth.

Between twelve and fifteen the beatings occurred every other day. During the two years before the tragedy most of the punishment was just slapping around but there were more beatings in which his father used his fists. Beatings with clenched fists occurred every couple of weeks and the longest period between beatings was about two weeks. His father would beat him for not cleaning the home basement the correct way or fast enough; for being disrespectful; for walking with his mouth open; or for any change in his facial appearance which could be interpreted as an expression of anger.

There were many incidents in the home that added to the youth's fear of his father. For example, his father concerned, without cause, that his daughter's boy friend might rape her, patrolled the grounds outside their home at night for a week, wearing a combat fatigue hat, carrying a .30 caliber assault rifle loaded with a thirty round clip. His father would hold a loaded handgun behind his back when answering the front door and the youth was afraid that one of his friends might be threatened or shot because his father was so unpredictable.

His father usually carried a loaded gun in the house and would even take it with him to the bathroom. In the living room he would place it under his thigh while sitting on the couch, but usually he sat on the floor and put guns around him. It was reported that he owned over sixty firearms. One night when the youth was ten years of age he went to the refrigerator but kept the light off as he did not want to wake up anyone. When he closed the refrigerator, he heard the click of a pistol being cocked, the light went on and his father was holding a pistol about eight inches from his face.

Two years later while they were out hunting rabbits his father deliberately fired three shots between two other rabbit hunters scaring them greatly. About 1 AM one morning while his father was handling a shotgun it discharged blowing a hole in the wall of the den and waking the youth who was so scared that he got out of bed and hid in a corner of his room. At first he thought there were burglars in the house but then his father appeared and said it was an accident.

Although verbal abuse by the father might not seem to be important in comparison with the physical abuse, nevertheless it surely affected the youth's self-esteem. Over the years the father constantly called him a pinhead, a shithead, a pimp, an arsehole, a queer and a faggot. His mother testified that her husband called his son and daughter little bastards and struck them on the head with some force when they were two and three years of age. She stated that she tried to protect the children but they said she would also strike them and would report misbehavior to her husband knowing that severe punishment would follow.

The youth concealed the beatings and bruises from his friends for many years but eventually he reported a beating to his ROTC instructor. The sheriff's department took pictures of his bruises and questioned his parents. Due to a lack of foster home facilities the youth was returned to his parents' home. Six months later after a severe beating and fearing yet another beating he waited in the garage of his home and shot his father with a shotgun as he walked from his car to open the garage door.

In a home where the use of metal spoons to eat soup was forbidden because it was too noisy, it is likely that the youth's behavior on many occasions was offensive to his father, but the excessive punishment was not a response to a pattern of antisocial behavior. The youth had no prior history of juvenile delinquency, alcohol or drug abuse. He distinguished himself by holding the rank of batallion adjutant in the ROTC and was highly regarded by his teachers.

His seventeen year old sister also reported a long history of physical abuse. "A lot of slapping, he'd punch me, grab ahold of my hair, he liked to grab me by the neck and shake me against the wall really hard sometimes. He beat me because I left the H out of my name while writing it on a lunch sack, for leaving crayons on the floor, for having the stereo on loud, for him to have it on was loud, for not cleaning up my room.

"He beat me whenever he felt I was being disrespectful to mum, use his belts, shoes, fists, hands, a black eye once or twice, I'd have welts and bruises for days. He'd brush our teeth so hard we couldn't eat for days. If I had a pimple he'd scrub it off." Between the ages of five and ten she recalled seeing her father kneeling on her mother's head, pinning her head down and beating her with his fists. Her father frequently called her names such as a shit, a nigger, a fucking slut, a fucking arsehole slut, a fucker, a bitch, a whore, a pig, a slob and a freak.

At least once a week between the ages of seven and twelve, her father fondled her breasts, buttocks and genitals. This stopped after her brother saw father touching her breasts and complained to his mother. Her last beating by her father was four days before his death. She also complained about her mother. As a child she would be punished twice, first by her mother and then by her father when he arrived home. "Mother would always report, she knew punishment would follow." She said that once her mother struck her several times knocking her down. Her head hit a towel rack and sutures were required to close the wound.

On the fatal day her brother rose at 5 AM to attend an extra credit class at 6:55 AM. His father demanded an explanation and responded to it with the comment "arsehole." When he arrived home at 4:30 PM he sensed that his mother was in a bad mood. At the meal table she started yelling at him about how rotten her life was and blamed him. She called him a punk, a bastard and a son of a bitch, then started throwing things at him. Yet she blamed him for the mess in the kitchen when his father arrived home. She also complained that he had called her a bad parent, but he had not said this.

His father beat him with his fists. Before his parents left to go to a restaurant to celebrate the twentieth anniversary of their meeting, his father told him "I'm disgusted with the shit you turned out to be. I don't want you to be here when I get back." He also said "I don't care what I have to do, I'm going to get rid of you. I don't know how but I'm going to get rid of you, you bastard."

He thought his father would beat him on returning home and he recalled an incident some months earlier in which his father mentioned that he could handle frustrations at work but not at home. His father said that one day he was going to hit someone so hard that he'd kill them and they would deserve it. As he said this he glared at his son who felt that this was a threat on his life. He felt trapped, he could not take it anymore, and it was like he was silently breaking down. That was when he started looking for the guns.

At his trial he testified that he told his sister he was going to kill his father and that she asked him if he was going to kill his mother. When he said no she asked him to kill their mother too. His father usually carried a gun and he recalled a film in which a man protected his home by placing firearms in every room. He placed weapons including two shotguns, three rifles and a .38 caliber pistol around the home and he showed his sister how to operate a .30 caliber M1 carbine in case she had to defend herself.

He changed into dark clothes and to keep up his courage he wore a drill whistle that he used as an ROTC officer. Armed with a shotgun he waited in the garage for his father to return home. He had thoughts of confronting his father, standing up to his father and telling him that there were to be no more beatings of him and his sister. He had thoughts of hugging his father and telling him that he loved him. He also had thoughts of killing him.

"It was time to defend myself, my family, everything, before I would just stand it, take it all. I never stopped and thought everything out . . . All this suppressed anger, I always kept it in, I never let it out, all my life it's been building. That night it came out."

At his trial he described his father's approach to the garage door. "I remember he was stomping. When he stomped down the hall he was really mad and really prepared to beat someone up, beat on one of us. I remember being a little kid, just sitting in my room. My dad stomping after me to hit me, that I could never stop him . . . This time I stopped him." He blew on his ROTC whistle and opened fire with a shotgun. Four of the six cartridges struck his father.

The district attorney pointed out that testimony on the physical abuse came only from the mother and her son and suggested that the extent of the abuse had been exaggerated. The youth was found guilty of voluntary manslaughter and sentenced to five to fifteen years in prison. He testified at his sister's trial that she did not help in the planning or the actual shooting of their father. She was found guilty of aiding and abetting manslaughter and sentenced to three to eight years in prison. The Governor of Wyoming commuted both sentences. The youth will probably have to serve a year in an Industrial Institute and his sister was placed on probation for one year.

Parents who batter their children expect and demand much from them. The children are expected to assume responsibilities within the home at a much earlier age than is usual in most homes. The consequence is that they appear to be unusually mature for their age despite their low self-esteem, but this is a pseudomaturity which conceals immaturity in many aspects of their personality development.

The battering parent feels insecure and unsure of being loved, and looks to the child as a source of reassurance, comfort and loving response (27). There is a reversal of the dependency role. Instead of the parent taking care of the child, the child is expected to respond to the emotional needs of the parent. The seventeen year old daughter in the above tragic example told me, "We were the adults and they were the children. Our parents were the ones who pulled tantrums. We didn't." Her sixteen year old brother told me, "It seemed like we changed roles. Dad kicked the cat in a fit of rage. I told him not to do it and he said the cat was in the way."

Satten et al. in a study of murder without apparent motive examined four men convicted of bizarre, apparently senseless murders. In the historical background of all cases was the occurrence of extreme parental violence during childhood. Duncan et al. found that among six prisoners convicted of first degree murder remorseless physical brutality at the hands of the parents had been a constant experience for four of them. Brutality far beyond all the excuses of discipline had been inflicted on them; often it was so extreme as to compel neighbors to intercede for the boy.

One father held up his nude little boy by the heels, belted him, then dropped him on his head to the floor. Recurrently some prisoners, when children, had been flung bodily across the room. Only by chance were some of them not fatally injured. The authors state that although such violence was a common factor in the four cases it should not be concluded that violence is the major factor in the causation of murder. Imitation and identification with violent parents, however, constituted the commonest pattern found.

The findings of such a high incidence of parental brutality in these two studies were not corroborated by Langevin et al. who reviewed the childhood and family background of 109 killers seen for psychiatric assessment and compared this group with nonviolent offenders and normal controls. Killers experienced somewhat more family violence than normal controls but they did not differ from nonviolent criminals in this regard. In my study of twenty homicide offenders, twenty psychiatric patients who had made homicidal threats and twenty Veterans Administration hospital psychiatric patients with no history of homicidal behavior, there were no statistically significant differences among the three groups with respect to parental brutality. Individual members of the groups were matched according to age, race, sex, parental social class, freedom from psychosis and (when applicable) relationship to the victim (19).

One should be cautious in drawing conclusions on the causes of murder from the study of dramatic case histories of small groups of murderers especially when no attempt is made to compare the childhood backgrounds with those of others who have not murdered. There is widespread belief that children who have been battered by their parents will become child batterers themselves. This may occur but this outcome is not inevitable.

Over sixty years ago Freud warned that so long as we trace a person's development backwards from its final outcome, the chain of events appears continuous and we feel that we understand the person's behavior. But if we start from the beginning, from the time of the person's birth then we no longer get the impression of an inevitable sequence of events. We notice at once that there might have been another result, and that we might have been just as well able to understand and explain it.

Thus a child who has been savagely and repeatedly beaten by his father may later kill someone or commit other crimes of violence. He may cruelly beat his own children or he may never lay a hand on them. His need to protect his children from the pain of physical punishment that he suffered may lead to the other extreme; he spoils his children and fails to discipline them in any way, even when correction is clearly necessary in the best interests of the child. Indeed he may become a social worker in a program to help battered children, or become an author of heart touching novels centered on the theme of child abuse. Any of these events could be attributed to the childhood beatings. The final outcome is dependent on the influences of other experiences in life.

PARENTAL SEDUCTION

The mother who continues to shower with her son until he is a sophomore in college may not be acting in his best interests. Such behavior, whether it is intended or not, may arouse sexual feelings that are usually held in check because of the taboo against incest. Anxiety is also aroused and this feeling may be accompanied by guilt and anger which can amount to murderous hatred. When murder occurs mother is seldom the victim, rather it is a substitute victim who resembles her in age, appearance, first name, mannerisms, or personality as in the following example.

I was asked to examine a young man who had strangled his pregnant girl friend. He did not know why he did it but he thought it was spur of the moment anger. There had been problems in their relationship. A year earlier in an angry moment he had torn up pictures of her, three months earlier he had a dream of killing her, "It happened just like the dream, just as I dreamed it." Two months previously he learned that she was pregnant. "In a way I was happy because I wanted to marry her and I wanted children, but somehow I felt I wasn't ready to settle down. I didn't want to face up to the responsibility of being tied down."

The murder occurred on the day that he was to leave her and move to Denver. She had accepted his plan to get a job in Denver then marry her or pay her child support, but that day she accused him of having girl friends in Denver, then she started telling him he did not love her. Each time she said this he told her he did love her. "She said this five or six times. This repetition or sequence really got me. She was standing up with her hands on her waist hollering at me. I told her not to say it and she kept saying it.

"By this time I'm standing up also to scare her out of this. I decided to shake her, it was like a record or a tape recorder. When I grabbed her to shake her she kept saying it and I made a threat to break her from saying it, to shock her, not to actually harm her. I said if you say it once more I'll kill you. The threat didn't help and the shaking didn't help so I took my hands and I grabbed her by the throat, putting pressure on, squeezing. I didn't want to do this but it seemed I couldn't stop.

"Her legs collapsed underneath her, I went down with her, I released my hands from her body, she was red in the face, choking and coughing. She was pretty mad, she was furious. After some time we made up, I said I was sorry, we proceeded to the bedroom, we shed our clothes, we started to proceed in the act of intercourse. I guess I wanted to more than she did. It seemed she just went along because she had a deep strong love for me. Partially or half-way through she wanted to (have intercourse) and I didn't. When I wanted to stop, she said again that I didn't love her.

"This really set me off. It seemed like part of me was thinking of doing something and part of me wasn't. I grabbed her by the throat and started applying pressure. I wanted to stop but it didn't seem as if I was able to. I was pretty well sure she was no longer breathing. I got up to get a cigarette and turned the TV on. I came back, it seemed like she moved on me. So I took the belt off my pants, put it around her neck and pulled it tight. I was exerting all the strength I had. I could still hear the sounds from her body. I was sure she was dead. I think it was air still in her body."

After watching TV he went to a tavern. A cocktail waitress he knew asked him if he was going to marry his girl friend. He replied "No, I'm a murderer, I killed her tonight." When he was told "Get serious" he replied "You better believe me, she's dead, there's blood all over the apartment." The waitress did not believe him and at closing time she agreed to have breakfast with him at a hotel. They stopped at her apartment to pick up her car keys.

While she was showing him her new apartment he stood close to her, then put his arms around her. It didn't seem to him that she resisted, but when he tried to kiss her she pushed him away and called him a little boy or a little man. This enraged him and he tried to strangle her. The woman later told police, "He put his hands on my throat and started squeezing and at first I wasn't scared because I felt that he would not really hurt me. He had a funny look on his face and things started going black and I remember thinking if he really did kill his girl friend, one more is not going to make any difference.

"I knew I had to get away from him and I found extra strength because of this and then I started screaming help me and we scuffled on the bed and I managed to throw him off between the wall and the bed, but he got ahold of me again and things started going black again. I had my coat on and he kept holding on to my coat and tore the collar off and the buttons. When he was on the floor I almost got away but he caught me again and threw me on the bed, I was kicking, scratching and screaming and we rolled off on the floor and I kicked him and got away from him . . . During the evening at least four times he told me that he had killed his girl friend and he would be going to jail."

During his psychiatric evaluation he revealed that whenever he saw his stepmother without her clothes on he felt sexually aroused. He had baths and showers with her until he was twelve or thirteen years of age. When his father was away from home he would sleep in her bed. While she was sleeping he would fondle her breasts and touch her genitals. His sexual arousal would lead to ejaculation. One time when she was wearing a bra and panties he was able to remove them without waking her. Another time when he was ten or eleven his stepmother had been drinking and that night he had intercourse with her, but she never opened her eyes. At a later interview he denied ever having had intercourse with her and said it was a dream.

He complained about his stepmother's bossiness and said that she wanted to keep him like a little boy, a little baby for eternity. In talking about her he used the word "they" as though all women were like his stepmother. "I wanted to be independent, they wouldn't let me. Like all women they wanted to be dominant." Of his stepmother he gave the example of his first opportunity to vote after reaching twenty-one. He said she refused to drive him to the polling booth unless he voted according to her instructions. Of his girl friend he said "She'd talk me out of watching TV programs I liked. I'd watch three or four of hers in sequence, then if I wanted to watch one of mine—wow!"

He complained that "If things go too smooth it seems women invent agitation or conflict" and he said that most women are "deceiving, ever enticing, hard to understand." On a sentence completion test he wrote **My greatest mistake** was killing my girl friend and not killing the second party. It seems a great mistake to have the second party go on living and enticing others." He told me "If this girl (the cocktail waitress) came in this room right now, I'd do anything I could within my power to take her life. Part of me wants to, part of me doesn't want to repeat this."

He said that the first time he met her she had a nightgown on, high heels and hose. It was clear that he saw her as proof of his viewpoint that women are deceiving, ever enticing and ultimately rejecting. "Wiggle here, wiggle there, help me with my zipper but don't touch; lead guys on then cut them off, like all women, like turn a light on and off that quick, when it came right down to it like a tease."

Easson and Steinhilber reported that among seven children and adolescents who showed murderous aggression, lack of privacy, physical overcloseness and, at times, the grossest seduction were repeatedly found. The mother of one thirteen year old boy, had for five or six years been in the habit of getting into bed with the boy and, face to face with him, massaging his back. The grandmother of a sixteen year old boy continued to sleep with him. The mother of another thirteen year old boy, still bathed him. She gave him details of her first intercourse, and her feelings during the intercourse when his sister was conceived. Whenever he asked if he could have intercourse with her, her standard answer was, "Yes, but it will be horrible."

In my study of twenty homicide offenders, twenty psychiatric patients who had made homicidal threats and twenty psychiatric patients with no history of homicidal behavior there were no statistically significant differences among the three groups in the incidence of parental seduction. Such parental seduction was recorded when the parent of the opposite sex slept in the same room or bed with a child to the age of five or beyond; exposed breasts or genitals; had sexual relations with marital partner or lovers in the presence of the child; discussed sex in a pathological manner or sexually assaulted the child (19).

PERMISSIVE PARENTS

Some parents are unduly permissive. A young boy was caught by his sister choking his brother who was blue in the face. The mother found out about this attack five days later, but felt then it was too late to do or say anything and she did not tell her husband, a physician. One week later the sister found the boy trying to strangle his younger brother with a belt. The school authorities immediately notified the parents who did nothing. The father felt it was part of growing up. A week later the boy was discovered trying to drown his brother by holding his head under the bath water. Only then did the parents take their son to a psychiatrist (9).

Parents may show, directly or indirectly, approval of violent behavior. A sixteen year old youth in a two year period hit his adoptive mother with a golf club, set her hair on fire, threw knives at her "in fun" and twice slashed her arms with a knife after mild reprimands. The adoptive mother passed off these assaults as "adventurous" and she smiled with obvious pleasure while describing them.

In yet another case described by Easson and Steinhilber, a thirteen year old boy who exhibited extreme aggressivity toward his parents and threatened them several times with a gun said, "I could always get what I wanted if I made enough fuss. Why didn't they stop me? They were scared of me. They didn't need to be. I am still small." He was allowed to keep his guns and knives despite his suggestion that his father should take control of them.

Parents who express strong condemnation of illegal behavior may nevertheless provide indirect encouragement of such behavior, through repeated expression of fear that a son or daughter will break the law. Usually just one child is selected as a scapegoat, perhaps a rebellious daughter or a son who resembles a relative with a bad reputation. An adopted child is a ready choice as the delinquent behavior can be attributed to heredity rather than to some failure of the adoptive parents. Johnson and Szurek suggest that these parents gain vicarious pleasure from the child acting out their own forbidden impulses. Another factor is the expression of hostile destructive impulses felt toward the child.

The father who shows baseless concern lest his son should become a criminal may find his expectations fulfilled. By repeated suspicious questionings and dire warnings, he transmits to the son a paternal concept of the youth behaving otherwise than acceptably. The writer has examined several persons, charged with serious bodily assault or murder, who were told repeatedly in their youth that they would end up in the gas chamber. Some of these predictions were made before the appearance of delinquent or criminal behavior.

A professional worker told Johnson that seventeen years earlier she visited her friends who had a nine month old baby boy. The worker took the little boy on her lap and when he reached up and put his hands around her neck, the child's mother with a really frightening expression said, "I hope my son won't be a killer." By the age of fifteen years that boy had committed murder. Carlyle in **Sartor Resartus** wisely comments, "In a very plain sense the proverb says call one a thief and he will steal."

The parent who indirectly encourages antisocial behavior may escape recognition because of his or her law-abiding reputation and position of great respect in the community, especially when parental control appears to be unusually strict, as in the following example. The mother of a sixteen year old youth charged with armed robbery was at a loss to explain his crime which involved an assault on the victim with a blunt instrument.

She herself was active in community organizations and was regarded as a pillar of respectability. She set very strict rules for her son and was both overcontrolling and overprotective. He had to keep her informed of his every move and she would often insist on accompanying him to school and to social and to sports activities rather than letting him go with his friends. Indeed a neighbor rebuked her for treating her son as if he were a three year old child.

The youth readily revealed a long history of delinquent behavior including repeated thefts over many years, at first from his parents and later from others. Although he complained of the strict rules set by mother, he added that often she would not say anything to him when he disregarded the rules. "I could get away with a lot of things." The father did not have a prominent role in the family, and the youth was able to circumvent his father's disciplinary measures by going to his mother to get what he wanted.

On interview his mother concealed much of the delinquent behavior previously reported by her son. When she was confronted, she claimed loss of memory, "it slipped my mind," but the incidents that slipped her mind included visits to the home by the police and serious criminal offenses unlikely to be forgotten under any circumstances. She admitted on further confrontation that her failure to mention this significant information about her son was intentional. She turned a blind eye to some indications of illegal behavior by her son as, for example, his possession of expensive articles from department stores. These items were obtained with stolen credit cards.

When asked how her son had been caught in a car theft, she said, "He left his school books in the car, how stupid can you be?" Her concern was over his stupidity in leaving clues rather than over his committing an illegal act. Unfortunately she had no recognition of her contribution to her son's illegal behavior and within a year he was involved in two robberies involving the use of firearms. In one robbery he shot at but fortunately did not injure his victim. The youth was later shot to death in an armed confrontation with a police officer.

CRIMINAL PARENTS

When a child is raised by criminal parents it is unlikely that he will have deep respect for the laws of society. Some families expect their sons to serve in the armed services, other families expect their sons to serve time in the state reformatory or state penitentiary. One mother kept a scrapbook with newspaper clippings on the criminal careers of all her sons. A father kept in his wallet all the clippings on his son's bank robberies. A man who had shot three police officers, killing two of them, was told by his father after his arrest, "That was good shooting son."

Ma Barker

"Ma overwhelmed her boys with affection and target practice."

Ron Goulart, *Lineup: Tough Guys*

Ma Barker tried to keep her sons away from liquor and women, yet encouraged them to commit robbery, kidnapping, and murder. Herman, the eldest son, was the first to be arrested. The charge was highway robbery. Herman did not live long enough to help his mother in her golden years of the 1930s. In 1927 he was wounded in a shootout with the police, and he killed himself to avoid arrest for the murder of a deputy sheriff in Wyoming.

Lloyd, the second son, while still young, was separated from his mother by a federal judge who gave him a twenty-five year sentence for mail robbery. Arthur ("Doc"), the third son, after serving thirteen years for the murder of a night watchman in a holdup, became a leading member of the Barker-Karpis gang. Within four years of receiving a life sentence for kidnapping he was shot and killed while attempting to escape from Alcatraz.

Freddie, the baby of the family and Ma's favorite, was with his mother when she died. They were both killed by federal agents in a shootout after Freddie refused to surrender. A machine gun was found in Ma Barker's hands and a .45 caliber pistol was found alongside Freddie's body. Freddie is believed to have killed at least six persons. As Alvin Karpis commented, "My great pal Freddie Barker was a natural killer." Freddie's mother rose angrily to the defense of her children whenever they were accused of wrongdoing. She protested their innocence regardless of the facts and blamed others for their shortcomings (18).

THE OEDIPUS COMPLEX AND MURDER

According to Greek legend, Laius, kind of Thebes, was warned by the Delphic oracle that his son would one day kill him. Later when his son was born, he pierced the infant's feet with a nail and left him to die on a mountainside. But a shepherd found the boy and named him Oedipus, because his feet were deformed. As a young man Oedipus learned his terrible destiny from the oracle at Delphi. He was told, "Away from the shrine, wretch, you will kill your father and marry your mother."

Oedipus believed that he could escape this fate by leaving Corinth, the home of the couple, whom he assumed to be his true parents. But in his travels he quarrelled with a stranger and killed him. The stranger was his father, Laius. Unaware that the first part of the prediction had been fulfilled, Oedipus continued on his way. When he killed the Sphinx, a monster with a woman's head, lion's body and eagle's wings, which had been terrorizing the countryside, he was rewarded with the kingdom of Thebes. He married Jocasta, the widow of Laius, unaware that she was his mother. On discovering his crime he blinded himself as punishment and Jocasta hanged herself.

The term Oedipus complex has been used to describe attachment of the child for the parent of the opposite sex, together with aggressive feelings toward the parent of the same sex. These forbidden feelings may be banned from consciousness; exceptionally the death wishes for the parent of the same sex find expression in murder. The victim may be either the hated parent or some parental figure whose behavior reactivates earlier feelings of overwhelming hostility.

Kessel suggests that Freud got it wrong and that it is the father—Oedipus's dad—who sees the child as the rival for the mother's affection rather than the other way round. The child, he points out, knows only the state into which it is born, but the father experienced sole rights to the affection of the woman before his rival appeared. Even in the legend it is Laius, the dad, who first tries to kill Oedipus, the son, and fails.

THE ORESTES COMPLEX

"I trow, my father, had I face to face
Questioned him if I must my mother slay,
Had earnestly besought me by this beard
Never to thrust sword through my mother's heart."

Euripides, *Orestes*

The tale is told in Greek mythology of the tragic hero, Orestes, whose father Agamemnon was murdered by his mother, Clytaemnestra, and her lover, Aegisthus. Orestes recognized his duty to avenge his father's death, but hesitated to kill his mother and only proceeded on his grim purpose when advised to do so by the oracle at Delphi.

He was helped by his sister, Electra, and both were charged with the crime of matricide. Pending the trial Orestes was prevented from washing his bloodstained hands. Both were sentenced to be stoned to death, but the sentence was commuted to one of suicide. The gods, however, intervened and Orestes and Electra escaped. Orestes during a period of madness purged himself of guilt by shaving his head, and placated the avenging Furies by biting off a finger in his torment.

In **Dark Legend** Wertham has described a case of matricide which resembles in some respects the legend of Orestes. Gino, a seventeen year old boy, stabbed his mother to death in her bed, in a New York tenement. The youth said he stabbed his mother thirty-two times with a table knife because she dishonored his family. Six years earlier, following his father's death, his mother had a succession of lovers. She neglected and ill-treated her children. When Gino became aware that his mother had a lover, he knelt down in prayer and made a vow that his right hand must be cut off at the wrist, if he did not kill her some day. At his father's grave he promised to avenge the family name.

It was five years before Gino fulfilled his oath and during this time he was a hard-working well-behaved youth. During the month before the tragedy he slept poorly, ate little and appeared to be preoccupied and absent minded. At this time he made the decision to kill his mother with a table knife. As the knife was blunt he asked his mother to sharpen it, and as she did so he thought, "You sharpened it for yourself." He had some difficulty in convincing a policeman that he had killed his mother.

Wertham has drawn attention to some striking similarities between the behavior of Orestes as recorded by the Greek dramatist, Aeschylus, and Gino's behavior. Like Orestes, he went to his father's grave for inspiration. Gino listened to the father-image that spoke to him in a dream, just as Orestes listened to the oracle of "our father—I mean not mine, but the great sun-god Apollo, who witnesses all these events." Both promised to avenge the father, both considered that the mother deserved to die and both contemplated suicide.

Gino faced the punishment and admitted his deed as openly and in almost the same words as Orestes, who said before the court in Athens:

> "I slew her. That is not to be denied . . .
> With sword-edge pressed against her throat . . .
> And to this hour I am well content with all . . .
> I fear not."

Gino told Wertham, "I killed her . . . I took her life away . . . I stabbed her in the neck . . . I was always happy since the day I killed her. I was glad I done it. I did not worry about it."

Hostility against the mother based on excessive attachment to her has been designated by Wertham as the Orestes complex and he lists six characteristics: excessive attachment to the mother-image; hostility against the mother-image; a general hatred of women; indications of homosexual potentialities; ideas of suicide; and an emotional disorder based on profound feelings of guilt.

THE SUPERMAN COMPLEX

The philosophy of the superman has been spelled out by Nietzsche. Contemptuous of Christian ethic, he substituted violence for love, evil for good. The masses should be subordinated to Siegfried, the biologically superior man, who tramples under foot the servile herd of the weak, degenerate and poor in spirit. Milk is for babes, the strong man should be soaked in blood and alcohol. "Evil is man's best strength. Man should be trained for war and women for the recreation of the warrior. All else is folly. Thou goest to woman? Do not forget thy whip."

The self-inflation, arrogance and belief in a superior power of evil, shown by some murderers, suggest the superman philosophy. But the fantasies are translated into action. Twenty year old Harlow Fraden, who poisoned his parents with a cyanide and champagne cocktail, compared himself with the Greek gods and believed that he was superior to the rest of humanity. He held long discussion on the philosophy of Nietzsche with his accomplice. "You speak about the norm. In my case it is something that passes the normal and the abnormal. Mount Olympus is a lonely place. So few of us are there. One wearies of continual hatred and contempt. My own idea of superiority may yet destroy me" (4).

The mass murderers of the Nazi SS organization, who exterminated thousands of Jews in the gas chambers of the concentration camps, cultivated the myth of the superman and extolled their own interpretation of the writings of Nietzsche. Hitler and Nietzsche, alike, damned democracy, pacifism and humanitarianism, although for quite different reasons. Both applauded the merits of racial purity, ruthless aggression and the will to power. The Fuehrer publicly acknowledged his debt to the philosopher.

Bertrand Russel comments, "It does not occur to Nietzsche as possible that a man should genuinely feel universal love, obviously because he himself feels almost universal hatred and fear, which he would fain disguise as lordly indifference. His 'nobleman'—who is himself in daydreams—is a being wholly devoid of sympathy, ruthless, cunning, cruel, concerned only with his own power . . .

"It never occurred to Nietzsche that the lust for power, with which he endows his superman, is itself an outcome of fear. Those who do not fear their neighbors see no necessity to tyrannize over them. Men who have conquered fear have not the frantic quality of Nietzsche's 'artist-tyrant' Neros, who try to enjoy music and massacre while their hearts are filled with dread of the inevitable palace revolution" (23).

Perhaps it is unfair to blame Nietzsche for murder. Captain James Purrington who murdered his wife and six children in 1806 before taking his own life, had his Bible opened to Ezekiel, chapter nine, "Slay utterly old and young, both maids and little children and women." Surely the Bible is not to blame for these murders?

Raskolnikov, the hero of Dostoyevsky's novel **Crime and Punishment,** divided mankind into ordinary men and the extraordinary men. The latter, the Mahomets and Napoleons, must by their very nature, their superiority, be criminals. The extraordinary man has a right—not officially sanctioned, of course—to permit his conscience to step over certain obstacles, to step over a corpse or wade through blood. Thus, Raskolnikov explains his murder of Ivanovna, the elderly woman money-lender. Raskolnikov is like a corruption of Nietzsche's superman. He tells his friend Sonia, "Power is given only to him who dares to stoop and take it . . ."

POWER

The weak and timid gain instant power with a .38 caliber revolver—

the power of life and death over others. Several armed robbers have boasted to me "I could give him his life or take it." A petty thief and small time burglar liked to brag about his crimes but he was never involved in any crimes of violence. Those police officers who knew him well did not regard him as a dangerous offender and were surprised when he was arrested on charges of armed robbery, kidnapping and murder. He picked up a hitchhiker, a Colorado University student, took him to a rural area and shot him with a pistol.

The twenty-one year old offender had obtained the weapon in a burglary and felt like a million dollars after finding it. He was only 5'6" in height and he had a Nazi swastika tattooed on his left arm. He mentioned his approval of the Nazis "Clean efficient people get the job done, no bullshit." The Nazi emphasis on ruthless aggression and power has a special appeal for those who are weak and fearful.

He played the role of a tough guy who was not to be trifled with. He boasted of his many fights in which he had injured ten to twenty persons, and he claimed to have ruptured a man's spleen. He told me he was going to murder his stepfather and said of his companion in the robbery and murder, "If I'd wanted to kill him, I'd have wasted him too." Referring to another psychiatrist he said "I just about slugged that bastard."

Apparently concerned that I might not have gathered that he was a dangerous person he threatened to kill me if I pushed him too far. One day when another prisoner was threatening to attack me, he shouted encouraging comments from his cell, thereby adding to a rather sticky situation. Later I explained to him that he was capable of better behavior.

The next day he apologized saying "I feel much better because you got mad at me yesterday and put me in my place. I respect you now, you told me to fuck myself yesterday, only you used nice words." This was a turning point in the psychiatric evaluation and for the first time he was able to talk about his tough outer shell and his inner feeling of weakness. "I talk bad shit like I'm a tough guy, I ain't I'm scared of everybody."

When he talked about the murder he made many references to his power over his victim. "He would do anything I told him to do." Unfortunately the victim did not do everything he was told to do and he was shot nine times. He continued his threatening, intimidating behavior in the state penitentiary and within a few months another of my acquaintances killed him.

PROOF OF MANHOOD

A fifteen year old youth together with his girl friend of the same age decided to obtain money for a vacation by holding up a cab driver. The youth, although of very superior intelligence (IQ 135) and physically strong in the upper part of his body, was crippled in his legs from polio and used half crutches. Their plan was to tell the cab driver to stop and hand over his money. Instead the cab driver sped down the street while the girl screamed at her boy friend "Shoot! Kill him! Don't be yellow, you weakling!" He hesitated briefly but then shot the man in the back. When the car crashed, the girl ran while he attempted to crawl away (20).

This direct instigation to homicide in a holdup was accompanied by direct threats to the manhood of this physically handicapped youth. Threats to manhood have many sources and the responses take many forms. Hemingway turns in his novels to the bullfight and the safari as means of resolving inner doubts. Alternative test situations include other dangerous occupations such as lion taming, perilous games like Russian Roulette and a criminal career as an armed robber or member of an organized crime group.

A tall well built assertive young man told me that his ambition was to become a hit man for the Mafia or Murder Incorporated and he complained to me about the difficulty in securing such employment in Colorado. Despite his outward appearance of self-confidence he was very unsure of himself. He joined the Marine Corps to prove he was a man. My efforts to help him were not successful and he became a well known bank robber. It was said of another famous bank robber, the Spanish bandit Sabate, that he robbed banks not simply for money, but as a torero fights bulls, to demonstrate courage (13).

Murder by homosexuals, especially by homosexual prostitutes, has been attributed to ambivalence, guilt, and shame over their sexual inadequacy. In killing their homosexual partner they are destroying the shameful part of themselves, or so it seems. A nineteen year old homosexual prostitute following a minor argument with the client over the fee strangled him. A few days later after he was accosted by an effeminate homosexual, he knew he would kill again. "I suddenly found myself hating the guy who accosted me, hating his flabbiness and softness, hating the fact that I needed him. I knew I was going to kill again. I did not care. I was getting rid of something mean and dirty about myself. I was getting even. I was getting back for not being wanted for myself" (1).

Torture and execution style slayings of bound victims seem to be more common in homosexual murderers.

NEED FOR ATTENTION

*"It is better to be wanted by the police
than not to be wanted at all."*

It is difficult to believe that a man would kill to obtain attention, however persons unlikely to be featured on television news programs or in newspaper headlines gain instant recognition by murdering a prominent citizen. Arthur Bremer, who had no interest in politics, decided to kill President Nixon but was unable to get close enough to shoot him. Instead he shot presidential candidate George C. Wallace, paralyzing him from the waist down.

In his diary before the shooting Bremer expressed fear that if something big happened in Vietnam on that day he would not get more than three minutes on network TV news. He compared Wallace with the late FBI director, J. Edgar Hoover, and indicated that killing Hoover would have provided more publicity. He also complained about the lack of publicity for those who threatened the President and suggested that they needed an organization such as **Make the First Lady a Widow, Inc.** with a national convention every four years to pick the executioner (3).

MOTIVELESS MURDER

The most puzzling murders are those without apparent motive. Satten and his colleagues reported four cases of apparently senseless murder. "For the most part, the murderers themselves were puzzled as to why they killed their victims. Attempts to reconstruct a rational motive were unsuccessful. In each case, there was no gain to the murderer by killing the victim, nor was there any accompanying crime. The victims were relatively unknown to the murderers, and the method of the murder was haphazard and impromptu. In no case did the murderer use a conventional weapon, but killed either with his bare hands or whatever could be immediately pressed into use.

"In all instances, however, the murder was unnecessarily violent, and sometimes bizarre, and there was evidence that the assaults on the bodies continued until long after the death of the victims. The most uniform, and perhaps the most significant, historical finding was a longstanding, sometimes lifelong, history of erratic control over aggressive impulses. For example, three of the men throughout their lives, had been frequently involved in fights which were not ordinary altercations, and which would have become homicidal assaults if not stopped by others" (24).

In their early years they were concerned about being considered sissies, physically undersized or sickly. As adults, despite their violent behavior, they still saw themselves as physically inferior, weak and inadequate. Three men stuttered in childhood and under stress in adult life. All showed sexual inhibitions and were afraid of women; two had overt sexual perversions. They had repetitive dreams of killing, burning or mutilating others and experienced no anger or rage during violent assaults or murder. There was no guilt, remorse or depression following their killings.

A case of apparently motiveless murder in the author's experience, showed some of the features above described. In Denver, one winter night, a middle aged man was beaten to death and his body was seriously mutilated. A twenty-two year old laborer, EM confessed to the crime.

The only reason that he could give the police for his action was, "All I can say is, well I wanted to do it." EM met his victim for the first time only a short interval prior to the assault and exchanged no more than a few words with the man he was about to kill. He offered to see his drunken victim to his lodgings. There was no attempt to rob the victim apart from taking a dime which he used to call the police. The senseless brutal nature of the crime and the complete lack of guilt or remorse are revealed in EM's account of his crime:

"I was supposed to go to work, but I was sick. The man I worked for said I could get my money around 4:30. I was paid at 4 PM. I went to a bar and kept on drinking beer and wine. I kept it up for quite a while. I knew it was starting to hit me. Kept on drinking till about 11 PM. I was pretty well drunk. I usually drink by myself, I don't like to be around people. I seen this guy right in front of the mission. I'd never seen him before in my life. I couldn't see his face, he was probably drunker than I. I wanted to get him. I don't know why but I wanted to. So I went up and told him I would help to take him home. But I knew then and there I wasn't going to do it, I wasn't going to take him home.

"I took him down an alley. It was about fifty feet inside the alley, a big hallway — you could put a car in there. I knew the place. He was leaning against me. I don't think he said more than three words to me the whole time he was with me. He said, 'I don't have any money.' I got to the spot where I wanted. I pushed him ahead a little bit, then I turned him around quick but not too quick as he would have fallen down. I hit him with my fist and knocked him down. Maybe he said something I couldn't make it out. I got a big board and broke it down the middle. I started hitting him in the face with it. I just wanted to I guess. I hit him three or four dozen times. The blood was kind of caught in his throat — he gurgled a bit, guess he couldn't talk. His head came up like he was coming to, so I kicked him in the face as hard as I could.

"I lit a few matches. He was bleeding good, I got a good feeling out of it. That's what I can't understanding feeling good watching a guy getting murdered. I found a broken wine bottle — before that I was mad enough I practically tore the clothes off him. I started jabbing him in the stomach with the bottle. I still wasn't satisfied so I started scraping him in the stomach with the edge. I stopped and picked up the board again. I started beating him in the face with the board. I don't know how many times. Then I hid the board. I thought I hid it but the cops got it. He looked dead. I couldn't feel no pulse. I wanted to beat him up.

"It wouldn't have made any difference, man, woman or child. I striked the matches to see what he looked like. The more I see his face, the more I wanted to beat him. I waited quite a long time before I light another match — 'cause, well, the guy wouldn't change too much a few more cuts and bruises. You should have seen that board, it was covered with blood. That's where I made my mistake — they would never have caught me if I'd known they could get fingerprints off a board. I hid the board, too. I spent about an hour beating him. When I called for the police, I thought it was a perfect crime. I went into the tavern next to the alley and told the boss I seen this guy in the alley and I couldn't feel his pulse, and I thought he was dead.

"I told him he better call the police. I told them I'd stick around as the police might want to ask me some questions which they did. The police took me back and we both took a look at him. They took me and locked me up. I thought they was just going to keep me till they investigated the crime. They said they had my fingerprints off the board, so I confessed. Tell me, can they get my fingerprints off the board? I'm not worried — there is nothing to worry about. As long as it don't bother me I don't see why it should bother anyone else.

"With this guy, I figured, heck, I could give him his life or take it away from him. I guess some people haven't got the stomach for it. It never did bother me. I don't mind seeing blood as long as it ain't mine. I could kill a Mexican and smile while I was killing. I know I'll do it again. I know it's wrong to kill somebody. The Bible says its wrong. Thou shalt not kill. I think I've broke every rule in the Bible. I know I done it but I don't care. Why should I care as long as it don't bother me and it don't bother me. They can only lock you up in prison or give you the electric chair. That don't worry me, I'm not afraid. After it (referring to the murder) I felt full and comfortable just like you had a good meal."

EM's father, an alcoholic cook, not infrequently returned home drunk, and on these occasions he would beat his wife. He showed no interest in his children except when they bothered him, and then he would thrash them with a belt. The mother was also described as an alcoholic. As a child EM always wanted to be left alone, not to be bothered by other people. Following the divorce of his parents he spent two years in an orphanage. Each of the parents married again and he lived alternately with his father and stepmother, and his mother and stepfather.

His stepmother neglected him and he spent his time roaming the streets. His stepfather, also an alcoholic, made life unpleasant for him and threatened to kill him. Similar threats were made on the life of his mother. When EM was sixteen years of age, his mother took him to a mental hygiene clinic, because he had threatened to kill her.

It is of interest that, as a child, EM stuttered until cured by a special teacher. He was reported to have a terrible temper and he was arrested many times for fighting. Once he beat up a cripple. "I'd never seen him before, he had a bum leg and crutches. He said something, I don't know what. I busted his mouth open. I wouldn't have stopped if my brother hadn't told me the police were coming. If he'd hit me with the crutch, I would have beaten him to death."

By his own admissions he had attempted murder on five occasions. In his daydreams he thought constantly of killing people in various ways; by twisting their necks with piano wire, shrinking their heads, cutting off their heads with a meat cleaver, using a pet gorilla and so on.

When the psychologist, Dr. Stuart Boyd, requested him to draw a man and a woman he readily complied, saying that drawing was one of his hobbies. He drew the top half of the man with swift sure strokes. The face was massive and powerful, the neck short and bull-like. The arms were heavily muscled, almost disproportionately so, with the fists clenched and club-like. The chest was barrelled with heavily defined pectorals. He drew a line at the navel and asked if he should continue.

When the examiner asked him to continue he became hesitant in his draftsmanship and produced hips and legs which give a definite impression of infantilism, and clothed the genital area in what looked like diapers.

The drawing shows his insecurity and inadequacy in relation to sexual function, feelings which may have driven him to develop himself physically, so that muscular strength and aggression have become of central importance with him. He must prove himself a man at all costs. It is perhaps significant that four months prior to the murder, he was circumcised and treated for an infection in his groin.

At his trial the writer stated that EM suffered from a psychopathic (sociopathic) personality and although he was not psychotic he was nevertheless legally insane. The jury agreed with this finding and EM was committed to a mental hospital.

When seen two years later he said that his one desire was to prove that he was well enough to be released. He claimed that at the time of his previous examination he had acted abnormally, on the advice of a prison guard, in order to be found insane. He said that his dreams about a "pet gorilla" were "a lot of bunk" and this may well be true. Furthermore, he denied striking matches to look at the corpse. When reminded that the police investigation showed numerous burnt matches at the scene of the crime, he asserted that he lit the matches "to see if I wasn't hurting him too bad." Because of the nature and extent of the terrible fatal wounds, this statement must be viewed with skepticism.

He also claimed that the motive for the crime was robbery. This does not explain why he should tear the victim's clothes off and lacerate the abdomen with a broken bottle, after the victim had lost consciousness. Quite apart from his wish to prove that he is well enough to be discharged from the hospital, he doubtless had a need to provide a satisfactory explanation for a cruel and senseless murder.

In some cases of so-called motiveless murder there may have been a motive, which escaped recognition.

REFLEX ACTION AND MURDER

The German criminologist Hans Gross one evening passed through an infrequented street and came upon an inn just at the moment that an intoxicated fellow was thrown out. He writes, "At the very instant I hit the poor fellow a hard blow on the ear, I regretted the deed immediately, the more so as the assaulted man bemoaned his misfortune, 'inside they throw him out, outside they box his ears.' Suppose that I had at that time burst the man's ear drum or otherwise damaged him heavily. It would have been a criminal matter and I doubt whether anyone would have believed that it was 'reflex action' though I was then, as today, convinced that the action was reflex.

"I didn't in the least know what was going to happen to me and what I should do. I simply noticed that something unfriendly was approaching and I met it with a defensive action in the form of an uppercut on the ear. What properly occurred I knew only when I heard the blow and felt the concussion on my hand . . . If I had done the greatest damage I could not have been held responsible — **if** my explanation were allowed; but **that** it would have been allowed I do not believe."

Thus the reflex crime is committed "semiconsciously": the subject feels he has to do the act, but has not the time to reflect upon it. Ellenberger comments: "The act is accomplished in the fashion of a reflex, and when one thinks of abstaining, it is already too late. As in the poem by Goethe, 'It was done before the thought.' The reflex act is unleashed by a particular situation which presents itself in an unexpected way. It is usually not difficult to explore its meaning: the explosion of a feeling hidden or obscured for a long time, the repetition of an earlier life situation, the sudden eruption of childhood memory, highly charged with affect, or several of these elements.

"Gross recounts that while a number of convicts were working on the construction of a new court house in Graz his attention was attracted to one of them, a murderer, whom he found particularly appealing. He learned from this man's history that his conduct had been exemplary before, as well as after, his crime. This son of a blacksmith had lost his father when he was young; the mother remarried a stingy, brutal man who had formerly been an employee of the father. The stepfather did all that he could to drive the boy away and to dispossess him of his heritage. The young man, who wished to remain in his familiar surroundings and who, besides, had fallen in love with the daughter of a neighbor, restrained himself in spite of the continuous brutalities of his stepfather. The crime exploded unexpectedly one morning, after years of continued martyrdom. Passing in front of the brick oven where the household bread was baked, the young man saw his stepfather about to draw out the embers, with his body almost completely in the brick oven. Seized with a sudden impulse, he violently pushed the man into the oven, slammed the door, and left. Death was rapid, and the murderer confessed without difficulty. Upon interrogation he gave the following explanation: 'I do not know how it came to pass. Pushing him in and closing the door happened as quickly as one can squash a mosquito. I had not thought about it, reflected upon it or wanted to do it, it seemed to happen spontaneously and it was not until I was in front of the house that I considered what I had done. It was then too late to repair that which had been done, and also I was paralyzed with shock, with the best intentions I could not have moved a limb.'

"This young man of Gross was considered well-liked and a person of good will, but it is clear that he had accumulated a terrible hidden hate against the tyrant who had long made him suffer so much. One might question whether a childhood memory had not played a role here: the death of the wicked witch whom the children pushed into the bake oven in the tale of **Hänsel and Gretel** which the young man must have heard often in his childhood.

"In his studies of reflexoid action, Gross focused largely on criminal ones. But it must not be forgotten that there are reflexoid acts of an heroic mold as well as those with a quasi-suicidal character. The young man who sees someone drowning and hurls himself into the water without knowing how to swim; or the one who, 'listening to nothing but his courage' throws himself in front of a frightened runaway horse and is knocked down, also perform reflex acts. Who knows how many heroic sacrifices in warfare and elsewhere might be attributed to this type of cause? . . .

"We see that a great many individuals, perhaps all of humanity, are endowed with hidden predispositions and latent capacities which can carry them, according to the circumstances, to fill the role of criminal or victim" (10).

PSYCHOLOGICAL DEFENSES AGAINST THE URGE TO KILL

"The bad do what the good dream."

Aggression is, next to sex, the most highly regulated and repressed of all types of human social behavior (26). Frequently it finds outlet in dreams, fantasies or words, rather than in action. Vicarious gratification of murderous impulses may be obtained by identification with the slayer in the murder mystery or gangster film. The writer and playwright also experience gratification in this manner. Hobbies provide similar outlets.

A prominent surgeon spent his vacations visiting the scenes of infamous crimes. On one occasion he gave a lecture based on his unusual hobby. He was so engrossed in his description of the mass murderer, Petiot, that he was apparently unaware of his frequent slips of the tongue. The audience listened with growing horror as he described in great detail the murderous exploits of Petiot. For too often the speaker said "I" when he should have said "he."

The gruesome slides used to illustrate the topic concluded with a striking portrait of Petiot with gleaming eyes and sneering face, hunched forward with hands across the chest. When the lights were turned on again the blurred outline of the slide was still visible on the screen behind the speaker, but it appeared to be an enormous malignant shadow of the speaker himself, with gleaming eyes and sneering face, hunched forward over the lectern with hands across the chest.

When hostility is directed against a loved person, its expression even in fantasy may be forbidden. So great are the taboos against murderous impulses that many of us cannot permit ourselves conscious awareness of these impulses. If homicidal urges threaten to break into consciousness great anxiety may result. This anxiety is a warning signal of the need for further defensive measures.

Overcompensation

A person may overcompensate for his unconscious homicidal impulses by showing great love not only toward his intended victim, but toward other persons as well. A young girl spoke only in glowing terms of her mother who was so active in the Parent Teachers Association and various social activities that she had little time left for her daughter. Recurrent nightmares in which she dreamed of her mother's death in automobile and plane accidents, betrayed underlying death wishes for the rejecting mother. A person with unconscious homicidal tendencies may show great indignation over aggressive behavior in others and become a militant pacifist, anti-vivisectionist, or vociferous opponent of both physical and capital punishment.

Obsessional Neurosis

In obsessional neurosis homicidal thoughts appear in consciousness but responsibility for them is disowned. The patient is at a loss to understand why he should be troubled by recurrent ideas of killing a close relative whom he loves. The idea is subjectively perceived as a foreign body, not really the product of the individual's mind. The father who has unconscious homicidal wishes to destroy his family may suffer from an obsessive need to check repeatedly to make sure that the gas jets on the stove are turned off. Thus, he may get up several times during the night to turn the gas jets on and then off. The obsession that the jets are on is accompanied by the fear that the household might be asphyxiated, and stems from unconscious hostility. Turning the jets off after turning them on symbolically undoes the forbidden tendency and relieves anxiety.

A meek, middle-aged minister of religion of irreproachable character sought psychiatric help because he would wake up his wife in the middle of the night and tell her that he wanted to stab her in the heart and "rip her guts out" with a knife. She did not take these threats seriously and would calmly tell her husband to turn over and go back to sleep again. He was, however, so distressed by his homicidal impulses that he was unable to continue in his profession as a preacher.

Hysteria

A defense against homicidal impulses is the development of a hysterical paralysis which prevents the act of murder. For example a very conscientious army sergeant developed a paralysis of his right arm, shortly after he was unjustly rebuked by his overbearing commanding officer on the parade ground. Psychiatric examination revealed long standing resentment toward this officer who reminded him of his brutal father. The hysterical paralysis of his arm served to prevent expression of his impulse to strike the officer.

Suicide

Murderous tendencies may be turned against oneself resulting in depression and suicide, or thoughts of suicide. As Menninger points out, one who nourishes murderous wishes also feels, at least unconsciously, a need for punishment of a corresponding sort. Dostoyevsky wrote a very famous illustration of this in **The Brothers Karamazov** in which it will be recalled that Dmitri, who did not kill his father, nevertheless seemed to demand punishment for himself as if he had done so. He accumulated and displayed all sorts of circumstantially incriminating evidence. He put himself through the horrible torture of the trial and permitted himself to be sentenced to life imprisonment, when he could easily have escaped it by the proper maneuvers in the courtroom. His brother, Ivan, was driven mad by the whole thing and angrily denounced the court, saying that it was absurd for them to make so much over this affair, since everyone in the courtroom was just as guilty as Dmitri. "Everyone of you has wished for your father's death," he cries to them. "Why do you persecute my brother, who has done no more than this?" But Dmitri knew that to have wished for his father's death as he had (he even went so far as to plan it) carried with it a burden of guilt almost as great as if he had indeed perpetrated the act (21).

Lindner has described the case of a forty-five year old alcoholic, who shortly before he committed suicide wrote: "My great struggle has been from doing her (mother) harm. Last week she had a 'spell' in the bathtub and I had to go to her aid. When I lifted her poor shrunken body from the water, I was seized with the tenderest feeling for her, but at the same time I actually had to fight against a desire to keep from pushing her under the water and drowning her. How could such great love and hate exist side by side? I wish I had the money to move away from her. I have to get away before one of us gets hurt."

Here is a dramatic portrayal of co-existing emotions of love and hatred, felt by a son for his mother. In Lindner's opinion the son's suicide prevented him from killing his mother. It is not rare for a rejected lover or marital partner to murder the object of his affections. Frequently the murderer, in these cases, has marked ambivalent feelings of love and hate. When love is spurned the contrasting feelings readily come to the surface. Homicide, suicide or both may result. Sometimes murder may occur as a form of disguised or displaced suicide. The victim is the image of the slayer himself, as the hated person.

Self-Betrayal

The person with homicidal tendencies may warn his intended victim, or others, of his murderous plans. The self-betrayal may be involuntary and represents one last defense against the urge to kill. Ramon Mercader, alias Jacques Mornard, drew attention to himself by many acts of folly, before he assassinated Trotsky in Mexico. It is indeed remarkable that this man, who had insinuated himself into Trotsky's entourage, did not arouse the suspicion of Trotsky's guards although they were daily expecting attempts on Trotsky's life.

"His psychic state was such that he said and did many things which should logically have led to his detection and exposure as a Soviet agent. Whether these 'mistakes' were part of a deliberate strategy of failure or were slips of the unconscious, they are equally significant . . . his practice of dropping little clues became more frequent as he was drawn into closer association with the Trotsky household" (16).

"The appointed murderer drew attention to himself by every conceivable mistake: travelling on a forged Canadian passport with the provocatively odd name of 'Jacson'; declaring himself to be the son of a Belgian diplomatist whose non-existence could easily be established; being unable to find his way about a town which he purported to visit twice a week on business; naming a different firm as his employer to each of several friends who were mutually known to one another; carrying a mackintosh (to conceal his lethal weapon) on a hot sunny day after constantly boasting 'his ability to go around bareheaded and without a coat in the foulest weather' and so on" (28).

William Heirens made a remarkable plea for help at the scene of one of his murders, when he wrote in lipstick on the wall of the livingroom, "For heavens sake catch me before I kill more, I cannot control myself."

THE MURDERER'S BEHAVIOR AFTER THE DEED

The murderer's conduct after his crime is of particular psychological interest. Confession, flight or suicide are among the choices of action open to the offender. Almost one-third of all English murderers take their own lives; this outcome is much less common in the United States. In **Macbeth** Shakespeare gives a dramatic portrayal of the mind under the pressure of remorse. Simenon in **The Murderer** records with stark truth and without mercy the gradual and inevitable spiritual disintegration of a doctor who has murdered his wife and her lover. In a masterly study of the sense of guilt gradually corroding the murderer's personality, Simenon makes us feel both horror and pity.

Some offenders make little effort to avoid legal execution; others, as in the following example, actively seek the death penalty.

Jack Chester, a young man who murdered his fiance in Boston in 1957, made every effort to ensure his execution. After the crime, this quiet-spoken youth had some difficulty in persuading a patrolman, who was directing traffic, that he had just committed murder. While awaiting trial he attempted suicide twice, once by setting his clothes on fire and another time by slashing his wrists.

He confessed that he had murdered his fiance by firing nine bullets at her through the door of her house and he regretted only one thing, that he had not saved one shell for himself. He seemed determined to leave nothing unsaid that might help bring him the death penalty. In view of his need to declare his guilt over and over again, his lawyers endeavored to prevent him from testifying at his trial. This strategy was upset at the last moment when the youth demanded to be heard. For ninety minutes he gave the court a detailed recital of the crime and he made a dramatic appeal for the death penalty.

"Before I go on any further, I want the members of the jury to understand one thing. I am not looking for your sympathy. I am not denying the fact that what I did was pre-meditated, cold-blooded murder. The only thing that, the only thing that I want to establish, is that at the time that I spoke with the District Attorney and the officers in the Brookline Police Station, I was very emotionally upset and that I wanted to go to the electric chair as quickly as possible. I have not changed my opinion." And again, before the jury withdrew for deliberation, he made the following statement: "It is my opinion that any decision other than guilty, guilty of murder in the first degree, with no recommendation for leniency, is a miscarriage of justice." When this verdict was indeed brought in Jack rose and said, "Thank you — it's what I wanted. I don't want any stay or commutation. The sooner it's over, the better." Later his attorney went to visit Chester in the Walpole jail, and observed ironically, "He looked marvelous — he had a good night's sleep — I never saw him look so good."

He refused to sign a petition for commutation of the death penalty. His lawyers, however, succeeded in making this request over his strenuous objections. The prospects of clemency were considered to be excellent, but before a decision was reached, Chester finally succeeded in achieving his wishes. He committed suicide in jail.

This tragic case is of great psychological interest as the young man blamed himself and his mother for the death of his father. At six years of age he left his home without his hat, despite his mother's demands and arguments. His father, at the mother's insistence, followed him out of the house, hat in hand, to persuade him to put it on. While running after the boy, his father slipped on the ice and suffered a head injury which resulted in his death one month later.

Just prior to the murder Jack thought of his father's death. Referring to his thoughts at this time, he testified at his trial:

"And then I thought, 'Jack, you don't really want to die, do you" And

I said, 'No.' And I said to myself, 'But are you going to let them get away with it?' and I said, 'No.' I said, 'Do you realize if you do this they will electrocute you?' And I said, 'Yes.'

"And then I thought of my father. I do not know why, it just shot through my mind for a minute. And I came to the conclusion that that was exactly what I deserved."

An offender, while ostensibly seeking to avoid detection may, nevertheless, behave in such a manner as to draw police attention to himself. Murderers who escape detection may yet inflict some form of punishment on themselves in order to atone for the crime. Even when detected, the slayer may unconsciously seek greater punishment than that inflicted by the court, as in the following case:

The writer gave evidence at a murder trial in which the question of insanity was not raised. My evidence was favorable to the accused who was subsequently found guilty of the lesser charge of manslaughter. The Assistant District Attorney who had prosecuted the case was somewhat bitter at the outcome of the trial. He thought that the accused had hoodwinked me and referred to me jokingly outside court, as the "felon's friend." An attempt was made in private to explain to the DA the basis of the psychiatric opinion expressed in court. However, the DA could see no redeeming features in the accused and regarded him as a cunning unscrupulous criminal with no conscience and no mental abnormality.

Both defense and prosecution attorneys became united in this viewpoint when, following conviction, the offender abused them both and accused them of withholding information, distorting the facts and behaving unethically. The court had expected the accused to become jubilant on escaping the gas chamber and to be very grateful to the attorneys who had defended him so ably. The prisoner's resentful attitude and ingratitude toward his attorneys came as a surprise. Although likely to escape with a short prison sentence and although he was obviously sane, the accused insisted on a further trial to determine his sanity. His whole attitude was very provocative toward the court. The prisoner's subsequent behavior in jail resulted in my being asked to see him again. At that time, he was in a depressed state but not psychotic. Some months later, the newspapers reported that he would have to serve his full prison sentence because of his uncooperative behavior in the penitentiary.

Some weeks after the trial, I was able to speak again with the Assistant District Attorney who by this time was beginning to have some doubts about his earlier opinion of the accused. It was agreed that the strange behavior of the man following conviction could not be explained on logical grounds. Indeed his behavior was such as to assure maximum punishment by the judge. The jury had found him not guilty of murder, but in his own mind his conscience demanded the punishment which had not been forthcoming from the jury. While ostensibly trying to escape all punishment, he behaved in a manner which suggested motivations to the contrary. The district attorney accepted this viewpoint and gave up his earlier attitude of disrespect for me and my opinion.

The murderer's return to the scene of the crime is seen by Reiwald as an attempt at atonement, an unconscious wish on the part of the murderer to give himself up to justice. One killer remained at the scene of the crime for nine months. In October 1941, seventy-three year old Phillip Peters was battered to death in his Denver home with a cast-iron stove shaker. All efforts to solve the crime were unsuccessful. In July 1942, a companion of the victim's widow saw a stranger in the house. No sign of the intruder was found by the police. Later that month two detectives made a surprise visit to the house and on hearing a noise they rushed upstairs. The rooms were unoccupied, but in a closet a man's legs were seen disappearing through a small 7" by 15" panel in the ceiling.

The detectives seized fifty-nine year old Theodore Coneys, an emaciated, unwashed man clothed in rags held together by string. He revealed that since August 1941, he had been living in the triangular shaped attic which was 27" high at the peak and 57" wide. Coneys, a skid row character, who usually lived in doorways and alleys, had called at the Peters' home in the owners' absence. After raiding the refrigerator he explored the house. On discovering a loose panel in the closet, he decided to "hole up" in the attic during the cold winter months. From time to time he stole small amounts of food from the kitchen.

On October 17, 1941, he slipped downstairs to brew some coffee after he thought Peters had left the house for dinner. Peters returned unexpectedly and when he threatened to call the police, Coneys beat him to death. Life in the attic must have been extremely unpleasant. During part of the winter the heat was turned off in the house and Coneys suffered from frostbitten feet. The detective who managed to enter the attic vomited because of the stench from the gallon cans brimful with human excrement. Previous search had not revealed the entry to the attic as Coneys had used side-bolts to lock the moveable panel firmly in place. The jury imposed a sentence of life imprisonment (5).

The mass murderer, Kurten, has recorded his pleasure in returning to the scene of one of his murders.

"Next evening I went back to the spot and thought over where I could bury the body. I thought how nice it would be if I had something of the kind to go and sit by when I took a walk. I dug a deep hole in a woody corner of the field. I took the body and laid it just as one would lay an ordinary corpse in a grave . . . I had a feeling of solemn tenderness all the time. I stroked her hair and shovelled in the first spadeful of earth very evenly and carefully . . . I went to the grave many times afterwards and kept on improving it. Later on I must have been to the spot at least thirty times, and every time when I thought of what was lying there I had a feeling of satisfaction" (29).

REFERENCES

1. Blackman, Nathan: Precarious sexual identity as a factor in sudden murder. *Med Aspect Hum Sex, 4*(8):72, 1970.
2. Bowlby, John: Forty-four juvenile thieves. *Int J Psychoanal, 25*:19, 1944.
3. Bremer, A.H.: *An Assassin's Diary.* New York, Harpers Magazine Press, 1973.
4. Cassity, J.H.: *The Quality of Murder.* New York, Julian Press, 1958.
5. Childers, J.E. and Snyer, J.: Death was a phantom lodger. *Denver Post,* Feb. 7, 1960.
6. Dollard, J., Miller, N.E., Doob, L.W., Mowrer, O.H. and Sears, R.R.: *Frustration and Aggression.* New Haven, Yale University Press, 1939.
7. Dostoyevsky, Fyodor: *Crime and Punishment.* Translated by Magarshack, David. London, Penguin Books Ltd., 1951.
8. Duncan, G.M., Frazier, S.H., Litin, E.M., Johnson, A.M., and Barron, A.J.: Etiological factors in first-degree murder. *JAMA, 168*:1755, 1958.
9. Easson, W.M. and Steinhilber, R.M.: Murderous aggression by children and adolescents. *Arch Gen Psychiat, 4*:27, 1961.
10. Ellenberger, Henri: Psychological relationships between criminal and victim. *Arch Crim Psychodyn, 1*:257, 1955.
11. Ferenczi, Sandor: *Further Contributions to the Theory and Technique of Psychoanalysis.* London, Hogarth Press, 1926.
12. Freud, Sigmund: Psychogenesis of a case of homosexuality in a woman. In *The Standard Edition of the Complete Psychological Works of Sigmund Freud,* Vol. 18. London, Hogarth Press, 1955.
13. Hobsbawm, E.J.: *Bandits.* New York, Delacorte Press, 1969.
14. Johnson, A.M. and Szurek, S.A.: Etiology of antisocial behavior in delinquents and psychopaths. *JAMA, 154*:814, 1954.
15. Langevin, R., *et al.*: Childhood and family background of killers seen for psychiatric assessment: a controlled study. *Bull Amer Acad Psychiat Law, 11*:331, 1983.
16. Levine, I.D.: *The Mind of an Assassin.* New York, Farrar, Straus and Cudahy, 1959.
17. Lindner, R.M.: The equivalents of matricide. *Psychoanal Quart, 17*:454, 1948.

18. Macdonald, J.M.: *Armed Robbery.* Springfield, Illinois, Charles C Thomas, 1975.

19. Macdonald, J.M.: *Homicidal Threats.* Springfield, Illinois, Charles C Thomas, 1968.

20. Malmquist, C.P.: Premonitory signs of homicidal aggression in juveniles. *Amer J Psychiat, 128*:93, 1971.

21. Menninger, K.A.: *Man Against Himself.* New York, Harcourt Brace, 1938.

22. Reiwald, Paul: *Society and Its Criminals.* New York, International Universities Press, 1950.

23. Russell, Bertrand: *A History of Western Philosophy.* London, George Allen and Unwin, 1948.

24. Satten, J., Menninger, K., Rosen, I. and Mayman, M.: Murder without apparent motive. *Amer J Psychiat, 117*:48, 1960.

25. Schilder, Paul: *Psychoanalysis, Man and Society.* New York, Norton, 1951.

26. Scott, J.P.: *Aggression.* Chicago, University of Chicago Press, 1958.

27. Steele, B.F. and Pollock, C.B.: A psychiatric study of parents who abuse infants and small children. In Helfer, R.E. and Kempe, C.H. (Eds.): *The Battered Child.* Chicago, University of Chicago Press, 1968.

28. Times Lit Suppl, April 15, 1960.

29. Wagner, M.S.: *The Monster of Dusseldorf.* London, Faber and Faber, 1932.

30. Wertham, Fredric: *Dark Legend.* London, Victor Gollancz Ltd., 1947.

CHAPTER 6

THE URGE TO CONFESS

*"Confession is a unique psychological
phenomenon difficult to explain,
inasmuch as it always works to the
detriment of the one who made it."*

Hans Gross

"The conscience is a thousand witnesses."

Richard Taverner, *Proverbs*

IN **Crime and Punishment** Dostoyevsky gives a dramatic portrayal of a murderer's need to confess his crime. Raskolnikov says to his mother, who visits him soon after the crime, "We will have time to talk to each other freely." Having said that he becomes embarrassed again and pale: "Again a short sensation of deadly cold passed through his soul, again it became entirely clear to him that he had just told a horrible lie, that he would never again be able to speak freely, that he must never again, never talk to any one at all." But as Reik points out when we are silent and do not care to say anything, unknown powers still force us to unconscious confessions.

Petrovich, the prosecuting attorney describes to Raskolnikov the strange behavior of the criminal shortly after the deed: ". . . He thrusts himself forward, giving his opinion unasked, talks continuously of things best left alone, revels in parables and asks why he is not arrested."

Not all criminals thrust themselves forward in this manner; nevertheless a surprising number of criminals sooner or later incriminate themselves. Lawes describes the case of Thomas Bohan the taxi driver who had held up a petty gambling establishment and had murdered one of the patrons to cover his escape. He fled to South America where he started life afresh and succeeded in becoming fairly prosperous. One night in an argument in a prominent cafe he warned a semi-drunken patron who had questioned his valor "Listen feller, I once croaked a guy in New York because he got too wise. You better watch your step." This remark led to his arrest. Before he was executed at Sing Sing prison he summed up the cause of his predicament, "You know, Warden, shootin' off a gun ain't dangerous. It's shootin' off your mouth." Lawes believes that at least 95 percent of Sing Sing's murderers either literally talked themselves into arrest, or gave themselves away through some careless act.

Even though the murderer may not volunteer a confession his total behavior may be such as to draw attention to himself as the guilty person. The plane bomber, Graham, who was responsible for the loss of forty-four lives, is a case in point. After identifying himself as the son of one of the victims, he told a business acquaintance how easy it would be to blow up a plane. He gave a thinly disguised description of the method he had employed and mentioned the irony of the crash. If the plane had not taken off twenty minutes late it would have crashed in the mountains and no one would ever have suspected sabotage. (At the time the possibility of sabotage had been raised in the newspapers.)

Graham did not hide or destroy the articles which he had taken out of his mother's suitcase to make room for the bomb. When told by his FBI interrogators that he could return to his home he offered to remain for further questioning and this led to his confession.

One offender, a watchmaker by trade who was later found guilty of murder altered nine of ten stolen watches so that they could not be recognized by the owner, and then pawned only that watch which he had not disguised. Glatman, the strangler, included in his photographs of one of his victims, his drivers license (to identify himself). Landru listed his victims in his notebook. Many murderers have kept highly incriminating diaries.

Haigh, the acid-bath killer, entered in his diary, alongside the sign of the cross, the initials of his victims. After he had been arrested in connection with the disappearance of his sixth victim, a wealthy elderly widow, he asked, "How can you prove a murder if there is no body." He had neglected to destroy a highly incriminating "shopping list" which included:

Drum

H_2SO_4

Stirrup pump
Gloves
Apron

Soderman has described the case of a French physician, Doctor Thevin, who was treating a patient for venereal disease with weekly injections. The patient on one of his clandestine visits to the doctor confided that he was carrying a large sum of money. Doctor Thevin impulsively substituted cyanide for the antivenereal drug. The body was locked in a closet in which his nurse was accustomed to hanging her coat. As the days went by the doctor made no attempt to dispose of the body. He attributed the increasing odor to some animal, perhaps a rat, which had died under the floor. Neighbors complained about the smell, but the doctor still did nothing. On the ninth day after the murder the nurse persuaded a neighbor to force open the closet and the half putrified body of the victim fell out.

A murderer made a fatal slip of the pen. He pretended to be a bacteriologist and purchased in this capacity cultures of dangerously infectious bacilli with which he eliminated persons with whom he was intimately connected. This man once complained to the head of the institute about the ineffectiveness of the cultures sent to him. In his letter, however, he made a slip of the pen, writing "In my experiments with human beings" instead of "in my experiments with mice and guinea pigs."

When the multiple murderer Madame de Brinvilliers was arrested, a full confession was found on her person. The confession was written in such horrifying detail that the publisher considered it necessary to print the volume in Latin.

Frequently criminals notify the police of their crime immediately or shortly after the murder. In other instances the confession may be delayed or hinted at only indirectly. The guilt which leads to confession is usually at its height in the first few days following the offense. Later the burden of guilt is relieved by various mental mechanisms. Recollection of the details of the crime undergoes change — the victim made some insulting remarks or reached in his pocket as if for a gun. Frankly psychotic defenses may be utilized. The victim was tormenting the assailant with poison gas, influencing his mind with radar waves or seducing his children. Immediately following arrest the assailant may give a detailed account of the circumstances of the crime only to repudiate his confession a few days later and to claim that it was a false statement elicited under threats by the police.

The murderer's return to the scene of the crime may originate in an unconscious wish to confess. Certainly this behavior may lead to detection as in the following case.

A thirty-six year old man and his common-law wife were arrested after they cashed checks belonging to a rich bachelor who had been missing for some weeks. The couple claimed that the missing man, before going on a trip to New Mexico, had given them permission to cash the checks and to live in his Denver home. Murder was suspected, but the body could not be located. When the suspects were questioned they mentioned repeatedly the name of a friend. When the friend was interviewed, she volunteered that she had spent an afternoon with the couple at a picnic ground in the mountains. She recalled that her host had shown unusual interest in a pile of rocks. Police investigation of the picnic site led to discovery of the burial site beneath the rock pile. The murderers later volunteered that they had camped overnight just forty paces from the victim's body on at least three occasions. The man was sentenced to death and his common-law wife to life imprisonment.

CONFESSIONS YEARS LATER

> *"My conscience has a thousand several tongues,*
> *And every tongue brings in a several tale,*
> *And every tale condemns me for a villain."*
>
> Shakespeare, *Richard III*

In 1860 the body of a four year old boy was found stabbed to death in the backyard of his parents' home. Suspicion fell on the nursemaid who was taken into custody. Within a week she was released and a Scotland Yard detective who had taken charge of the investigation arrested Constance Kent, the victim's sixteen year old stepsister. She was also released as there was insufficient evidence to commit her to trial. Indeed it was generally considered that she had been wrongfully accused. Constance Kent entered a convent. Five years later she confessed to the Mother Superior of the Order that she had killed her stepbrother as an act of revenge on her stepmother. She was sentenced to death but the death sentence was commuted to life imprisonment and she was released from custody twenty years later.

In 1971 a middle-aged man walked into a newspaper office in Manchester, England and calmly told a reporter that nineteen years previously he had killed a prostitute in Liverpool. While drinking with her on a piece of waste land he battered her to death. After his confession he obtained considerable relief from irritability, sleeplessness and nightmares. The judge, who passed a lenient sentence of one year in prison, felt that retribution had been adequately visited on the offender in the form of years of unhappiness (5).

In 1983 near Chester, England a man excavating peat near the home of a fifty-seven year old airline official Peter Reyn-Bardt discovered a woman's skull. It was reported that Reyn-Bardt confessed to the police that twenty-two years earlier he had strangled his wife and dismembered her body after "she threatened to expose my homosexuality, blackmail me and disgrace me . . . It has been so long I thought I would never be found out." In court he testified that he remembered grabbing his wife by the shoulders and shaking her, but could remember nothing else until he saw her dead on the floor. He admitted to dismembering her body.

The supreme irony of his confession is that the skull turned out to be that of a woman who died in the year 410! Experts reported that the skull had been preserved in the peat bog for over sixteen centuries. Reyn-Bardt was found guilty of murder and sentenced to life imprisonment.

In 1944 Edward Cameron, a thirty year old farmer, disappeared from his home in Raeford, North Carolina. His wife said that he just stepped out the backdoor and never returned. In 1979 the couple's oldest daughter during psychiatric treatment for emotional problems recalled hearing her parents quarrelling and later seeing her father's body partially submerged in excrement in the family outhouse. At the time she was nine years of age and she did not tell law enforcement officers because she was afraid they would listen to her then leave her alone with her mother.

The sheriff obtained a search warrant and excavated the location of the old outhouse. Human bones were found and the next day sixty-nine year old Winnie Cameron walked into the woods near her farm and fatally shot herself with a revolver. She left a written confession that she had killed her husband thirty-five years previously.

UNUSUAL CONFESSIONS

Gribble has reported an unusual confession by an English murderer. In August 1951, nineteen year old Herbert Mills, a self-styled poet of Nottingham, rang a London newspaper and offered to report a murder which the police did not know about in return for $700. He was asked to ring back in half an hour during which time the police were informed. When apprehended by the police he readily told them that he had found a dead woman on some waste ground, but denied responsibility for her death by strangling.

During the police investigation of the murder Mills attempted without success to sell stories about the crime to a number of newspapers. Then he made an appointment to see the crime reporter of the newspaper which he had rung to report the murder. This story was exclusive, it was a confession to what he had thought would be the perfect crime. Psychiatrists reported that he was legally sane and he was sentenced to death.

In 1950, Donald Hume was arrested for the murder of Stanley Setty, a London used car dealer. Setty's headless and legless body was found in a swamp near the Thames estuary and it was obvious that the torso, which was packed into a blanket, had been dropped from a plane. Scotland Yard officers went to every small airfield near London asking if anyone had seen a pilot loading large parcels into a plane. Hume, an amateur pilot, confessed that he dropped two large packages, one with Setty's torso and the other "probably with his head and legs." He insisted that the packages had been brought to his apartment by three men whom he knew only as "Mac," "Jolly" and "The Boy." They paid him $440 for the funeral.

At his trial his wife testified that she was with him on the night of the murder, and that it would have been quite impossible for him to murder and cut up a body without her knowing it. He was acquitted on the charge of murder, but was found guilty of being an accessory after the fact of Setty's murder and was sentenced to twelve years imprisonment. Following his release, in 1958, he sold a London newspaper his confession of Setty's murder. He described in detail the murder, mocking Scotland Yard because under British law he could not be retried. Later that year two bank officers were shot and wounded in armed holdups. It is suspected that Hume was the assailant on both occasions. In January 1959, Hume wounded a bank teller and killed a taxi driver during a bank holdup in Zurich. The Swiss Court sentenced him to life imprisonment.

FALSE CONFESSIONS

False confessions of murder are not uncommon, especially in those unsolved murders which attract considerable newspaper publicity. The

Black Dahlia murder is a case in point. Twenty-two year old Elizabeth Short, a fast-living young woman acquired the soubriquet Black Dahlia because of her penchant for black dresses and black underclothing. On January 15, 1947, her nude body, cut in half at the waist and mutilated with twenty stab wounds, was found in a vacant lot in Los Angeles. More than thirty persons have confessed responsibility for her death, but the crime has yet to be solved. A wish for publicity and notoriety is evident in some of these confessions.

Too forceful or unethical interrogation may result in false confessions. The story is told that SS leader Himmler, while visiting a concentration camp, found that he had lost his pipe. A search followed but on returning to his car, he discovered it on his seat. "But sir," protested the camp commandant, "six prisoners have already confessed to stealing it."

Borchard has reviewed the cases of sixty-five persons convicted in America and England and afterwards proved innocent. He states that it is a common phenomenon for certain types of people, when subjected to interrogation, accusations or suggestions from persons of stronger will, to ultimately succumb and accept the conclusions of the more powerful intellect. The following case of spurious confession to murder has been summarized from Borchard's carefully documented account.

Louise Butler was accused by her daughter and niece of having murdered another niece who lived with her. Louise at first denied the accusations, but after a few days in jail she suddenly confessed that she had killed her niece and with the aid of a friend, George Yelder, had tied an old automobile casing to the body and thrown it into a river. Yelder denied having committed the crime and Louise repudiated her confession. Both defendants were found guilty and were sentenced to a life term in the Alabama State Penitentiary. Within a week after they had been sent to the penitentiary the niece was found alive at the home of relatives in a neighboring county.

It is not unusual for a murderer to include in his confession false statements, thus the murder may be acknowledged but sexual assault and sadistic acts are denied. The presence of an accomplice is concealed or undue blame is placed on another participant in the crime. Vigilance is required to detect false statements as in the following example.

A young man who confessed to beating his two and a half year old son to death was evaluated after his plea of not guilty of murder by reason of insanity. On my first interview he told me that at breakfast on the day of the crime he made his child drink five ounces of rum and cola. He described various assaults which took place between 10:30 AM and 3:30 PM when he started mouth to mouth resuscitation.

"I had to drive to get the mail and I hit him in the stomach two or three times. I guess it was just because he was falling asleep or maybe I wanted to hear him cry. I guess I stood on him in the livingroom. I was standing on him for about twenty seconds and he threw up his breakfast.

"I hung him up in the closet (suspended from a crossbar) with a piece of rope, a tie from his bathrobe. I hung him up by his hands then by his feet, spun him around, hit him in the stomach . . . I guess I hit him in the stomach a couple of times. Then I shut the door a couple of minutes and came back and hung him the other way. I guess I took him in the bathroom and held his breath on him, my hand over his face so he couldn't breathe.

"I shoved him in the toilet I guess and closed the seat down on him. I don't know if it was head first or feet first. Then I took him out of there and stood him up and hit him and knocked him down. I think he hit his head on the cabinet. Then I stomped on him with my foot a couple of times. He was having a hard time breathing after that. I didn't quite know what was wrong with him. He looked real funny, his eyes rolling around."

My immediate reaction of distress on listening to his detailed account of such cruel behavior distracted my attention from indications of untruthfulness. On reflection I was puzzled over his striking his child for sleeping in the car. Abusive parents seldom strike sleeping children rather their anger is provoked by crying, soiling or acts of disobedience. Furthermore he had not mentioned, either to the police or to two defense psychiatrists who had reported a finding of legal insanity, the incident in the clothes closet. It occurred to me that he was exaggerating the extent of his brutality in order to convince psychiatrists that he was insane. Such indeed was the case.

On checking autopsy records I found that the child's blood alcohol test was negative and there were no marks on the wrists or ankles which would have resulted from the child's suspension from a crossbar in the closet. On checking several toilets I found that it would be impossible to shove a child of his age in the toilet and close the toilet seat. After reviewing my report to the court his attorneys withdrew the plea of insanity.

CRIMINAL INTERROGATION

Certain factors are likely to induce confession. It is advantageous to create feelings of anxiety and guilt and to induce or enhance a state of mental conflict. Every effort is made to take advantage of the pressure of conscience. Dostoyevsky in **Crime and Punishment** recognizes the importance of these factors. Petrovich makes the following significant comments to the suspect Raskolnikov:

"If I should consider one man or another to be guilty of some crime, why I ask you should I trouble him too soon, even if I had in my possession evidence against him? There may be cases, of course, where it may be my duty to arrest a person immediately, but there may be cases of quite a different character. Yes, indeed! So why shouldn't I let my suspect run about the town for a bit? . . . And if I put him under lock and key a bit too soon — even though I were certain that he was my man — I'd most probably be depriving myself of the means of obtaining more evidence against him. And why? Because I'd give him, as it were, a definite status, I'd, as it were, satisfy him psychologically and set his mind at rest, so that he'd slip through my fingers and retire into his shell. He would realize at last that he was really and truly a suspect . . .

"Were I not to arrest him or trouble him, but were he to know all the time, or at least suspect, that I knew everything and was keeping him under close observation day and night, and were I to keep him in this state of continual terror and suspense that he was under suspicion, why I assure you, he'd lose his head and come to me himself . . . He won't run away from me psychologically — ha ha! What a way of putting it, eh! He won't run away from me, even if he had some place to run to, because of a law of nature. Ever watched a moth before a lighted candle? Well, he, too, will be circling round and round me like a moth round a candle.

"He'll get sick of his freedom. He'll start brooding. He'll get himself so thoroughly entangled that he won't be able to get out. He'll worry himself to death. And what's more, he'll provide me himself with a nice, easy mathematical problem like twice two — if I give him enough rope. And he'll keep on describing circles round me, smaller and smaller circles, till — bang! he'll fly straight into my mouth and I'll swallow him! And that, my dear sir, is very satisfying indeed, ha, ha, ha! Don't you think so? Raskolnikov made no answer. He sat pale and motionless, still peering into Porfiry's face with the same intense concentration. 'The lesson is a good one,' he thought, turning cold."

A person suspected of homicide is likely to be in a very anxious and emotional state during the period immediately following his arrest. He may be locked by himself in a cell for a few hours in order to heighten his anxiety and apprehension. The interview should be in privacy in a bare room with table or desk and chairs, without a telephone, glass partition or window. The suspect's attention should not be distracted by a telephone call, diplomas on the wall and activities outside the room. His chair should be alongside rather than behind the desk and it should be no less comfortable than the questioner's chair.

The interrogator's approach will be determined by the circumstances of the murder and the personality of the suspect. A false start may be disastrous. The suspect should first be evaluated carefully to determine his strength and weaknesses. Every man is proud of something whether it is his intellect, sense of honor, loyalty to companions, muscular development or physical appearance. Attention should be directed toward his source of pride. An uncooperative soldier suspected of strangling his girl friend responded quickly when his biceps were felt and favorably appraised. A poorly educated but intelligent slayer confessed after his interest in books and wide range of knowledge were remarked upon.

First offenders, as well as those who kill in the heat of anger without planning and not for financial gain, are susceptible to a sympathetic approach, especially when they are burdened by feelings of remorse and guilt. The suspect should be encouraged to tell his side of the event and the detective should indicate his understanding of adverse pressures on the suspect including possible provocation by the victim. Harsh words such as murder, stab and rape should not be used.

A direct, confident, forceful approach — "I'm here to talk to you about the crime you're involved in," may be successful even with career criminals who at first refuse to say anything apart from "If you've got it, file it." Such a response should not discourage the interrogator, although there will be offenders who will not cooperate. Few murderers have faced criminal interrogation with the composure of the multiple murderer Landru. After a particularly gruelling interrogation he appeared silent and pensive. When the interrogator remarked to Landru that he seemed preoccupied — "I am," Landru sighed deeply, "and who could help being so? Alas, my thoughts are engrossed by the electoral situation of this unhappy country."

The suspect may be disconcerted by the detectives' unexpected attitude. There is an adage, "Treat a duchess like a whore, and a whore like a duchess." Resort is sometimes made to a combination of an authoritarian brusk senior interrogator and a more understanding kindly junior officer. When the senior officer leaves the room his assistant, who had previously remained silent, apologizes for his colleague's manner and sympathizes with the suspect. The suspect is drawn into confession in order to show up the impatient unfriendly interrogator. A kindly remark or thoughtful gesture may succeed where other methods have failed. A police chief while inspecting the detention cells stopped to chat with a murder suspect about matters unrelated to the crime. The conversation turned to a fatherly discussion of their children. Suddenly the suspect broke down and blurted out a full confession.

The most usual means of obtaining a confession from a guilty person, according to Louwage, is to let him trap himself in a net of lies. "Generally the prisoner who is guilty will build up an edifice which, as the interrogation proceeds, becomes more and more shaky, for nothing is more difficult than to lie, even for those who have worked out a scheme in advance. The suspect must improvise as he goes along, for he soon feels that his questioner knows far more than he had suspected. To modify or think out another scheme on the spur of the moment, especially on a shifting foundation, is not a thing that everyone is capable of doing. All that need be done is to note the explanations, and when they have been made, show the prisoner the discrepancies, comparing them with either others made by himself or those made by witnesses or facts shown by clues." Even if the suspect does not confess, his false statements may count against him when revealed to the jury.

The criminal who does not wish to confess may do so unwittingly. Gross points out that the desire to fool others has its limitations, thus simple yet significant gestures may contradict false statements. For example, a man said he lived very peacefully with his neighbor and at the same time clenched his fist. The latter meant ill will toward the neighbor while the words did not. Gross gives another remarkable example involving a girl suspected of killing her newborn child.

"The girl told that she had given birth to the child all alone, had washed it, and then laid it on the bed beside herself. She had also observed how a corner of the coverlet had fallen on the child's face, and thought it might interfere with the child's breathing; but at this point she swooned, was unable to help the child and it was choked. While sobbing and weeping as she was telling this story, she spread the fingers of her left hand and pressed it on her thigh, as perhaps she might have done, if she had first put something soft, the corner of a coverlet possibly, over the child's nose and mouth, and then pressed on it. This action was so clearly significant that it inevitably led to the question whether she hadn't choked the child in that way. She assented, sobbing" (4).

The interviewer should be very observant and watch for both verbal and nonverbal communication which may show the need for further inquiry. Slightly hesitant speech for the first time, a change in the tone of voice or rate of speech, twisting of a lock of hair, a flush rising from the base of the neck or a sudden downward look may all suggest that the whole truth is not being told. A sudden interest in something in the interviewing room may point to deception as in the following example:

A middle-aged chronic alcoholic man, who pleaded not guilty by reason of insanity to a charge of murder, was friendly and cooperative on psychiatric examination. He spoke freely and when questioned directly on any subject he replied without hesitation. It was noted that he appeared somewhat ill at ease when describing his school record. The subject was therefore raised again at a later interview and once more he appeared somewhat discomforted. His answers were not as spontaneous as previously. He turned half away from me and appeared to be interested in the contents of a glass medicine cabinet. In view of his change in demeanor, I assumed that he was withholding some information.

He denied this, but became more obviously distressed, and then suddenly with considerable abreaction he revealed that at the age of twelve he had seen his father shot and killed by a revenue officer. He rushed inside, picked up his father's loaded shotgun, went outside and killed the revenue officer. His placement in a reform school had interfered with his schooling. On his release from prison he had traveled to another state, married and settled down.

This man had been successful in keeping this information a secret from his wife for their thirty years of married life. The earlier murder conviction was not on his police records, but was confirmed by correspondence with the reform school.

Much depends on the persistence and skill of the detective. Confession is good for the soul and every effort should be made to persuade the suspect to reveal himself. Society attaches great importance to acknowledgment of guilt. Reik points out that confession is the criminal's first step on his way back to society. The criminal shows in his confession his intention to re-enter society by declaring himself deserving of punishment. The outsider is on his painful detour back to the family of man (10).

LIE DETECTOR TESTS

The person who falsely denies his crime may betray himself by involuntary bodily responses as for example an increase in his pulse rate or changes in his pattern of breathing. The lie detector technique was foreshadowed in the 14th century by the Decameron, which tells how King Agilulf of Lombardy, coming home late one night, dropped in on Queen Theodelinda. She demanded to be informed why he appeared again only five minutes after saying "Goodnight." The monarch surmised that he had been impersonated by a nocturnal marauder. In order to avoid scandal he decided to say nothing and handle the case by himself. Going through the sleeping quarters of his retinue, he cautiously listened to every man's heart. One was going like a trip hammer. Because of his horror of scenes, Agilulf didn't kill the man on the spot, but merely marked him for identification by cutting off a bunch of hair. Realizing that he had been marked for a quiet death the next morning, the man saved himself by taking a pair of shears and marking all of the servants in the same manner. Unable to pick out the guilty man, the king had to drop the matter (6).

Lie detector machines record changes in respiration, pulse, blood pressure and other physiological changes in the suspect during interrogation. These instruments should more properly be called stress-detectors. The detection of lying is made by the person who operates the machine.

The use of the instrument, or even the mere suggestion of its use, may have a strong psychological effect on the suspect and thereby induce confession. The abnormal changes recorded by the machine, in response to crucial questions, when demonstrated to the subject may be sufficient to convince him that further denial is fruitless. As innocent persons, especially those who have guilt feelings regarding some other crime or behavior forbidden by conscience, may show abnormal records and as the guilty person may not betray himself on the machine, the technique has obvious limitations.

An evaluation of polygraph testing in criminal investigations by the U.S. Office of Technology Assessment showed that countermeasures, including physical movement or pressure, drugs, hypnosis, biofeedback and prior experience in passing an exam may lead to a false report that a person did not commit the crime. In a review of twenty-four studies meeting minimum acceptable scientific criteria, it was found that correct guilty detections ranged from about 35 to 100 percent. Overall, the cumulative research evidence suggests that when used in criminal investigations, the polygraph test detects deception better than chance, but with error rates that could be considered significant (9). Much depends on the skill of the polygraph examiner. Some examiners claim accurate detection rates of 95 percent.

TRUTH SERUM

Much publicity has been given to the use of drugs in obtaining confessions from suspected criminals. The term "truth serum" suggests the existence of a drug with the remarkable property of eliciting the truth. The reputation enjoyed by truth serum is based on spectacular newspaper reports rather than on carefully documented case reports in professional medical or legal journals. The description truth serum is misleading as the drug used is not a serum, and it does not always lead to the truth. Formerly scopolamine was used, but today a barbiturate drug, such as sodium amytal, is usually employed. The test may not be performed unless the suspect willingly gives his consent. The drug is injected slowly into a vein in order to induce a relaxed state of mind in which the suspect becomes more talkative and has less emotional control. This technique is variously called truth serum test, narcosis and narcoanalysis. The mental state produced is not unlike that seen in acute alcoholism.

It is well known that a person under the influence of alcohol may reveal information which he would not disclose when sober. Barbiturates are preferable to alcohol because results are obtained in a shorter time, under more uniform conditions which are easier to control and which are more conducive to satisfactory interrogation. The intravenous injection of a drug by a physician in a hospital may appear more scientific than the drinking of large amounts of bourbon in a tavern, but the results displayed in the subject's speech may be no more reliable. The drugged person may be just as boastful and untruthful as the alcoholic.

There are many recorded instances of the successful use of drugs in obtaining confessions. These well-publicized and dramatic successes probably account for the misguided public belief in the effectiveness and reliability of drugs as a means of obtaining confessions. Law enforcement agencies, no doubt attracted by the misleading term "truth serum," not infrequently request physicians to administer drugs to suspected criminals. There is the danger in such a practice that narcoanalysis might be substituted for the painstaking, time consuming inquiries which form the basis of competent police investigation.

As Sir James Stephen stated in 1883, referring to a practice of police officers in India, "It is far pleasanter to sit comfortably in the shade rubbing red pepper into a poor devil's eyes than to go about in the sun hunting up evidence." Although occasional spectacular results in criminal investigation have been credited to narcoanalysis, it is very doubtful whether the technique has been of value in more than a few isolated but highly publicized cases.

It might be thought that no problems would arise from the use of drugs on persons who are, in fact, innocent. Unfortunately, persons under the influence of drugs are very suggestible and may confess to crimes which they have not committed. In Hawaii, a murder suspect under the influence of drugs falsely confessed to writing the ransom note, but later the real murderer was discovered. False confessions under drugs may lead to a miscarriage of justice. A false confession may also interrupt the criminal investigation at a crucial time and enable the real criminal to escape detection. The test has been recommended as a valuable method of exonerating the innocent suspect, but the test is not sufficiently reliable for this purpose.

A confession made under the influence of drugs is inadmissible in evidence because of the rule against involuntary confessions. Some guilty suspects confess while under the influence of drugs. These confessions might appear to favor the use of truth serum tests. However, the suspect who is determined to lie will usually be able to continue the deception even under the effects of drugs. The confident criminal relishes the prospect of making self-serving statements in the pseudo-scientific atmosphere of the truth serum test. The person who is likely to confess will probably do so as the result of skillful police interrogation, and it should not be necessary to use drugs. Narcoanalysis is of value in restoring memory, when there is genuine amnesia for the crime, as in the following case.

A thirty year old man entered a plea of not guilty by reason of insanity in response to a charge of murder. Previously he had been discovered in his apartment unconscious with knife wounds in his throat and abdomen. His wife had been murdered, death resulting from a cut throat. On regaining consciousness in the hospital, he told detectives that he could not recall what happened after an epileptic attack during an argument with his wife. Psychiatric examination showed him to be a cooperative but somewhat apprehensive, rather dependent person of normal intelligence.

He agreed to narcoanalysis and under the influence of sodium amytal his amnesia was resolved. He described the argument with his wife in which he declared his intention to divorce her and obtain custody of the children as his wife was neglecting them. His wife shouted that the boy was not his, but his brother's child and the dispute became very heated. Suddenly his wife picked up a knife and stabbed him several times in the chest and abdomen. In the struggle he obtained the knife and attacked his wife. He recalled thinking that he was mortally wounded and that his wife would probably escape punishment for his death. He decided to cut his own throat as he was in severe pain and as he thought that he was dying anyway.

The story was told with considerable release of emotion. Following the interview, the amnesia returned. At the trial, the psychiatric testimony, including the results of the narcoanalytic examination, was helpful in giving an account of the events on the night of the tragedy and revealed the extreme provocation. In giving evidence, I stated frankly the unreliability of narcoanalysis, my opinion that the man was telling the truth was based on observation of the patient's behavior under narcosis and on the total psychiatric examination.

A criminal may choose to simulate a recovery of memory under drugs in order to form a basis for a subsequent insanity plea. The following is a case in point:

A twenty-nine year old man was arrested in Denver, while in possession of a stolen car. The trunk of the car was bloodstained and had an unpleasant odor of decomposing flesh. The owner of the car had been missing from his home in California for some weeks and it was suspected that he had been murdered. The suspect claimed amnesia from the time he escaped from a California mental hospital two months previously, until he found himself in a Denver hospital for treatment of a bullet wound, received while trying to escape from the police. Prolonged questioning by the police failed to reveal any further information, although he made several untruthful statements.

He agreed to narcoanalysis and this was performed over a five hour period during which 1.5 gm of sodium amytal were injected. While under narcosis he described his escape from the hospital and his subsequent meeting with the missing man. One evening he left this man in the car while he went to buy some food. On his return he discovered the owner of the car with his head "bashed in." He was frightened that he would be blamed as he had a criminal record. He drove to an isolated spot in New Mexico where he buried the body, which was later found in the location he had described.

He displayed little emotion and no remorse as he described these events. Indeed he was very selfpossessed and he appeared almost to enjoy the examination. From time to time he would request that more amytal should be injected. In view of his previous untruthfulness and his behavior while under narcosis it was considered that he was not suffering from a genuine amnesia. Incomplete psychiatric examination suggested that he was a sociopathic personality. He later confessed to the crime and entered a plea of insanity, which was subsequently rejected by the jury.

In summary, criminal suspects while under the influence of barbiturate drugs, may deliberately withhold information, persist in giving untruthful answers, or falsely confess to crimes which they have not committed. Narcoanalysis is of doubtful value when used for the purpose of obtaining confessions to crimes. It is sometimes of value in restoring memory when there is genuine amnesia for the crime. Careful psychiatric examination will show whether the amnesia is feigned or genuine.

REFERENCES

1. Borchard, E.M.: *Convicting the Innocent.* New Haven, Yale University Press, 1932.
2. Dostoyevsky, Fyodor: *Crime and Punishment.* Translated by Magarshack, David. London, Penguin Books, 1951.
3. Gribble, L.R.: *Murders Most Strange.* London, John Long, 1959.
4. Gross, Hans: *Criminal Psychology.* Boston, Little Brown, 1939.
5. Hepworth, M. and Turner, B.S.: *Confessions: Studies in Deviance and Religion.* London, Routledge and Kegan Paul, 1982.
6. Johnston, A.: The magic lie detector. In Leonard, V.A. (Ed.): *Academy Lectures in Lie Detection,* Vol. II. Springfield, Illinois, Charles C Thomas, 1958.
7. Lawes, L.E.: *Meet the Murderer.* New York, Harper and Brothers, 1940.
8. Louwage, F.E.: Some remarks on police interrogation. *Internat Pol Rev, 8*:114, 1953.
9. Office of Technology Assessment, U.S. Congress: *Scientific Validity of Polygraph Testing: A Research Review and Evaluation.* Washington, D.C., U.S. Government Printing Office, 1983.
10. Reik, Theodore: *The Compulsion to Confess.* New York, Farrar Straus and Cudahy, 1959.
11. Soderman, Harry: *Policemen's Lot.* New York, Funk and Wagnalls Company, 1956.

CHAPTER 7

MASS MURDERERS AND
SERIAL MURDERERS

"So shall you hear
Of carnal, bloody and unnatural acts,
Of accidental judgments, casual slaughters."

Shakespeare, *Hamlet*

THE PLANE BOMBER, arsonist and train wrecker can by a single act cause the loss of many lives. As these offenders are often detected they seldom have an opportunity to repeat their crimes. Similarly the offender who, within a few minutes or hours kills many persons, is usually shot down by a police special weapons attack team, executed after trial, or confined for many years in a penitentiary or a mental hospital. These offenders who kill many persons in one location at one time are called **mass murderers.** In contrast the **serial murderer** kills repeatedly over many years in many different localities.

MASS MURDERERS

From time to time there are reports in the newspapers of persons who go berserk and kill or assault anyone they encounter. Berserk, a wild Norse warrior, grandson of the mythical eight-handed Starkadder, never fought in armor but in his **ber sark** or bear skin. His name was applied to a predatory group of brawlers and killers who disrupted the peace of the Viking community between 870 and 1030 A.D.

Berserks, according to Schubeler, were men who at certain times were seized by a wild fury, which, at the moment, doubled their strength

139

and made them insensible to bodily pain, but which also deadened their humanity and reason, and made them like wild animals. This fury, which was called 'Berserksgang,' occurred not only in the heat of battle, but also during laborious work. Men who were thus seized performed things which otherwise seemed impossible for human power. This condition is said to have begun with shivering, chattering of the teeth, and chill in the body, and then the face swelled and changed its color. With this was connected a great hotheadedness, which at last went over into a great rage, under which they howled as wild animals, bit the edge of their shields, and cut down everything they met, without discriminating between friend or foe. When this condition ceased, a great dulling of the mind and feebleness followed, which could last for one or several days (11).

Amok is a Malayan word that refers to a sudden, brief outburst of homicidal violence. Captain Cook on his first voyage round the world reported that amok had prevailed from time immemorial. The affected person armed with a curved knife (kris) or a chopper (parang) indiscriminately cuts down anyone in his path—relatives, neighbors, strangers and animals. Ten or more persons may be killed and so great is the amok runner's fury that he is often killed on the spot because he cannot be safely restrained. In former times a two forked prong on a long handle was kept in police stations for the special purpose of pressing an amok runner against a wall or tree so that he could be captured without having to grapple with him (14).

The violence may be preceded by a period of brooding over some untoward event, such as the death of a friend, an insult or humiliation, however there may be no warning signs. Amok, like "berserksgang" is followed by exhaustion. There is usually loss of memory for the violence although the person may report talking to the devil. In one case a friend in a plea for his life asked an amok runner if he recognized him. The runner replied, "Yes, but my spear doesn't know you" and stabbed the friend in the chest and stomach. The assailant was himself stabbed to death, but before he died he said that he did not know what he was doing, that his head went round and the devil told him to do it (15).

After an English judge suggested that amok runners should be apprehended and hanged legislation was passed and the amok rate dropped markedly. Amok still occurs and the weapons now include rifles and grenades. Sudden senseless mass murder is not confined to Malaysia where folk beliefs and social expectations of the behavior of the amok runner probably contribute to the nature and incidence of amok.

Underlying psychiatric disorders in mass murderers include sociopathic personality, schizophrenia and paranoid disorders. An example of a mass murderer with long-standing paranoid delusions is Wagner, the German schoolteacher of good reputation. In September 1913 at the age of thirty-nine he murdered his wife and four children. The next day he set fire to houses and barns, killed cattle and shot everyone he met. Altogether he killed fourteen persons and seriously wounded twelve before the police seized him when he had to reload his pistols. He had 198 bullets in his possession and he was disappointed that he had not been able to slaughter more citizens before his capture.

It had been his intention to kill his brother and his family, then burn down their house as well as the house in which he had been born. As a final step he had planned to proceed to the royal castle in Ludwigsberg, overpower the guards, set fire to the castle, and die in the flames or jump off its walls, thereby terminating his own life (3). He had mailed a confession of his intended crimes to a large newspaper for publication as an editorial. Wagner, the son of an alcoholic father, who died when he was two years of age, and a promiscuous mother, was a clever youth with a reputation as a girl chaser. At the age of twenty-six, while drunk, he committed an act of sodomy. Later he had paranoid delusions that others knew about this crime, talked about it and held him in contempt. He believed that his murders were justified because of the suffering inflicted on him by this gossip. Shortly before his death in a mental hospital in 1938, twenty-five years after his murders, he said, "I could not live on the outside amongst people. It would be intolerable torture to hear them talk about me. Even here, in the institution, I heard them talk six months ago, that I was a sodomist" (3).

Another mass murderer without a prior criminal record, who also had paranoid ideas that the neighbors were making derogatory remarks about him, is Howard Unruh. At the age of twenty-eight this tall pharmacy student, a loner preoccupied with religion, was living with his parents in Camden, New Jersey. He became upset when a gate was stolen from a high fence that he had erected around the yard of his parent's home, and on September 7, 1949, he walked down the street armed with a Luger pistol.

Within twelve minutes he killed fourteen persons and wounded three others. Victims included the owner of a shoe repair store, a drugstore owner, his wife and mother, a barber and the six year old youth whose hair he was cutting, a two year old boy looking out of a window, a man in the street who went to aid one of his victims and two women in a car stopped at a traffic light.

After he returned to his parent's home, a reporter asked him on the telephone, "I want to know what they are doing to you?" He replied, "They haven't done anything to me yet, but I am doing plenty to them." When asked how many persons he had killed he replied, "I don't know yet. I haven't counted them, but it looks like a pretty good score." Eventually he surrendered to the police and he was later committed to the New Jersey State Hospital. In 1984, not to the delight of his neighbors, he was released.

One wonders whether psychiatric consultation might have saved Wagner and Unruh from killing so many people. In March 1966 Charles Whitman, a twenty-five year old student of architectural engineering at the University of Texas in Austin, Texas consulted a psychiatrist because he was upset over his parent's separation. In a two-hour interview he stated that he had beaten his wife several times and although he was making intense efforts to control his temper, he was worried that he might explode. He revealed that he was thinking about going up on the University Tower with a deer rifle and start shooting people.

In August 1966 he went to his mother's apartment where he stabbed and shot her. On his return home he stabbed his wife. In a note addressed "To whom it may concern," he recorded the deaths of his first two victims and expressed love for his mother and hatred for his father. The following day he carried three rifles, a shotgun and other firearms to the observation deck of the 307-feet-tall University Tower. From this vantage point he shot forty-four persons killing fourteen, before he was killed by police officers. At autopsy, which he had requested in a note written before his rampage, a small brain tumor was found but it was considered that this did not cause his homicidal behavior.

On July 17, 1984, Mrs. Etna Huberty telephoned a mental health clinic in San Ysidro, California to ask whether her husband James had obtained an appointment. She said that he had guns and was going to kill someone. It was reported that she was told to call the police but did not do so because her husband had previously made remarks about killing that she did not take seriously. She called another health center and once again was told that her husband had not been given an appointment, however a later review of the health center records showed that a Mr. Suberty had requested an appointment.

After spending the next day with his wife and daughters at the zoo, Huberty changed into camouflage fatigue trousers and a black tee shirt. On leaving his apartment he told his wife, "I'm going to hunt humans."

Huberty armed with a rifle, shotgun and pistol entered a nearby Mc-Donald's hamburger restaurant about 4:00 PM. He shouted, "I'm going to kill you all" and began shooting staff, customers and persons on the street. He killed twenty-one persons and wounded nineteen before a police marksman shot him to death at 5:15 PM. The fatalities included three eleven year old boys who were shot as they rode their bicycles up to the restaurant.

Huberty, a forty-one year old unemployed security guard, who had moved from Ohio to California was described by former neighbors as a brooding ill-tempered loner, a survivalist who hoarded food, kept menacing guard dogs in his yard and boasted that he had a loaded gun in every room of his home. In his twenties he studied to become a funeral director, obtained a diploma from a mortuary school and worked for a short time as an apprentice embalmer in a funeral home.

It is a comparatively simple matter for a mass murderer to blow up an airplane in flight by placing a time bomb in a passenger's luggage or in air freight. There is always the risk that the departure time may be delayed or that the luggage may be placed on another flight, but the chances of fatal outcome for the intended victim and his fellow passengers are not small. The risk of detection is reduced if the explosion occurs over an ocean hundreds of miles from land.

The first known example of this form of crime occurred on May 7, 1949, when a Phillipine Air Lines plane, a converted C47, crashed into the Phillipine Sea twenty-five minutes after it had taken off from Daet enroute to Manila. The nine passengers and four crewmen lost their lives. A fisherman who witnessed the crash reported that the plane was not on fire, but that its tail had been sheared off. The only parts of the aircraft recovered were pieces of the toilet seat into which had been driven pieces of alloy from the rear baggage compartment. All the luggage and air freight loaded at Daet had been placed in the rear compartment.

Crispin Verzo, an employee of Fructuoso Suzara who was one of the victims, was arrested along with two other men. The three men were convicted of placing a time bomb in a wooden box which they had consigned on the plane. Verzo was said to have been in love with his employer's wife. His death sentence was commuted to life imprisonment and his assistants' death sentences were commuted to seventeen years in prison.

Five months later on September 9, 1949, a Canadian Pacific Airlines DC-3 exploded and crashed twenty minutes after it had taken off from

Quebec. Twenty-three persons lost their lives. If the plane had not been five minutes late in taking off it probably would have crashed as the bomber had planned in the broad St. Lawrence River. Traces of dynamite were found in the baggage compartment. Subsequent police inquiries were successful in locating all but one of the persons who had consigned air freight on the plane. The missing person who had consigned a twenty-six pound box which was said to contain a religious statuette was identified by the taxi driver who had driven her to the airport. Subsequent inquiries revealed that Joseph Guay, a jewelry salesman, whose wife was one of the victims had persuaded a crippled watchmaker friend to make a timing mechanism. A former mistress of Guay, had purchased ten pounds of dynamite and had taken the time bomb to the airport. Guay who wished to marry another woman saw his wife off at the airport, and while there insured her life for the journey, (a one flight policy despite the fact that a return flight policy is no more expensive). He was careful to ask who would be the beneficiary in the event of anything happening on the journey. All these conspirators were hanged for the crime.

The aim of some plane bombers has been suicide without regard for the lives of others on the plane. In January 1960, a dynamite blast caused a plane crash at Bolivia, North Carolina killing thirty-four persons. The Civil Aeronautics Board reported that a dynamite charge was exploded by means of a dry cell battery within the passenger cabin, and at a point beneath the extreme right seat of seat row number seven. No attempt was made to fix the blame for the explosion, but the board noted that a New York attorney, who carried more than a million dollars worth of accident and life insurance policies was in close proximity to the dynamite charge when the detonation occurred.

John Gilbert Graham

On November 1, 1955, John Gilbert Graham, a twenty-three year old night mechanic drove his mother to Stapleton Airport in Denver, Colorado. Her luggage was thirty-seven pounds overweight and she did not want to pay the $28.00 surcharge, but her son told her that she would need all her luggage for her visit to Alaska. If she had removed articles from her luggage to avoid the extra payment she would have discovered her son's time bomb which consisted of a timer, hotshot battery, blasting caps and twenty-five sticks of dynamite.

On his mother's request Graham took out three insurance policies each with a different beneficiary. He failed to complete properly two application forms and had to throw them away. The policies were to have been for $6,250 but by mistake he deposited extra coins in the machine for his policy, thus giving it a value of $37,500. After the plane left he had dinner with his wife and child in the airport restaurant. During dinner he became nauseated and vomited in the restroom. Eleven minutes after leaving Denver the four engine airliner exploded and crashed with the loss of forty-four lives.

Graham's behavior following the plane crash seemed almost designed to draw attention to himself as the plane bomber. In order to make room for the bomb in his mother's suitcase he removed gifts purchased by his mother for her grandchildren in Alaska. He did not hide or destroy these gifts but left them in a chest of drawers in the bedroom used by his stepsister when she came to Denver for their mother's funeral. His explanation that their mother did not have space in the suitcase for the gifts seemed improbable as there were other items, such as boxes of ammunition and shotgun shells, which their mother would be more likely to leave behind.

He told his family before the funeral that the explosion on the plane would have set off these shells, "Can't you just see those shotgun shells going off in the plane every which way and the pilots and passengers and grandma jumping around." This callous inappropriate comment would not be expected from a grieving son. On November 10 he told an employee of a garage which had repaired his pickup truck that he had once worked for the Civil Aeronautics Administration and an old friend in this agency had told him that the center of the plane on which his mother had died had been blown to only small strips of metal.

He went on to say how easy it would be to blow up a plane and estimated that it would require two gallons of nitroglycerine and a timing mechanism which could be placed in a suitcase and slipped on the carts which carry baggage to the planes. He mentioned the irony of the crash. If the plane had not taken off twenty minutes late it would have crashed in the mountains and no one would ever have suspected sabotage (6).

On November 13 after prolonged questioning by FBI agents he confessed, he was arrested and charged with the crime. During the interrogation the agents told him that he could return home and later he asked himself "a million times" why he did not accept the offer. I examined him following a plea of insanity. He insisted that he was innocent and said that he confessed falsely because he could not stand the questioning; when he told the truth and was not believed, he thought "to heck with it;" he was manhandled and threatened with bodily injury. There was no evidence of threats and the principal questioner was smaller than Graham.

In his confession to the FBI he had distorted many facts in the optimistic belief that by disproving these inaccuracies in court he would be acquitted. His hopes of acquittal were dashed when his attorney discovered where he had purchased the dynamite, timer and battery. He became depressed and made a suicidal gesture. He asked me to do him a favor. His wife believed his claims of innocence and he wanted me to tell her that he committed the offense. His original intention was to blow up his drive-in restaurant which was not a financial success. When his mother refused to stay with him until Thanksgiving he decided to blow up the airplane on which she was travelling. He told me:

"I tried to tell her how I felt about it. She just said she wouldn't stay, she wouldn't give me any reason at all, no reason why she didn't want to stay. I thought it was the last time she was going to run off and leave me. I wanted to have her to myself for once. Since I was just a little kid she'd leave me with these people, those people, I wanted to get close to her, everytime I'd get close to her she'd just brush me off like I was a piece of furniture, as if I didn't mean more to her than nothing. If she gave me money I was supposed to realize that was enough. I just wanted to do things with her, to sit down and talk to her—just like everybody else's mother would do.

"I just had to stop her from going—yet it seemed I had to be free from her, too. She held something over me that I couldn't get from under. When the plane left the ground a load came off my shoulders, I watched her go off for the last time. I felt happier than I ever felt before in my life. I was afraid to do anything without asking her and yet I wanted to go ahead on my own without having to ask her. Down deep I think she resented me, little things she would do to aggravate me. It's such a relief to tell somebody what I did. It was such a terrible thing I couldn't bear to tell anybody. I deserve to be taken out and shot. I can't find an excuse for something like that."

In subsequent interviews, he was alternately callous and remorseful regarding the tragedy. "I just felt if it killed somebody that was tough. When your time comes it comes. It seemed the odds were big enough, there was more fun that way. I just didn't think about the other people on the plane. I don't think it's hit me yet. I guess I thought I could keep it all inside of me and forget about it. I finally decided I couldn't live with it myself."

A review of his life history showed that he knew little about his father who left his mother when he was eighteen months of age. His mother who had a daughter by a previous marriage then went to live with her mother and returned to work. There was a childhood history of bedwetting, stealing and firesetting. When Graham was six his grandmother died and he was placed in an orphanage. His school records noted that he felt his mother did not love him because she had put him in an institution.

When he was nine his mother married a wealthy rancher but she refused his repeated pleas to live at home. Several times he ran away from the school to his stepfather's ranch but each time he was returned to the orphanage. Two years later the institution insisted that his mother take him. While living on his stepfather's ranch he knocked his mother down some steps in an argument and he nearly beat a cow to death with a club after it had kicked him.

At sixteen with the help of his mother he claimed that he was eighteen and enlisted in the Coast Guard. Within six months he went absent without leave and he was discharged. He was described in Coast Guard records as an exceedingly immature, dependent person with strong ties to his mother. Poor judgment and impulsive behavior were seen in his sleeping on watch, stealing food and returning to work drunk. Unstable antisocial behavior continued on his return to civilian life. He had difficulty holding jobs as a truck driver and construction worker.

He forged over forty checks for $4,500 and was placed on probation for five years. In Texas after crashing through a road block at high speed he was arrested and sentenced to sixty days in prison for bootlegging and for carrying a concealed weapon. He told me that he set fire to a garage causing $100,000 damage because he had been refused a discount on car repairs. He told FBI agents that an explosion one night in his drive-in restaurant occurred after he disconnected a gas pipe from an oven. The escaping gas was ignited by a pilot light on a water heater.

During the psychiatric evaluation he was friendly and courteous. He admitted a brief attempt to fake insanity by claiming that people were trying to poison him. The diagnosis was sociopathic personality (Chapter 10). The insanity plea was withdrawn, and he was convicted of murder. He opposed any appeal of the death penalty and he was executed in the gas chamber of the Colorado State Penitentiary.

SERIAL MURDERERS

The serial murderer just keeps on killing year after year. Some victims are selected because their absence is likely to pass unnoticed, or if noticed there are no close relatives likely to raise a hue and cry. Haarman sought out children who had run away from home. Juan Corona killed twenty-five vagrants and migratory workers. Landru picked middle-aged spinsters and lonely childless widows. His downfall came through a carelessly selected victim, a girl who had a sister and friends with initiative (5). Petiot killed Jews who took steps to conceal their identity as they were fleeing from the Gestapo. Mafia hit men who kill other members of organized crime groups know that relatives will not rush to the police to make accusations of murder.

The occasional disappearance of a prostitute attracts little attention. The serial murderer knows that when a young single girl fails to come home for dinner or does not appear at her job as a bank teller, there will be a police investigation. However he reduces the risk of detection by concealing the body or by selecting a complete stranger as his victim. Whenever a body is found suspicion falls on the spouse, lover, friend, enemy or business partner but there may be no link between the victim and the serial murderer. Perhaps a woman was seen getting in a stranger's car but the witness did not notice the license plate and cannot even describe the stranger in any useful detail.

The multiple murderer is frequently reticent regarding the number of his victims and he may confess only to those crimes which have already been detected by the police. On the other hand he may exaggerate his total score in the hope of facilitating acceptance of a plea of not guilty by reason of insanity. Thus it is difficult to obtain reliable figures of the number of victims of multiple murderers. Brief accounts are given below of a number of notorious murderers, most of whom killed thirty or more people.

Gilles de Rais, 1404-1440

Pride of place in the ranks of multiple murderers must be accorded to Gilles de Rais, nobleman, Marshal of France, personal bodyguard of Joan of Arc, exhibitionist and homosexual sadist. He is alleged to have tortured and killed over 800 boys, although Montague Summers states that 200 were killed, of whom 120 were identified. Even the smaller figure far outstrips the more modest accomplishments of most serial murderers. Like many of his less accomplished colleagues he combined murder with the outward forms of religious observance. Thus, he was careful to order Masses for the children he had murdered. It had been asserted that he offered to the devil the blood of little children in hope that he could call up the prince of darkness.

At his trial he stated, "I do not know why but I, myself, out of my own head without the advice of anyone, conceived the idea of acting thus, solely for the pleasure and delectation of lust; in fact I found incomparable pleasure in it, doubtless at the instigation of the devil. This diabolical idea came to me eight years ago. I found a latin book on the lives and customs of the Roman Caesars by the learned historian called Suetonius; the said book was ornamented by pictures, very well painted, in which were seen the manners of these pagan emperors, and I read in this fine history how Tiberius, Caracalla, and other Caesars sported with children and took singular pleasure in martyring them. Upon which I desired to imitate the said Caesars and the same evening I began to do so following the pictures in the book . . . for a time I confided my case to no one; but later I took the mystery to several persons, whom I trained for this sport. The said individuals aided in the mystery and took charge of finding children for my needs. The children killed at Chantoce were thrown into a vat at the foot of a tower, from which I had them taken out . . . they were burned in my room except for a few handsome heads I kept as relics. Now I cannot say exactly how many were thus burned and killed but they were certainly to the number of six score per year."

Evidently the tendency to blame illustrated books for murderous behavior was as fashionable in the 15th century as it is today. At the age of thirty-six, Gilles de Rais was first hanged and then burned for his crimes. It is of interest that this wealthy seigneur squandered his fortune on the production of theatrical performances for which people were paid to attend and fined for nonattendance. Gilles spared the boys with the best singing voices and kept them for his choir.

William Burke, 1792-1829

> *"Up the close and down the stair,*
> *But and ben with Burke and Hare,*
> *Burke's the butcher, Hare's the thief,*
> *Knox the boy that buys the beef."*

> Old Song

In the 18th and early 19th century the demand for dead bodies for dissection purposes in medical schools far exceeded the legitimate sources of supply. In order to meet the needs of anatomists, "resurrectionists" used to rob recent graves. Not a few body snatchers found it more convenient to murder than to desecrate graveyards. The infamous Irishmen Burke and Hare, who sold bodies to the Edinburgh anatomist Dr. Robert Knox, are reputed to have killed thirty-two persons. A small number compared with their colleague in London, John Bishop who had killed some sixty persons before his career was cut short on the gallows.

Burke and Hare's first sale involved the body of a lodger in their apartment who had died from natural causes. He was in arrears in his rent and no doubt the body snatchers felt justified in turning their loss into a profit. Encouraged, presumably by the ease of the transaction they expedited the departure from this world of another lodger who was also in arrears in rent. Prospective victims were lured into their lodgings, plied with alcohol, suffocated so that the body showed no evidence of violence, concealed in a tea chest and delivered to Dr. Knox in Surgeon's Square. When taken into custody Hare informed on his partner and was pardoned. Burke was executed.

Henri Désiré Landru, 1869-1922

"Landru . . . a ruthless and efficient killer,
but urbane and witty, always the intellectual
master of the situation, a man with certain
qualities of greatness."

Grierson Dickson, *Murder by Numbers*

The "Bluebeard" Henri Landru upon promise of marriage obtained the possessions of a number of women whom he later murdered. In Paris newspaper advertisements, Landru described himself as a widower, age forty-six with a comfortable income, affectionate and serious who would like to meet a lady of the same age with a view to matrimony. The lady need not be well off, but she should be willing to go abroad with him. The 283 replies which he received were classified in his notebook as follows:

1. To be answered **poste restante**.
2. Without money.
3. Without furniture.
4. No reply.
5. To be answered to initials **poste restante**.

6. Possible fortune.
7. In reserve. For further investigation.

"Landru was the ardent lover, and would write pages to grizzled old washerwomen in the fifties, who had inherited a few thousand francs, about their lily-white hands, their soft eyes and their gentle hearts. Landru would capture the affection of women such as these, promise marriage and bind them to him. Then he would suggest that they should allow him to sell their old furniture, for it would no longer be wanted when they were married. He was careful, wherever possible, to secure a legal transfer from them. By assuring them that he could obtain four times the interest that they were receiving from the bank, he induced them to hand their deposits to his care" (8).

The exact number of victims is not known, but from entries in his notebook the police were able to charge him with the murder of ten women and the son of one of these women. The vital notebook, which sealed his doom on the guillotine, included names of his victims, the dates of their deaths, the cost of their entertainment and the value of their cash and possessions. This frugal Frenchman was careful not to waste money and sinister entries in his notebook record the purchase of railway tickets to his country home — one single 3.95 frs; one return 4.95 frs.

Tiny fragments of human bone and teeth were found in ashes from his kitchen stove but they could not be identified as belonging to any of the women who had vanished. There was not a single witness who could testify as to how or when the murders were committed. Indeed in the opinion of Commissioner Jean Belin of the Sûreté, Landru would never have been convicted if he had succeeded in his attempt to throw away his notebook while being driven to police headquarters for questioning.

The skeletons of three little dogs were found near his home and Landru admitted strangling them with wire because, as he said, it was the easiest and pleasantest way of dying. Belin suggested that Landru strangled his victims with thin wire nooses after first doping them in order to prevent resistance. There was a book in his home dealing with poisoners and poisoning. When this was mentioned in court Landru blandly remarked to the judge that surely "reading is not a criminal offense."

The police were able to trace about 100 of the women listed in his notebook and most of them had been his mistresses or casual lovers within a period of just over four years. He told one woman that he was a police inspector. The defense attorneys suggested that Landru had shipped the missing women to brothels in South America. A suggestion which brought forth the devastating prosecution comment, "What? Women of over fifty? Women whose false hair, false teeth, false bosoms, as well as identity papers, you, Landru, have kept and we captured?" (2)

Scant details are available of the early life of this self-assured bearded, bald, round shouldered man of unimpressive appearance. In his childhood he was a choirboy. His known criminal record begins at the age of thirty-one when he was sentenced to two years imprisonment for fraud. Further sentences totalling nine years followed, and in 1914 he was sentenced in his absence to four years imprisonment. His career of murder started that year. Two years previously his father committed suicide.

At his trial he showed his wit and quick humor to the enjoyment of the court if not to his own advantage. Dickson has recorded responses he was supposed to have made to an attentive audience. When he entered the dock and saw the stacks of stained sideboards and seedy settees of his victims, he said: "Ah, we will now have an auction sale. Monsieur le President (the Judge) will perhaps act as auctioneer."

Asked to comment on his intimate relations with so many women, he made a considerable understatement: "The ladies whom you call my fiancées knew what they were doing, seeing that they were all"—he paused—"of age."

Asked about individual women he would reply, "I am a gallant man and will say nothing," or, "I could not think of revealing the nature of my relations with MMe Gullin without the lady's permission," which was a pretty safe offer.

Asked about certain entries in the **carnet noir,** he said, "Perhaps the police would have preferred to find on page one an entry in these words, 'I, the undersigned, confess that I have murdered the women whose names are set out herein.' "

Asked to comment on several disappearances, he said, "And are there no others who have also disappeared without anyone being accused of their death?"

Reminded of neighbors' complaints about the villa at Vernouillet, he said, "Is every smoking chimney and every bad smell proof that a body is being burned?"

Maitre Moro-Giafferi, who defended him, startled even his own client with the fantastic suggestion that Landru was not really a murderer but merely a white slaver, and had shipped all his elderly wrinkled widows off to South American brothels. The judge asked sarcastically,

"But what about the boy Cuchet? Is he there too?" To which Landru said, unanswerably, "He joined the Belgian Army at the outbreak of war. For all I know he may be the 'Unknown Soldier.' "

When he entered the roomy dock for the last time, to hear the jury's verdict, Landru gazed round at the many sweating and dishevelled women spectators who had been packed tightly for hours. He bowed and said, "I wonder if there is any lady present who would care to take my seat" (4).

Fritz Haarmann, 1879-1925

The precise number of victims of Fritz Haarmann, the ogre of Hanover, is not known; he himself stated, "It might have been thirty, it might have been forty, I don't remember." The court which sentenced him to death found him guilty of twenty-four murders. In any event one may question the decorum, but certainly not the truth of the inscription which he requested for his tombstone, "Here lies mass murderer Haarmann."

The family background is remarkable. His father was an ill tempered mean locomotive stoker; his mother, seven years older than his father, became bedridden following his birth. Three sisters were prostitutes, a brother was convicted of a sex offense and another brother was the only sibling with a respectable reputation. Fritz as a child used to dress in his sisters' clothing and took pleasure in household tasks. At seventeen he was sent to a mental hospital after he had been accused of offenses against children. At this time he was considered to be feebleminded and not responsible for his criminal acts. It has been suggested that Haarmann's hatred for his father, with whom he had frequent fist fights, was displaced onto his victims.

Escape from the mental hospital was followed by a period of service in the Army and frequent periods of incarceration in prison for theft, burglary, larceny and sexual offenses. Following World War I he became an active operator on the blackmarket. By killing children and young men he was able to combine sexual perversion with financial profit from sale of their clothes and (it is believed) their flesh in the form of blackmarket sausages. Haarmann, a police informer, used to pose as a detective and would either entice or use his authority as a "detective" to persuade his victims to come to his apartment. A younger homosexual partner, Hans Grans participated in some of the murders.

At his trial he denied having committed three of the twenty-seven murders with which he was charged. When accused in court by the father of one missing boy he said, "I have my tastes after all. Such an ugly creature as, according to his photographs, your son must have been, I would never have taken to. You say that your boy had not even a shirt to his name, and his socks were tied on to his feet with string. **Pfui Deibel.** You ought to have been ashamed to have let him go about like that. Poor stuff like him there's plenty. Just think what you are saying. Such a youngster was much beneath my notice" (2).

According to Dickson, his last request was that he might be allowed to "pass one merry evening in the condemned cell — an environment hardly lending itself to gaiety — and to have coffee, hard cheese and a cigar with his last meal. After which he said he would curse his father and regard his execution as his wedding, a remark not without psychological significance. He also requested that on his birthdays his fellow murderer, Hans Grans, should lay a wreath on his grave."

Marcel Petiot, 1897-1946

The French physician, Marcel Petiot claimed to have killed sixty-three persons, thirty-three collaborators and thirty German soldiers, for the Resistance movement during the German occupation of France in World War II. He was unable to prove that he was a "Resistance executioner" and was decapitated after he had been convicted of twenty-four of the twenty-seven murders with which he had been formally charged.

Petiot might well have escaped detection if his neighbors had not called the fire brigade because of a thick cloud of foul smelling smoke coming from his house. The fireman discovered a burning body in the furnace as well as several more awaiting cremation. Petiot blandly explained to police officers at the scene that the bodies were those of collaborators executed by the Resistance movement and promptly disappeared. He was later apprehended after he had written to a newspaper, under an assumed name, denying his guilt.

Posing as a member of a Resistance escape group, he undertook to help others, mainly Jews fleeing from the Gestapo, to escape from France. Prospective victims were told to bring all their cash and valuables. The need for secrecy was emphasized and they were cautioned not to reveal the plan to anyone. It is believed that he injected poison into his victims in a small soundproof room off his consulting room, and that he observed the death struggles by means of a peep-hole between the two rooms.

A married couple became suspicious when told by Petiot that they would need vaccinations so that they could enter Argentina after their escape from France. They did not proceed with their plans to escape and the husband later testified in court that Petiot had told him, "These injections will render you invisible to the eyes of the world." Petiot on hearing his testimony told the court, "I see it all now. The mad doctor with his syringe. It was a dark and rainy night. The wind howled under the eaves and rattled the windowpanes of the oak-panelled library—". At this point he was interrupted by the judge, "Petiot, please!" (9)

As a child Petiot tortured animals. Like many serial murderers, Petiot had committed other forms of crime; theft as a schoolboy, sale of narcotics as an army medical orderly and theft as a physician. A pregnant servant girl in his bachelor household disappeared without trace. In 1930, three years after his marriage, it was rumored that he was responsible for the murder of an elderly wealthy patient. One of his chief accusers was unwise enough to seek medical treatment for rheumatism from Dr. Petiot. Shortly after taking the drugs prescribed for him he died. Dr. Petiot conveniently performed the autopsy and found that he had died from natural causes. Shortly afterwards he was found guilty of pension fraud, for this he was removed from office as mayor of a small town and sentenced to three month's imprisonment. In 1936, he was found guilty of theft of a book from a book shop and it was recommended that he should seek psychiatric treatment.

When Petiot went to the guillotine Dr. Paul, the coroner who had witnessed hundreds of executions, said that he had never before seen a man show such perfect calm. "Most people about to be executed do their best to be courageous, but one senses that it is a stiff and forced courage. Petiot moved with ease, as though he were walking into his office for a routine appointment" (9).

John Wayne Gacy

"I'm bisexual, not homosexual."

John W. Gacy

In 1980 John Wayne Gacy, a thirty-seven year old building contractor, was convicted of murdering thirty-three young men and boys in his home at Des Plaines on the outskirts of Chicago. The last four victims were thrown over a bridge on an interstate highway into the Des Plaines River. By this time the crawlspace beneath his home with its musty smell was overcrowded with twenty-eight bodies covered by earth and lime. Another body wrapped in plastic sheets was under the garage floor.

Gacy came under suspicion, not for the first time, after a fifteen year old high school student failed to return home on the evening of December 11, 1978. He had last been seen talking to Gacy about a job. When the police checked to see whether Gacy had a criminal record they discovered that he had been convicted in Waterloo, Iowa in 1968 on a charge of sodomy and sentenced to ten years in the Iowa Men's Reformatory.

At the time of his arrest in Iowa Gacy age twenty-five, was working for his father-in-law as manager of Kentucky Fried Chicken outlets. He was active in the Jaycees and sought election as president, he was also a police buff and had a portable flashing red light on his car. At night he invited youths to his home for alcohol and homosexual activities. His favorite practice was to have a youth perform oral sex on him. He was arrested after he attempted to handcuff and force one youth at knifepoint to perform sexual acts. Gacy hired another youth to beat up and possibly kill this victim.

A presentence psychiatric evaluation showed that Gacy was an antisocial personality of bright normal intelligence (IQ 118). His wife divorced him while he was in the reformatory where he was active in the Jaycees, obtaining a "Sound Citizen Award." In 1970 a consultant psychiatrist diagnosed him as a passive-aggressive personality and recommended his release stating, "The likelihood of his again being charged with and being convicted of antisocial conduct appears to be small" (12).

On his release from the reformatory in June 1970, after serving twenty-one months of his ten year sentence, Gacy went to live with his mother in Chicago. In May 1971 he married for the second time but he had many young male visitors and in 1976 the marriage ended in divorce. His wife used to complain about the odor not only in the crawlspace but also in the bathroom and hallway. She thought there must be dead mice in the crawlspace. Her husband responded by spreading lime.

Gacy claimed that he did not force any of his victims to come to his home where all of the murders occurred between 3 AM and 6 AM. The first victim was stabbed to death and the others were strangled with a rope which was tightened with a stick. A couple of times he had to tighten the knot more than once because the victims showed signs of reviving. On two of three occasions he had "doubles"—nights when he killed two persons as in the following example described by Sullivan.

"Gacy told of bringing two youths home one night. He told one of them he would tighten the rope around the boy's neck three times, so he would get an erection, then Gacy would blow him. Gacy twisted the rope until the youth died. He went into the other room and told the other boy his friend was dead. The boy didn't believe him. Gacy led him, handcuffed, to the other room and strangled him in front of the body of his friend" (12).

He handcuffed, sexually assaulted and threatened to kill many young men. Before releasing the lucky victims he warned them that if they went to the police he would hunt them down. He added that it was pointless going to the police as the police would not believe them. Many of these young men were homosexual prostitutes and some of them believed Gacy's claim that he was a police officer. He had a police badge and his car was equipped with a red spotlight as well as a CB radio.

At least five victims complained to the police. As early as 1972 a youth reported that he had resisted Gacy's attempt to assault him sexually and succeeded in escaping. Gacy was arrested but the charges against him were dismissed after the youth was caught attempting to extort money from Gacy in return for dropping the charges. A youth who had been kidnapped at gunpoint in 1977 while waiting for a bus told police that Gacy anally assaulted him with a dildo, threatened to kill him, choked him, held him under water until he passed out and urinated on him. Gacy was arrested but he denied using either force or a firearm and claimed that the incident was a sex-slave act by mutual consent. The felony charges against Gacy were rejected by an assistant state's attorney.

When talking to police Gacy would brag about his political connections. He showed Des Plaines' police officers his picture taken with President Carter's wife, who signed the photograph, "To John Gacy, Best Wishes, Rosalynn Carter." Despite his extensive homosexual activity Gacy claimed that he was bisexual and not homosexual. He expressed hatred for homosexuals, especially homosexual prostitutes. He described a drag queen who danced for him as real weird, adding that God didn't put people on earth to do that. While strangling this victim, Gacy read the Twenty-Third Psalm to him (12). At trial Gacy was found legally sane and was sentenced to death.

Dennis Nilsen

An English homosexual murderer, Dennis Nilsen, had the same disposal problems as Gacy: overcrowding of bodies under the floorboards of his apartment and the stench of decaying flesh. Deodorant sticks were not much help so he placed one body in a huge bonfire in his garden and also burned some rubber to cover the smell of burning flesh. The neighborhood children gathered to watch the blaze. Later he used a pot to boil flesh from the skulls of his victims. He cut their flesh into small pieces which he flushed down the toilet.

One victim, a skinhead, had many tattoos, including a line around his neck with the inscription "Cut here." Nilsen did just that when dismembering him (16). Cutting up the bodies was a tiresome chore. Nilsen said, "The victim is the dirty platter after the feast and the washing-up is a clinically ordinary task . . . the flesh looked like just any meat one would see in a butcher's shop and having been trained in a butchery I was not subject to any traumatic shocks" (10).

It is not wise to flush victims down the toilet because it does clog the sewers. Other tenants complained that their toilets would not flush. The plumber, who knew his smells, on checking the sewer alongside the house commented "I know that isn't shit." He used a flashlight to show Nilsen and another tenant what he thought was flesh in the sewer. That night Nilsen was busy removing pieces of flesh from the sewer, but he was seen returning from the garden, and the next day the police talked to him in his apartment, about the problem of human remains in the drains.

Doubtless the strange smell in the apartment prompted the question "Where's the rest of the body?" But there was not just one body, there were parts of two bodies in two plastic bags in his wardrobe. Indeed Nilsen readily confessed that there had been fifteen or sixteen bodies. It is difficult to keep track of the exact number after the first few murders. All the murders occurred while he was under the influence of alcohol. All the victims were young men, strangers that he met in taverns, all with one exception had no permanent address, and all had been strangled between 1978 and 1983. Some were homosexual and a few were male prostitutes. Only two of his victims had been reported missing.

He would undress, wash and dry the bodies of his victims, and he either masturbated or had sex between the thighs of six of the victims. In addition to the fifteen murders there were seven attempts at murder, but these were usually not reported to the police. One victim who went to a hospital with a deep red mark around his neck and across his throat, as well as bloodshot eyes was told that his injuries were consistent with strangulation. He told the doctors he was mugged by a stranger. In one police investigation Nilsen denied any attempt at strangulation. In another police investigation the officers thought there had been a homosexual encounter and that neither person was a reliable informant. Many men who went to his apartment were not assaulted.

Nilsen was thirty-seven at the time of his arrest. He had worked as a butcher in the Army, then he became a police officer but resigned after one year to become a government employee at a job center. He never saw his father who deserted his mother and their three children. As a child he was quiet and withdrawn. His mother recalled that something prevented her from cuddling him. He was a loner but needed company and would sometimes take a corpse from beneath the floorboards and prop it up to watch TV with him. He used to put talc on his face and body to look like a corpse and gaze at his body in a mirror. After he started killing he had real corpses to join him in his mirror watching.

Lucas and Toole

Henry Lee Lucas claimed to have killed about 360 persons between 1975 and his arrest for murder in Texas in 1983, at the age of forty-six. A shabbily dressed roofer who obtained his clothes from rescue missions, Lucas roamed across the country in older model cars and pickups, robbing, raping and killing. His illiterate, homosexual lover, Ottis Elwood Toole, also a roofer and drifter, made the more modest claim of 125 murders. Both men have exaggerated the extent of their murderous activity.

In some cases there is evidence that Lucas was a thousand miles away the day before or the day after a murder that he confessed committing. He travelled long distances in a short time. Furthermore his work records may be misleading as supervisors would falsely list him as working in return for part of his paycheck. In at least one murder in Colorado law enforcement officers are confident that he made a false confession. Lucas now states that he has killed only three persons: his mother in 1960, Becky Powell, a girl with whom he travelled in 1982 and Kate Rich, an elderly woman with whom he stayed in 1982.

Lucas said that he made false confessions to investigators from thirty-five states to avoid transfer from a county jail to death row at Huntsville State Penitentiary and to make fools of law enforcement officers who were eager to clear unsolved murders off their books. On the other hand Lucas is reported to have taken investigators to grave sites that were as much as seven years old. Lucas admitted killing many women who were hitchhiking or who had car trouble. Some victims were kidnapped from convenience store parking lots. Robberies and residential burglaries were followed by homicides. Victims were stabbed, shot, strangled or beaten to death.

He would have sexual relations with the bodies of dead female victims. Some bodies were mutilated and burned. He is reported to have said "I was death on women. I didn't feel they needed to exist. I hated them. I killed them, I was doing a good job too."

Both his parents were alcoholics and both beat him. His father, who lost his legs in an accident, died when Henry was fourteen. His mother was domineering and according to news reports was a prostitute. Once she beat Henry after she caught him watching her have sexual relations with a lover. His mother, her boyfriend, his sisters, brothers and himself all slept in the same room of their two room house. Sometimes she dressed him in girl's clothing. It was reported that he was cruel to animals. As a youth he was accidentally blinded in his left eye by his brother.

As a teenager he stole radios from cars. At nineteen he was sentenced to the state prison in Virginia for burglaries. He escaped from a road gang but was captured and returned to prison. At the age of twenty-three he stabbed his mother to death following an argument.

"I don't know why I committed this crime. My mother and I got into a fight and it just turned out that way. We'd been to a bar together and both of us had a few bottles of beer. We argued about going back to Virginia. I felt I could do better in Michigan. She called me every dirty name she knew. She said I'd had sex with my sister and that really made me mad. It finally made me so mad I hit her. She started to fall down. When I went to pick her up I realized she was dead. Then I noticed I had my knife in my hand and she had been cut. I got scared and drove to Virginia. It was a terrible thing to do and I know I have lost the respect of my family, but it was just one of those things and I think it had to happen."

He was arrested, convicted of murder, and given a sentence of twenty to forty years. Altogether he served ten years in a prison and in a mental hospital. A year after his release he was sent to prison for five years for the attempted kidnapping of a fifteen year old girl. When asked why he threatened the girl he told the judge, "Just the urge I get sometimes to scare people." In 1975 he married at the age of thirty-six but in 1976 his wife sued for divorce, claiming that Henry had molested her two daughters.

Ottis Elwood Toole, eleven years younger than Lucas, had an alcoholic father and a mother who suffered from mental illness. He was very attached to his mother and after her death in 1981 he would often go to her grave and lie on top of it. As a child he set fires and often ran away from home. He liked to dress in girl's clothing. Although he attended special education classes for seven years he is illiterate. Despite two marriages he has been a homosexual all his life. There have been many arrests for window peeping, indecent exposure, obscene telephone calls, auto theft, larceny and arson. He is a pyromaniac, obtains sexual excitement from watching fires and masturbates at the scene. One man died in a fire set by Toole, who is now on death row at the Florida State Penitentiary.

Lucas and Toole travelled long distances across several states after a murder. For the most part there was no link between them and their victims as they seized strangers on an impulse to rob, sexually assault and kill. Victims were white, black, hispanic, rich and poor, young, middle-aged and elderly. Many were hitchhikers or drifters like themselves. They changed their vehicles, weapons and methods of killing frequently so that their crimes lacked a common thread. There were similarities: a pattern of stab wounds in the upper back, nude bodies with the socks left on and the bodies were often not concealed but were left in a remote area. It is not surprising that they were able for a long time to get away with murder.

THE TYPICAL MULTICIDE

Dickson has coined the term multicide to describe the series-killer, who plans and carries out murder after murder over a considerable period. Based upon his study of more than forty multicides, he has attempted to visualize a fairly typical multicide during his killing period, as he might appear to a casual business or social contact.

"He is probably a small, dapper, well-dressed man in his forties. He is a fairly sociable type, speaking quietly and correctly, perhaps with a trace of self-satisfaction at his own achievements, but with an undeniable charm of manner. He is abstemious, probably a teetotaller and non-smoker, he does not swear and the vicar of his parish probably believes him to be a good Christian.

"If in casual conversation he mentions some modest scholastic successes he may be a killer for profit; but if his school days appear to be a painful memory he is more likely to be a sexual pervert. In either case he is unlikely to say much about his war service, which was probably rather noticeably unheroic. He is still less likely to talk about civil experiences during his twenties, because he almost certainly spent a few spells in prison before he was thirty. His conversation will accordingly be more concerned with the present than with the past, and he may introduce anecdotes illustrating the business acumen which he rather erroneously believes himself to possess.

"On the subject of his domestic affairs he will be reticent; if he has a wife he probably parted from her years ago; but in the background he may have a woman friend who offers him not sex but sanctuary — someone to whom he can go when he does not like to be alone with his thoughts. He is very unlikely to have much sense of humor. He is probably rather mean in small financial transactions. It must be reluctantly agreed that the multicide is a type we are apt to meet in shop or office . . . such a horrifying ordinary little man that in his lack of outstanding qualities lies the secret of his success (4).

The FBI profiles of organized and disorganized serial murderers are reviewed in Chapter 13.

REFERENCES

1. Belin, Jean: *My Work at the Sûreté*. London, George G. Harrap, 1950.
2. Bolitho, William: *Murder for Profit*. London, Dennis Dobson Ltd., 1953.
3. Bruch, Hilda: Mass murder, the Wagner case. *Amer J Psychiat, 124*:693, 1967.
4. Dickson, Grierson: *Murder by Numbers*. London, Robert Hale, 1958.
5. Douthwaite, L.C.: *Mass Murder*. New York, Henry Holt, 1929.
6. Galvin, J.A.V. and Macdonald, J.M.: Psychiatric study of a mass murderer. *Amer J Psychiat, 115*:1057, 1959.
7. Levin, Jack and Fox, J.A.: *Mass Murder: America's Growing Menace*. New York, Plenum Press, 1985.
8. Mackenzie, F.A.: *Landru*. New York, Scribners, 1928.
9. Maeder, Thomas: *The Unspeakable Crimes of Dr. Petiot*. Boston, Atlantic Monthly Press Book, 1980.
10. Masters, Brian: *Killing for Company: The Case of Dennis Nilsen*. London, Jonathan Cape, 1985.
11. Schubeler, F.C.: Berserks, cited by Fabing, H.D., On going beserk, a neuro-chemical inquiry. *Amer J Psychiat, 113*:409, 1956.
12. Sullivan, Terry with Maiken, P.T.: *Killer Clown*. New York, Grosset and Dunlap, 1983.
13. Summers, Montague: *The History of Witchcraft and Demonology*. Secaucas, New Jersey, Citadel Press, 1974.

14. Teoh, J.I.: The changing psychopathology of amok. *Psychiatry, 35*:345, 1972.
15. Westermeyer, Joseph: Amok. In Friedmann, C.T. and Faguet, R.A. (Eds.): *Extraordinary Disorders of Human Behavior.* New York, Plenum Press, 1982.
16. Wilson, Colin and Seaman, Donald: *The Encyclopedia of Modern Murder, 1962-1982.* New York, G.P. Putnam's Sons, 1983.

CHAPTER 8

SEX MURDERS

"And therefore, since I cannot prove a lover, . . .
I am determined to prove a villain."

Shakespeare, *King Richard III*

A SEXUAL FACTOR is clearly apparent in many murders — for example the husband who kills his unfaithful wife or her lover, the rapist who kills to subdue his victim or to escape detection and the sadist who murders prostitutes. Even though the circumstances of a murder may not suggest a sexual motive, deeper study will sometimes reveal that sexual conflict underlies the act of aggression. Certainly a sexual element is present in all sadistic murders.

SADISM

The term sadism is derived from the name of a French nobleman, the Marquis de Sade, infamous for his crimes and the character of his writings. Fourteen years of his life were spent in prison, but his crimes were not as terrible as those described in his stories of sexuality, cruelty and torture. Sadism is more than mere delight in cruelty. Sadism is a sexual perversion in which sexual gratification is obtained from the infliction of pain and degradation on other persons and animals. The development of sadistic impulses has been related to childhood experiences of brutality in relation to sex.

The sadist may ejaculate on bludgeoning, stabbing or strangling his victim. There need not be any sexual contact. The murderer Vincenz Verzeni experienced sexual sensations as soon as he grasped his victims by the neck. It did not matter whether the women were old, young, ugly or beautiful. Usually simply choking them satisfied him and he then allowed his victims to live. When sexual satisfaction was delayed he continued to choke his victims until they died. Verzeni reported that his feeling of pleasure while strangling women was much greater than that which he experienced while masturbating (6).

When there is a sexual assault the sadist may find it necessary to degrade, injure or torture his victim in order to maintain his erection. Retarded ejaculation may prevent completion of the sexual act so that no sperm are found in the victim. The serial murderer Gacy urinated on some of his victims. Some wives of sadists tolerate binding, biting and choking but draw the line at beating, cutting and stabbing. In these circumstances the sadistic husband resorts to fantasies of mutilation and torture to avoid impotence.

The sadistic murderer who does not attempt sexual assault may masturbate over his victim or into the victim's underwear. He may force a stick or some other cylindrical object up the vagina or rectum of the victim. Mutilation may occur before and after death. Often there are repeated stab wounds of the chest, or massive skull fractures from the use of a rock or hammer. Breasts, genitals and intestines are removed. Some sadists drink the blood and eat portions of the victim's flesh.

The murderer Andreas Bichel said of one of his victims, "I opened her breast and with a knife cut through the fleshy parts of the body. Then I arranged the body as a butcher does beef, and hacked it with an axe into pieces of a size to fit the hole which I had dug up in the mountain for burying it. I may say that while opening the body I was so greedy that I trembled, and could have cut out a piece and eaten it" (6). Sadists will torture and disect animals as well as human beings. Cats and dogs disappear from the neighborhood.

Myra Hindley

It is not only men who gain sexual pleasure from inflicting pain on others and acts of cannibalism. A married man with numerous scars from cuts on his arms explained that before sex his wife would make him cut his arm. During intercourse she would become sexually excited by sucking blood from his wound. The female sadist may enlist a lover to help her kidnap victims for torture and murder. Myra Hindley is an example of the female sadistic murderer. In 1966 at the age of twenty-three Myra and Ian Brady, her twenty-seven year old boyfriend were tried in

England for three sadistic murders. There was evidence of abnormal sexual activity involving all three victims shortly before they died (5).

During the investigation of the axe murder of a seventeen year old homosexual youth by Brady in Hindley's presence the police were told Brady had claimed that he had killed three or four persons and the bodies were buried on the Pennine Moors. The police found a twelve year old girl who had visited the moors with Brady and Hindley. She showed the police the area where she had been taken and a search revealed the grave of ten year old Lesley Ann Downey who had been missing since Christmas 1964.

Four days later the police found in the spine of Myra's white prayer book, a souvenir of her first communion, and left luggage tickets for two suitcases stored at Manchester Central Railroad Station. In these suitcases were books on sadism and sexual perversion as well as photographs of Lesley Ann Downey showing her naked in obscene pornographic poses. There was also a frightening tape recording of this child screaming and pleading with Hindley and Brady not to undress her and to allow her to return home. There were repeated instructions by Hindley and Brady for the child to put something, possibly a gag, in her mouth. An additional indication of the sexual aspect of the attack on the child was that both adults had removed their clothing.

Other photographs showed Hindley and Brady posing on the moors. The police enlisted the aid of farmers, shepherds and members of rambling and rock climbing clubs to identify the scenes, and within days each photograph had a twin photograph taken by the police (5). At the site of a photograph showing Myra Hindley holding a puppy police discovered the grave of John Kilbride, a twelve year old boy who had disappeared in November 1963. The body was fully clothed, but the trousers and underpants were rolled down to the thighs indicating sexual interference (5). Pathologists were unable to tell from the decomposed bodies how the children died but they were probably strangled to death.

At first the police thought that Brady was the dominant partner but their opinion changed during their interrogations. They were able to get Brady to reveal incriminating information but Myra Hindley remained silent. As one detective commented "She said nothing. No remorse. No compassion. No human feeling. Nothing." The only time she showed any reaction was when the Downey tape was played to her. She said she was ashamed. At the trial she gave her evidence in a flat, emotionless manner, declining her counsel's suggestion that a few tears would not go amiss (8). Although she gave nothing away under cross-examination she was found guilty of two murders and of being an accessory to a third murder. Brady was found guilty of three murders. Both were given life sentences.

Peter Kurten, 1883-1931

The monster of Dusseldorf, as Peter Kurten was described, is a prime example of the male sadistic murderer. He gained sexual excitement from killing men, women, children and animals. At the age of thirteen Kurten first became aware of the connection between cruelty and sex when he became sexually aroused while stabbing sheep. At fourteen he ejaculated while strangling a squirrel. He also ejaculated watching big fires and he had an orgasm looking at blood gush from a man run over by a streetcar.

His wife complained about his lack of interest in sex and she usually took the initiative. She had to help him get an erection and he could not maintain it unless he had fantasies of violence. With other women he was unable to perform sexually without ill-treating the woman or resorting to cutting, stabbing or striking with a hammer. He ejaculated on sucking the blood of mortally wounded victims. Kurten told Karl Berg, M.D., the Medico-Legal Officer of the Dusseldorf Criminal Court, that if he had the means he would have killed masses. He described his feelings on committing his crimes:

"Sometimes even when I seized my victim's throat, I had an orgasm; sometimes not, but then the orgasm came as I stabbed the victim. It was not my intention to get satisfaction by normal intercourse, but by killing. When the victim struggled she merely stimulated my lust . . . That I wasn't out for normal sexual enjoyment you can tell from the Scheer case. That was a man . . . The man was staggering. He bumped into me. He was drunk. I stabbed him with the scissors. At the first stab in the temple he fell down. Then at once I got sexual excitement, and the more I stabbed the more intense it became. I gave him a severe stab in the neck and I heard distinctly the faint gushing of his blood. That was the climax. Then came the ejaculation. I stopped stabbing and just rolled the body over the bank" (2).

Kurten murdered or attempted to murder over forty persons. At the age of nine he drowned two playmates in the Rhine. His first murder as an adult was committed at the age of thirty in a burglary. Like some other serial murderers he varied his methods of killing—strangling, stabbing and assault with a blunt instrument—to convince the police that several murderers were responsible for his crimes. Some victims were raped. He derived considerable satisfaction from the newspaper publicity given to his crimes and he wrote letters in disguised handwriting to the press and to the police giving them information about his murders. He liked to return to the graves of his victims.

In his childhood, as well as in adult life, he was a firesetter and was cruel to both children and animals. He set fire to haystacks, buildings and a forest. Gasoline was used to burn the body of one victim. There were at least twenty-two fires as well as attempts to burn an orphanage. His sadistic behavior may well have been the result of his childhood experiences of brutality in relation to sex.

He was afraid of his brutal, alcoholic incestuous father and would often hide from him. His father's wages were spent on drinking and the family lived in poverty. "We all lived in one room. You will appreciate what effect that had on me sexually." He observed his parents having sexual relations and commented, "When I look back and think of the married life of my parents today I really think that had they not been married one would have had to think of it as rape" (2). His father was sentenced to eighteen months in prison for incest with his eldest daughter.

In 1931 at the age of forty-eight Peter Kurten was found guilty of nine murders as well as seven attempted murders and was sentenced to death. He wondered about his execution and asked Doctor Berg whether, his head chopped off, he would still hear the gushing of blood. That would be for him, he said, the pleasure of all pleasures.

RAPE AND MURDER

The great majority of rapists do not murder their victims. Force used to subdue the woman may result in death, although this outcome may not have been intended by the assailant. Pressure on the neck, insufficient to cause strangulation, may cause death from reflex causes. The offender, either deliberately or in panic, may kill in order to avoid detection as in the following case.

A twenty-five year old man who was not on speaking terms with his wife, spent Saturday afternoon drinking with a buddy. He had been feeling depressed that day because of a quarrel with his wife. During the evening he returned home to obtain his rifle, but exchanged no words with his wife. After visiting several bars he drove to a lake where he swam for about an hour. After this he shot one or two rabbits that were caught in the lights of his car. He drove around aimlessly and finally drove alongside a dam. On a sudden impulse he shot at the headlights, tires and windows of a car which was parked there. "I guess I was angry, I can't remember now what it was. It wasn't exactly anger, I kind of felt tense." He did not think there was anyone in the car and he was surprised to find two young couples huddled inside.

At gunpoint he robbed the men of their wallets; and as he feared they might attack him while he was turning his car around, he decided to take one of the girls as a hostage. The girl he chose, a slim attractive blonde, on his instructions drove his car farther into the mountains. After about forty-five minutes they were forced to stop because of a flat tire. He then raped her. While he was changing the tire, the girl ran down the road which was illuminated by the headlights.

"I hollered at her to stop. She didn't, I panicked, got scared or something. I fired twice. With a rifle I'm an expert, I aimed right at her head—her blonde hair showed out better than anything else—that's what I shot at. I wanted to stop her, I didn't want her to run away. I went out, she was kind of kicking, one of her legs was moving, I shot her again. I felt her pulse. If I felt it once, I felt it a dozen times. I must have killed her instantly. I knew I had to hide her then. As far as thinking about the law, I wasn't thinking about the law; I never thought about the consequences till it was all over. I've imagined that this is all a bad dream. I knew I done this, but I can't make myself believe I did it."

After burying the body some 800 feet up a steep slope in the mountains, he remained there for three or four hours wondering what he should do. He then drove to Wyoming where he decided to return to his home in Colorado and "get it over." He realized, correctly, that his car would be traced and he was arrested the following day. Within thirty minutes he confessed the crime and later he led the officers to the burial spot as he thought his victim deserved a decent burial.

On psychiatric examination he cooperated readily. He appeared depressed over his situation and he expressed considerable remorse for his crime.

A rather taciturn man he described himself as a person who preferred to get on with the job rather than talk about it. "I never speak my opinion on anything. I just go along with the crowd. I'm not one to judge other people. What other people do is their business. It's hard to get me mad, I seldom argue." Review of his personal history revealed that he was smaller than other children of his age and this always made him "feel out of place." He complained that the older school children used to pick on him. At ten years of age he became very friendly with a blonde girl; they always liked to do things together. It was agreed some years later that they would marry when they were old enough. At the age of seventeen he returned home after a week's absence to learn that his girl friend had married another man. At first he could not believe the news and when he realized it was true he became very angry. "I could have strangled her at the time; I really got mad at her. After she jilted me I didn't have anything to do with blonde girls."

A year later he married a girl who was about the complete opposite of his former girl friend in appearance and character. The marriage was not a success. There were three children of the marriage. As his wife did not want any more children he underwent a sterilization operation. Although he denied any regrets about this operation, the psychological effects of this operation may have been of some importance.

Although he blamed himself for the failure of the marriage, he complained that his wife was moody and sexually cold. There had been no sexual relations for the three months preceeding the tragedy. They seldom argued, but for periods of up to a week at a time they would hardly exchange a word. Following one argument he fired seven or eight shots at his mother-in-law's picture which was hanging on the wall of the living room. Following another argument he drove to the dam where he later abducted the girl, and swallowed the contents of a bottle of his wife's sleeping tablets. He was discovered unconscious and rushed to the hospital.

It is significant that his victim closely resembled his former girl friend. He claimed that the resemblance did not occur to him until after his arrest. It is likely that his crime had unconscious determinants in his anger at his rejecting wife and his deep resentment toward his former childhood sweetheart. It is of interest that twice following arguments with his wife he drove to the same dam: the first time his hostile impulses were turned on himself in the form of a determined attempt at suicide; the second time his anger found expression in shooting up an apparently unoccupied car and later in rape and murder. He was found guilty of murder in the first degree and sentenced to life imprisonment.

Albert DeSalvo, 1931-1973

"Albert was truly a remarkable man . . .
He was completely lovable to every individual
while working for me. Never was there any deviation
from the highest proper sense of things."

— DeSalvo's employer

On June 14, 1962, a fifty-five year old woman was found strangled to death in her Boston apartment. On June 30, two women, one sixty-five years old and the other sixty-eight, were strangled to death in the Boston area. There was no evidence of rape, but all three women had been sexually molested and a bottle had been forced into the vagina of one victim. On August 19, a seventy-five year old woman was strangled, and on the following day a sixty-seven year old woman was also strangled. By this date the older ladies in Boston had good reason to fear the Boston strangler. In December two girls in their twenties were strangled and sexually assaulted.

The slayings continued in 1963 and 1964. One girl was only nineteen. The victims were strangled in their apartments which showed no signs of forcible entry. They were discovered with a nylon stocking or other article of clothing tied around the neck, nude or partially undressed with evidence of rape or sexual molestation. There were variations on this theme. One victim had a broomstick in her vagina. Two victims were stabbed, and one had twenty-two wounds in her throat and left breast. ("She made me feel unclean the way she talked to me.") She had also been strangled. The body of one victim was covered with the bedclothes. ("She treated me like a man.") Some victims had been gagged and tied.

On October 27, 1964, a young woman was attacked in her apartment, gagged, tied to her bed and molested sexually. Her assailant, who was armed with a knife, left after extracting a promise from her that she would not tell anyone. She informed her husband and the police, who arranged for an artist's sketch of the man based on her description. The sketch resembled thirty-two year old Albert DeSalvo, who was known to the Cambridge police as the "measuring man."

Three years earlier, following his arrest as a housebreaker, he admitted that he had been measuring women on the pretext of determining whether they had suitable figures for employment as models. He was given a psychiatric examination in a state hospital and a diagnosis was made of sociopathic personality. In May 1961 he was sentenced to two years imprisonment for assault and battery (which was the charge used in connection with his measuring activities) and for attempted burglary. In his youth he had been a window peeper. In 1955 he had been arrested for molesting a nine year old girl but was released when the girl's mother refused to press charges. Two months later he was arrested for peeping and charged with disorderly conduct; however, the charge was dropped.

DeSalvo was questioned about the strangulation murders but he denied involvement and was committed to the Bridgewater State Hospital for pretrial psychiatric examination. While in the hospital he confessed to his attorney that he had committed thirteen homicides in the Boston area and in nearby Lawrence. The first homicide occurred two months after his release from prison in 1962. Subsequently he made a detailed confession to John Bottomly, Assistant Attorney General of Massachusetts, who had been appointed to coordinate the search for the Boston strangler. He also confessed that he had raped many of his homicide victims and claimed that he had sexually assaulted between eight hundred and one thousand women.

DeSalvo was sentenced to life imprisonment for assault with a dangerous weapon, assault with intent to commit rape and other charges related to his October 27, 1964, attack on the young woman whom he did not kill. He was not charged with the thirteen homicides because his confession was obtained under conditions which precluded use of the confession in evidence against him. In November 1973 he was stabbed to death in his cell, presumably because of his involvement in drug dealing.

Gerald Frank in **The Boston Strangler** has provided a fascinating encyclopedic account of DeSalvo, his crimes and the extensive prolonged police search for the strangler. This search was complicated by false accusations (some Boston women suspected their husbands) as well as by false confessions made by men who had memorized newspaper accounts of the crimes.

Frank notes that despite the climate of fear in Boston during this period, women continued to permit strangers to enter their apartments. DeSalvo would press the buzzers of an apartment house. The woman who opened the door first became his victim. He would say that he had been sent to do some work in her apartment. If she hesitated or refused to let him in, he would say, "If you don't want the work done, forget it" or tell her to call the apartment house manager. These comments served to reassure the suspicious victim. One fifty-eight year old woman, apologizing for her caution, mentioned the danger posed by the Boston strangler. She was the eleventh victim.

DeSalvo, who was diagnosed at Bridgewater State Hospital as having a sociopathic personality disorder marked by sexual deviation with prominent schizoid features and depressive trends, had a rather unusual home background. His father, who used to go around with prostitutes in front of his children, had been arrested five times for assault and battery on his wife. One time he broke her fingers. He had also been arrested for nonsupport, larceny as well as breaking and entering and had served time in jail. The children were frequently beaten by their father, according to Albert, who mentioned that his sisters "always had blacked eyes." Albert was involved in sex play with girls at ten years of age and he was seduced by a married woman at the age of fifteen.

While serving in the Army, he married a German girl. (He was a military policeman and the Army's middle-weight boxing champion of Europe.) He claimed that his wife frequently refused to have sexual relations with him; she in turn mentioned that he wanted to have sexual intercourse from four to six times a day. He complained that she "would put me down in front of others, make me feel like nothing in front of friends and give me an inferiority complex" (4). DeSalvo, like many other serial murderers, did not smoke or drink.

NECROPHILIA

Necrophilia refers to a desire for sexual intercourse with dead bodies. Krafft-Ebing in his **Psychopathia-Sexualis** describes with equanimity many brutal rape murders in which the victims were disembowelled or otherwise treated unkindly. His dispassionate attitude does not extend to necrophilia which he refers to as horrible and monstrous. Yet this is a crime without pain or suffering for the victim. There is the risk that if a suitable cadaver is not readily available the necrophiliac may pick up a knife or garrotte to obtain a fresh corpse for himself.

Some necrophiliacs seek employment as morticians, morgue assistants or grave diggers in order to satisfy their perverse needs. A grave digger who dug up the bodies of young girls said that as living women felt nothing but repulsion for him it was quite natural that he should turn to the dead who never repulsed him. This man who was retarded had no sense of smell, which must surely be an advantage for necrophiliacs.

A man with necrophiliac fantasies extolled the virtues of a corpse as a sexual partner. He described with relish the feeling of power and security that he could enjoy in making love to a corpse; it is there when wanted, you put it away when finished with it, it makes no demands, it is never frustrating, never unfaithful, never reproachful; persecution and guilt, he said, could be quite done away with. In his sexual relations with women he demanded immobility and compliance (9). A corpse is not going to criticize premature ejaculation, loss of erection or other sexual failures. There is no risk of pregnancy and no possibility of the victim making a report to the police.

Cases of homosexual necrophilia have been reported. A twenty-two year old married homosexual male had fantasies of a sexual relationship with a male wholly in his power—a man completely drugged or drunk, completely unconscious, a man powerless in the stocks, or, best of all a man who was dead. While his wife was in the hospital he took a male friend up into the mountains on a pretext, shot him in the head, indulged in anal intercourse and other sexual activities, then threw his body down a mine shaft. Later he said, "I do not think anything would have stopped me. I was mad with power, I had him in my power and nothing could stop me." He was sentenced to fifty years in prison (1).

Edmund Emil Kemper III

> *"If I killed them, you know, they couldn't*
> *reject me as a man. It was more or less*
> *making a doll of a human being."*
>
> Edmund E. Kemper III

Edmund Kemper is an excellent—perhaps deplorable would be a better word—example of a necrophiliac who killed women in order to have sexual relations with them. There were warning signs in his youth that all was not well. He cut off the heads and hands of a sister's doll, he cut off the head of the family cat and killed neighborhood dogs. A sister who thought he liked a second grade teacher suggested that he kiss her and he replied that he would have to kill her first. He would stage his own execution in which he had his younger sister lead him to a chair, blindfold him, and pull an imaginary lever, after which he would writhe about as if dying in a gas chamber (7).

In 1964 at the age of fifteen he was sent to live with his paternal grandparents. He thought his grandmother was bossy like his mother and had fantasies of killing her. When she told him not to shoot birds he shot and stabbed her, shot his grandfather, then telephoned his mother to tell her they were dead. After his arrest he regretted that he had not taken the opportunity to undress his grandmother. During his five years confinement at the Atascadero State Hospital he learned that the real target of his homicidal anger was his mother rather than his grandmother.

Ed was able to obtain employment with the California State Highway Department but he continued to have difficulty getting along with his mother. Although six feet nine inches tall with very superior intelligence (IQ 136), he lacked confidence in himself and felt inadequate around women. He did have sexual relations once with one woman but she refused to have anything further to do with him. Ed began to offer rides to university student hitchhikers but resented the superior attitude of these students. There were thoughts of raping them but first he had to kill them. "I had fantasies about mass murder, whole groups of select women I could get together in one place, get them dead and then make mad passionate love to their dead corpses. Taking life away from them, a living human being, and then having possession of everything that used to be theirs. All that would be mine. Everything" (3).

Between May 1972 and February 1973 he killed six students. It embarrassed him that while handcuffing one victim, the back of his hand brushed against one of her breasts and he apologized. The girls were strangled, stabbed or shot, then taken to his apartment or his mother's apartment. A body would be hidden in a closet and when mother left for work the next day he would have sexual intercourse. There was oral as well as vaginal sex with some victims. He said he cut their heads off to delay identification but it gave him a sexual thrill. One head was buried in his mother's garden facing his room so he could talk to it.

In April 1973 he killed his mother by hitting her with a hammer and cutting her throat. He used her head as a dart board and flushed her larynx down the garbage disposal. It was reported that he sexually assaulted his mother's corpse. An elderly friend of his mother was also killed. A full account of his crimes is provided by Margaret Cheney in **The Coed Killer**.

After the last two homicides he drove to Pueblo, Colorado where he telephoned the Santa Cruz police to confess his crimes. The Pueblo police who arrested him found in his car a 12 gauge shotgun loaded with three rounds, a .30 caliber carbine rifle loaded with thirty rounds, a .3006 caliber rifle loaded with five rounds, a cartridge belt with 100 rounds and additional ammunition. He said he wanted to turn himself in before he did something like shooting innocent people that he might happen to pass by. He was sentenced to life in prison.

VOYEURISM AND EXHIBITIONISM

It is commonly stated that the sex offender does not progress from minor to major sex crimes. While it may be true that persons convicted of voyeurism (peeping), exhibitionism (indecent exposure) and fetishism (sexual gratification from high-heeled shoes, pantyhose or other female clothing), seldom commit violence or murder; nevertheless some offenders commit both minor and major sex crimes. The author has examined several persons charged with murder who gave a history of voyeurism or indecent exposure. In all these cases the sexual perversion occurred in the setting of severe sociopathic personality disorder. Heirens, the seventeen year old college student who confessed the murder of a six year old girl and two women, suffered from sexual perversions including fetishism. At nine years of age he began stealing women's underclothing, and at one time was found in possession of forty panties.

REFERENCES

1. Bartholomew, A.A., *et al.*: Homosexual necrophilia. *Med. Sci. Law, 18*:29, 1978.
2. Berg, Karl: *The Sadist.* Authorized translation by Olga Illner and George Godwin. London, Acorn Press, 1938.
3. Cheney, Margaret: *The Coed Killer.* New York, Walker and Company, 1976.
4. Frank, Gerold: *The Boston Strangler.* New York, New American Library, 1966.
5. Goodman, Jonathan (Ed.): *Trial of Ian Brady and Myra Hindley.* Newton Abbott, David and Charles, 1973.
6. Krafft-Ebing, R.F.: *Psychopathia Sexualis.* Chicago, W.T. Keener and Company, 1900.
7. Lundee, D.T.: *Murder and Madness.* San Francisco, San Francisco Book Company, 1976.
8. Melvern, Linda and Gillman, Peter: Behind the mask of a killer. *Sunday Times,* (London), April 18, 1982.
9. Segal, H.: A necrophilic phantasy. *Int. J. Psychoanal., 34*:98, 1953.

CHAPTER 9

MADNESS AND MURDER

> *"His madness was not in the head*
> *but in the heart."*
>
> Byron, *Lara*

THE PROMINENCE given to the insanity plea in murder might suggest that murder and madness go hand in hand. Yet the studies of Guze and his associates of criminal offenders in Missouri showed that the only psychiatric disorders found more frequently among criminal offenders than in the general population were sociopathic (antisocial) personality disorder, alcoholism and drug dependence. The incidence of schizophrenia was only one percent. Even if every criminal offender found not guilty by reason of insanity during the study was assumed to be schizophrenic and was included in the figures, the three percent incidence of schizophrenia would account for only a very small part of the criminal population.

SCHIZOPHRENIA

> *"Have we eaten on the insane root*
> *That takes the reason prisoner?"*
>
> Shakespeare, *Macbeth*

Approximately 50 percent of all mental hospital patients suffer from schizophrenia or split mind. The splitting of the mind does not create a Jekyll and Hyde dual personality. Instead there is a disintegration of the personality revealed by inconsistency in thought, emotion and behavior.

The world of reality is replaced by a world of fantasy. The patient becomes preoccupied with his distorted perception of the world around him and tends to withdraw from relationships with other persons. The disturbance in thinking may not be readily apparent to the untrained observer or it may be so bizarre as to leave no doubt of the presence of psychosis.

The emotional disorder may show itself in a coldness of response to others or it may extend to inappropriate responses such as unfeeling cruelty, or hilarity in a tragic situation. Hallucinations and delusions, when present, may overshadow other symptoms, and may lead to strange behavior. Crimes of violence, including homicide, may usher in or complicate a schizophrenic illness. The onset may be sudden or insidious. The illness may commence with complaints of a physical nature such as headaches or abdominal pain. Relatives may note the appearance of irritability, sensitivity, social withdrawal, depression or growing eccentricity. There is a great variety of clinical pictures.

The paranoid schizophrenic may believe that he is being followed, that announcements are being made over the radio about him, that passers-by accuse him of sexual or other crimes, or that a gang is plotting to kill him. In paranoid disorders similar persecutory delusions occur, but the personality of the patient is better preserved than in schizophrenia. The person suffering from paranoid delusions may seek to protect his life by killing or attempting to kill his imagined persecutors as in the following cases.

A thirty-five year old man charged with the murder of his wife, claimed that she had been hypnotizing him for some months, and that he was in an hypnotic trance when he shot her. Indeed, he wondered whether his wife was really dead, as he did not hear the gun go off, and he thought that she might have hypnotized him into believing that he had killed her. He was arrested after he had driven his car with the body of his wife to the police station. A paranoid schizophrenic with delusions of grandeur and persecution, he boasted that he knew the location of all the gold mines in the country. He stated that his wife had tried to obtain this information from him through hypnosis, and that just prior to the shooting she had accused him of homosexual relations with another man.

A fifty-one year old white divorced man threw a bomb into a house, killing one of the occupants. On psychiatric examination he insisted that he was the innocent victim of a frameup by the Brotherhood of Railroad

Trainmen because of his failure to join the organization fourteen years earlier. During the last three years he had been subject to persecution. Several times dope was blown in his face making him sick for days. The first time he was in a caboose and the next thing he remembered was finding himself in an office building in the company of a man and a blonde who robbed him of $255. He appealed to the railroad, the sheriff and a private attorney for help without success.

He was convinced the other railroad men were talking about him and after an attempt was made to kill him by shaking him off a tank car he obtained a job putting hot rubber into a rolling machine in a rubber factory. While working on the job something hit him and he collapsed. On regaining consciousness he overheard someone say "Big Bill (a railroad switchman) blew him." Some months later he heard someone say that Big Bill had bragged that he went to the rubber factory to "put that SOB through the rolling machines." The man was clearly suffering from paranoid delusions. The owner of the house into which he threw the bomb was one of his imagined persecutors.

In the simple type of schizophrenia the patient loses interest in everyday affairs, becomes apathetic and is content to sit around home all day. Attempts to prod him into activity usually excite little response, but may result in impulsive assaultive reactions. A twenty-three year old simple schizophrenic was removed from a mental hospital by his family against medical advice. At first he could be persuaded to take care of himself and to perform simple household tasks. Later he became morose and irritable, spending his time slumped in a chair staring into the distance. His father remonstrated with him and the patient attempted to throttle him. A few days later when his mother persisted in her attempts to persuade him to go for a walk he threw her down, seized a wringer, and bludgeoned to death his mother, grandmother and sister. He made no attempt to avoid arrest and on return to the hospital he was mute and appeared to have no interest in his surroundings. Many skid row denizens and hoboes are simple schizophrenics who eke out an existence on the fringe of society.

In the catatonic form of schizophrenia, attacks of extreme excitement with violent assaultive behavior may precede or follow a dull stuporose state in which the patient says little or nothing at all and remains motionless in the same posture for hours at a time.

THE DANGEROUS CHRONIC PARANOID
SCHIZOPHRENIC

There are many chronic paranoid schizophrenics in the community but few of them kill. Those who do kill usually have had delusions of persecution for several years. Mowatt found that thirty-nine male murderers had been delusional for an average of four and a half years before committing murder. Six female murderers had been delusional for an average of nine years before killing. Within an eight month period in 1979-1980 in Colorado four chronic paranoid schizophrenics, who had been delusional for an average of seven years, each killed a complete stranger. One of these men was shot and killed but records were obtained on him. The remaining three schizophrenics who were charged with murder, were examined by the author and by Seymour Sundell, M.D., forensic psychiatrist for the Denver Manager of Safety. Our review of these men's illnesses may provide clues to the dangerous chronic paranoid schizophrenic.

1. The Stabbing of a Bus Driver

A twenty-one year old, single janitor, who had received psychiatric treatment intermittently over a period of five years, falsely believed that attempts had been made to kill him. Early one morning he decided to obtain a gun to protect himself. He drove his car through the locked entrance doors of the Denver Bear Valley shopping center mall, drove down the mall and through the doors of a sporting goods store. His intention was to take a .32 caliber pistol which he had looked at on a previous visit to the store. He seized a rifle but threw it down because he could not find any ammunition. After smashing a showcase he took a hunting knife and then drove four miles to the Englewood Cinderella City shopping center to obtain a firearm from another sporting goods store.

Once again he attempted to drive through the entrance doors into the mall, but his aim was not good and he hit a wall of the shopping center, wrecking his car. He thought that someone in the parking area was going to kill him and he believed that the area was swarming with undercover agents of the FBI and Central Intelligence Agency. These agents were trying to provoke him to do something wrong so they could arrest him. He also thought that they were going to kill him because he knew about corruption in high office and he thought that a bus parked nearby was put there for a purpose.

"I entered the bus. I told the bus driver to get out of the seat, he didn't get out of the seat so I stabbed him. He was a hindrance preventing what I think is right, so I stabbed him twice in the chest and twice in the back. He ran. I tried to start the bus. It wouldn't start." While leaving the scene he was arrested.

In his conversation there were many references to religion and the conflict between good and evil, between Christ and Satan. In support of his belief that it was alright to kill he mentioned that Moses, Samson, King David and others had killed. He had many paranoid delusions, for example that his father and brother were going to kill him and that the FBI and CIA were against him. There were also grandiose delusions that he was King David and that he was God. Previous violence included two arrests for assaulting his brother.

2. The Shooting of a Secret Service Agent

A thirty-one year old unemployed single man first came to the attention of the Secret Service in January 1974 when he appeared on two successive days at the White House requesting to speak to Mrs. Nixon about an invasion from outer space. He also wanted to offer his services to solve illegal drug trafficking because he was the James Bond type. Following admission to a hospital he was diagnosed as a paranoid schizophrenic. In 1976 he made a telephone threat to blow up the White House and later that year he appeared at the Nixon residence in San Clemente, California requesting to see the former President.

He complained that President Nixon had threatened him on television and had wanted to kill him since he was twelve years old. God had selected him to start a revolution which would follow the shooting of Nixon, but he was not the one to shoot Nixon. He claimed responsibility for bombing a propane plant in Minnesota, and he had a map showing the locations of propane plants in the United States, but upon inquiry it was found that he was not knowledgeable about explosives. Once again he was admitted to a hospital. Unlike the other schizophrenics in this group he appears to have cooperated in treatment but when discharged from a hospital he would not follow his promise to obtain further therapy.

Over the years he was in and out of hospitals in various cities across the United States. He had fixed paranoid delusions that Nixon wanted to kill him, that the FBI and police had shot at him, that the FBI had wiretapped his telephone, that the CIA had kidnapped his mother and had killed him with electronic bugging equipment but he was resurrected. He also had delusions of grandeur, for example he believed that he and his brother were the co-makers of heaven and earth, that he was the leader of a race of gods and that he was bulletproof.

He once said of himself "I am a Neo-Nazi, I am a time bomb" and he was certainly armed and dangerous. During an interview with a Secret Service agent he held a loaded .357 caliber revolver in his hand but eventually he was persuaded to surrender it. Another time a .357 caliber revolver was found where he had hidden it in the hospital parking lot. He also handed over to a counselor a machete with an eighteen inch blade. In August 1979 he was walking down a street in Chico, California with a semi-automatic rifle which was taken from him because he was obviously mentally ill.

On January 14, 1980, he went to the Denver office of the Secret Service and complained that Nixon had been threatening him. He stated that the government was trying to kill him. Without warning he shot an agent who was leaving the office. The mortally wounded agent shot him once and another agent shot him four times. He died at the scene.

3. The Stabbing of an Airline Passenger

A twenty-eight year old, single, unemployed man without warning and without saying anything stabbed to death a young man who was standing in a ticket line at Denver's Stapleton International Airport. The victim had completed his service in the U.S. Navy and had left San Diego to return to his parents' home in Iowa.

His assailant explained on psychiatric examination "I stabbed a guy at the airport, I wasn't sick. I was mad because I didn't have a place to stay. My mother was going to put me out of the house. People at the airport were plotting against me and my predecessors. People dressed up in police uniforms. They were keeping me from coming in contact with them. I noticed he had a corduroy shirt and blue jeans. He dressed like my legal aid attorney. I wanted to make sure that the legal aid people knew about the predecessors. They were trying to look like them."

He explained that his predecessors were people like himself in other persons' bodies. "I'm not supposed to tell people that I'm superman from the planet Krypton. If I tell people that they'll hold me here for the rest of my life . . . You're not going to stop me from going to Krypton. I want to be President of the United States and head of the Police Department." He admitted that on previous admissions to hospitals he thought that he was Jesus Christ and an android from another planet, from a galaxy.

This man had a thirteen year history of mental illness. He spent over five years in mental hospitals because of paranoid delusions and hallucinations accompanied by assaultive behavior. At the age of fifteen he defaced a portrait of his sister by scratching on the eyes and teeth with a pen. He struck his stepfather and threatened to kill other persons including a woman he falsely believed to be his wife. One time he threw a 200 pound concrete block through the window of her living room. He had thoughts of killing his psychiatrists. Seven months before the homicide a Denver Police captain wrote a letter to one of this man's doctors expressing concern about his dangerous propensities.

4. The Shooting of a Police Officer

The fourth homicide was by a forty-seven year old, divorced, unemployed electrician who had a five year history of paranoid schizophrenia. He first became ill in early 1975, when he thought that people were putting poison in his food, and was treated in a state mental hospital. The following year he was admitted to a Veteran's Administration hospital but left against medical advice. He had delusions that people were watching him, could read his thoughts and had placed electronic bugs in his apartment. He threatened his family, accused his wife of infidelity and beat his seventy year old father.

There were repeated admissions to mental hospitals. He complained of radiation burns from his eye glasses and he accused the police of causing radiation burns and blisters on his feet. In addition he believed that Senator Edward Kennedy tried to make his wife a prostitute and that later the police killed her. When he discovered that his son's soccer coach was a police officer he cut up his son's picture of the coach. In his opinion the only two police officers in the history of the United States who were not "Communist, KGB, satan, bullshit police" were Matt Dillon and Erskine, an actor in a television series on the FBI.

In April 1980 he was asked to leave a convenience store because he kept telling other customers that they were communists. A police officer, who responded to the store manager's request for assistance, persuaded him to leave the store. As the officer was walking to his patrol car the man shot the officer with a revolver which he had concealed in some papers. The mortally wounded officer shot his assailant who later claimed that the officer shot him first. "It was a set-up. He knew I was Jesus Christ, he was Satan." The man had previously been arrested for carrying a concealed weapon. The police had kept his revolver but a judge ordered that it should be returned to him. Three months later he used it to kill the police officer.

Danger Signals

Dr. Seymour Sundell noted that these four chronic paranoid schizophrenics who killed, shared the following seven features.

1. **Prior Violence.** All four men had assaulted other persons prior to their homicides and two had made homicidal threats. Law enforcement agencies had taken firearms from two of these men.
2. **Persistent Fixed Paranoid Delusions.** All these men had persistent fixed delusions of persecution. In three cases the delusions involved both family members and the police, FBI, Central Intelligence Agency or Secret Service. Three men believed that attempts either had been made or would be made to kill them.
3. **Persistent Fixed Delusions of Grandiose Identity.** All four men thought they were God, Jesus or a super power.
4. **Persistent Intense Feelings of Resentment and Anger.** In all four men these feelings were related to their delusional beliefs.
5. **Action in Response to Paranoid Delusions.** All four men took some action such as making homicidal threats, assaulting persons, or damaging the property of persons involved in their delusions; filing lawsuits to stop alleged harrassment; appealing to a law enforcement agency for protection from an imagined persecutor that might be another law enforcement agency, and carrying firearms or other weapons for protection.
6. **Lack of Insight.** All four men lacked awareness of their severe mental disorders.
7. **Refusal to Cooperate in Treatment.** In view of their lack of insight it is not surprising that three of these men refused to cooperate in therapy. When these persons seek help it is usually to obtain treatment for physical disorders caused by their persecutors, to obtain overnight lodging or to avoid arrest on criminal charges. All four men failed to seek follow-up therapy after discharge from hospital. At least three refused to take antipsychotic medication.

The above findings prompted a review of the illnesses of thirty chronic paranoid schizophrenics who had been examined by Dr. Sundell or myself. Twenty had been charged with murder and ten with attempted murder. There was a prior history of violence in 85 percent of the murderers and in 40 percent of those who attempted murder. In some other respects the two groups were very similar and figures will be given for the thirty subjects.

It is not surprising that these thirty chronic paranoid schizophrenics had a high incidence of fixed paranoid delusions. It is surprising that 80 percent had delusions of persecution by the police, FBI, Central Intelligence Agency, U.S. Secret Service or the KGB (intelligence agency of the Soviet Union). Furthermore, 93 percent had **persistent intense feelings of resentment and anger** related to their paranoid delusional beliefs. Acts of violence, damaging the property of imagined persecutors, filing lawsuits, appealing for police assistance, or carrying weapons for protection were present in 80 percent of the subjects.

Thirty-three percent had persistent delusions of grandiose identity (God, Jesus or a super power). There was a 97 percent incidence of lack of insight and 93 percent refused to cooperate in treatment. In most of these patients this refusal to cooperate persisted over the years. A basis for comparison is provided by a study of fifty-one paranoid schizophrenics in Washington, D.C., which showed that 80 to 89 percent had delusions of persecution, there were no figures on either delusions of grandeur or delusions of grandiose identity, 80 to 89 percent had lack of insight and 70 to 79 percent were unwilling to cooperate (13).

Murder by chronic paranoid schizophrenics is likely to increase because of the worldwide trend toward closing mental hospitals. Consequently chronic paranoid schizophrenics are either quickly discharged from mental hospitals or are refused admission. This policy of reducing the number of mental hospital beds seldom, if ever, includes provision for alternative outpatient treatment together with automatic regular follow-up evaluations of those paranoid schizophrenics who do not cooperate in treatment.

Indication of a trend toward a higher incidence of murder by schizophrenics is provided by Taylor and Gunn's survey of the records of 1,241 male prisoners in London. They found a higher prevalence of schizophrenia among men convicted of homicide and arson than would be expected in the general population of London.

DEPRESSION

"Tell us, pray, what devil
This melancholy is, which can transform
Men into monsters."

John Ford, *The Lover's Melancholy*

Severe depression may lead to murder and suicide. The victims are almost invariably members of the slayer's family. The husband who is so depressed that he can see no hope for the future may take his life in order to avoid further misery. His depression may be so severe that he believes that his wife and children also face such a bleak future that life has no meaning for them. Convinced that he is conferring an advantage on them by cutting short their lives, he may kill them one by one before taking his own life. Auditory hallucinations in the form of imagined voices of God or the devil may instruct him to commit murder. The shock resulting from these murders may relieve his depression with the result that the patient survives to face charges of murder.

A major depression in later life is characterized by the gradual onset of feelings of depression and anxiety, loss of interest in social activities, together with complaints of bodily ill health, and insomnia. The hypochondriacal symptoms, commonly consisting of complaints of abdominal discomfort and constipation, lead to a fruitless search for physical illness. Tragically the underlying depression may pass unrecognized by family and physician. The suggestion of a Caribbean cruise or vacation serves only to deepen the depression as the patient unconsciously seeks punishment rather than reward. The danger of suicide is great.

As the disorder progresses, frank delusions of ill health, poverty and sinfulness may appear. Thus, despite excellent health, comparative wealth, high moral standards and previous good conduct the patient becomes convinced that he is suffering from cancer, that he is ruined financially and that he has committed terrible crimes for which he deserves to die. Frequently, these patients are rigid obsessive persons who do not readily express anger. The last person one might expect to commit murder.

A fifty-five year old dentist had not felt well for several months. Because of forgetfulness, difficulty in concentrating and lack of confidence he began to cancel business appointments which led to a reduction in his income. Although his financial position was sound he worried that his income would be insufficient to meet his expenses. He was very concerned over his wife's ill health and he slept poorly despite medication for sleep. Gradually he became more depressed. He was convinced that his friends were avoiding him. Fleeting thoughts of suicide led him to give his guns to a friend for safekeeping.

One night the voice of the devil told him to kill his wife, child and himself. Through prayer he was able to overcome this impulse which he did not reveal to anyone. However, he sought treatment and arrangements were made for his admission to a hospital. At the last minute he decided that it was his duty to remain at home to help his sick wife take care of their young son. Three nights later, unable to sleep, he paced up and down his home brooding over his troubles. He felt that the whole world was crashing about him and he decided to commit suicide.

"It looked as though I was going to lose what I owned, what I'd saved. The taxes were coming in with a vengeance. I didn't want my family to go in want; it suddenly occurred to me if I got rid of them and me it would clear things up. I knew it was wrong and it wouldn't solve anything. I got thinking maybe it would be better if we all went together. I didn't want to leave them so they'd be all by themselves. My wife always said she didn't want to live without me. She told me that many times. I paced the floor and paced the floor and kept thinking about it. It seemed like the devil had hold of me.

"I felt terrible, I got the idea I should blow the lightswitch so my wife and son couldn't turn the light on. It entered my head that this turned everything off including the furnace. I went downstairs, it was running. I thought the gas would blow up the whole neighborhood so I turned the switch on again. I decided maybe I was worthless, I knew I was worthless. I went downstairs and got a hunting knife out of a box. I kept wandering around wondering what I was going to do. I thought I would gash myself with it across the jugular vein.

"I kept thinking about the bills coming, the house taxes. Piling up, piling up in my mind. I knew I couldn't keep doing that. I thought everything was going to fall around my head. I know it could be a catastrophe in a short time. My son wouldn't be able to stand the stigma, my wife wouldn't have the things she was used to. The voice of the devil told me to kill them."

That night he killed his wife and son with a claw hammer. Although he had planned to kill himself he seemed to have no energy to do this and some hours later he telephoned the police who found the two victims beaten to death in their beds. In jail he imagined that someone would shoot him in the back with a machine gun and he warned people in the corridor to keep away as they might be hurt by the gunfire.

On admission to a hospital he was in a state of severe depression. He socialized very little with the other patients as he was convinced that he would have an adverse effect on them and make them sick. Both in jail and hospital he heard voices which accused him of being a skunk and told him to commit suicide. The jury found him not guilty by reason of insanity and he was committed to a hospital. His depression responded to treatment and three years later he was discharged recovered.

Another form of depression, which may appear at an earlier age and recur at intervals is characterized by decreased speech and activity. In contrast to the ceaseless pacing to and fro, constant wringing of the hands and talkativeness of some persons with a major depression, one finds the patient slumped and silent in his chair with his head down. His answers to questions are delayed and his speech is slow.

There may be a history of a prior manic episode. The manic patient is hyperactive and distractible. He may have grandiose ideas about his wealth, his accomplishments, and his plans for the future. His mood is elated and he feels on top of the world, but he becomes irritable if crossed. Often he squanders his money, uses poor judgment and may indulge in uninhibited behavior including sexual escapades. He is not likely to kill others except possibly unintentionally through reckless driving. In the depressed phase there is a risk of suicide and homicide.

ORGANIC BRAIN DISEASE

> *"Now see that noble and most sovereign reason*
> *Like sweet bells jangled, out of tune, and harsh."*
>
> Shakespeare, *Hamlet*

Dementia

In the later years of life, when mental and physical health is beginning to fail, physical changes in the brain weaken the critical faculties, destroy memory, impair judgment and diminish self-control. Sexual and aggressive drives, previously held in check, may find expression in inappropriate sexual remarks, sexual assaults on children, or homicide.

Restlessness at night is common in the aged and the dementing senile, in his nocturnal prowlings, may set fire to the house or leave the gas taps on, with fatal outcome for the other members of the household. Although arteriosclerotic changes in the arteries of the brain and senile degeneration of the brain cells are primarily responsible for the onset of progressive dementia, psychological factors also contribute to the clinical picture.

Elderly persons who lead lonely, insecure, dependent lives are likely to develop depressive or paranoid symptoms. Depressive preoccupations lead to self-murder, while paranoid ideas or delusions frequently underlie homicidal assaults. The cantankerous, suspicious, insecure pensioner is prone to misinterpret the motives of people who enter his property and may not hesitate to shoot intruders, as in the following cases:

An eighty year old man who was employed as a watchman at a mine discovered a group of boy scouts climbing over some trestles near the entrance to the mine. Apparently he became alarmed when a dog started barking at him. He seized his rifle and started firing at the boys, one of whom was killed. When the sheriff arrived he said that a boy had fallen down and hurt himself. After adding that the boy wouldn't bother him anymore, he started laughing. Psychiatric examination revealed that he was suffering from an early stage of senile dementia.

A seventy-four year old widower, a former deputy sheriff, was arrested for the murder of his only friend, a much younger man. The friend had told him he had purchased a bolt action .22 rifle and the patient criticized this type of rifle as being unsatisfactory for shooting rabbits. He noticed a "terrible frown" on his friend's face and when the friend expressed the wish to show him the rifle, he demurred. Nevertheless, his friend produced the gun and demonstrated its action, holding the rifle pointed at the patient's chest. He ordered his friend to point the gun the other way, but his friend merely lowered the gun and continued to frown. Convinced that his friend was going to shoot him for his criticism, he thought what a terrible thing it was for a friend to kill a friend. He then thought "it's him or me," drew a pistol from his pocket and shot his victim twice.

His family reported that for some years he had shown an avid interest in rape and assaults on elderly persons. He had frequently commented on the danger to elderly people and had stated that he would kill anyone who touched a young girl or attempted to hurt an older person. He had been in the habit of obtaining and secreting firearms about the house. Whenever he left the house he would carry a firearm. He felt that he did so legally as he left the revolver butt sticking out of his pocket and he was not therefore carrying a concealed weapon. Five years prior to the fatal shooting, he had been arrested for shooting in the knee a man who had "attacked him." At this time the court admonished his family to keep guns away from him. He was fined $400 but the fine was suspended.

While in the hospital for psychiatric examination, he became very angry and threatened to kill a mentally ill patient, who made a suggestive remark to a nurse. He was preoccupied with fear of physical assault by a younger person. His memory and judgment were impaired, he was emotionally labile and showed evidence of arteriosclerotic brain disease. The jury found him not guilty of murder by reason of insanity.

Head Injury

Profound changes in personality may follow severe head injury. A conscientious hard-working man becomes lazy and shows complete lack of initiative; an amiable placid person becomes irritable, morose and subject to explosive outbursts of rage. Frustration arising from forgetfulness, difficulty in following conversations and inability to grasp problems, results in great anger. Suspicion that he is being imposed upon, coupled with awareness of difficulty in adequately representing his own interests may lead to homicidal assault by the handicapped person, as in the following case.

A thirty year old man received a serious head injury in an automobile accident and remained unconscious for five days. Recovery was slow and he was transferred to a mental hospital as he was mentally confused. After one month his parents insisted on taking him home, but he was so difficult to look after that they used to lock him in his room at night. It was almost two years before he recovered sufficiently to return to work as a laborer. He was handicapped by headaches and other symptoms which made work difficult for him. There were frequent arguments at home and at work and he was unable to hold a job for more than a few weeks at a time. He fought his brother, knocked his father's teeth out, struck his mother on several occasions, and hit his younger brothers whenever they disagreed with him. A month before his arrest on a charge of murder, he knocked his sister down and pulled some hair from her head when she criticized him for being untidy.

The fatal assault, three years after the accident, occurred following a heated argument with a garage owner over the cost of repairs to his car. He had been unable to pay for the repairs and was resentful because the mechanic, who had retained possession of the car, was reported to have driven it around town. The argument was terminated when he assaulted the mechanic with a tire iron. The assault was unusually violent and the victim's skull was shattered by repeated blows. His self-control clearly had been impaired by brain injury and the jury returned a verdict of not guilty by reason of insanity.

THE INSANITY PLEA IN MURDER

"Another day, another dollar."
Comment of Hinckley's attorney to
reporters after jury's verdict.

The plea of not guilty by reason of insanity is likely when the murderer's guilt is not in doubt and he faces the death penalty. In many jurisdictions, not only in the United States but also abroad, the tests of criminal responsibility are based on the M'Naghten Rules formulated in England in 1843. M'Naghten was not a judge but a deluded paranoid person, who in 1843, was tried for the willful murder of a Mr. Drummond. He believed that he was being persecuted by various people including the Pope and the British Prime Minister, Sir Robert Peel. In an endeavor to right his imaginary wrongs he decided to kill the Prime Minister but shot the secretary to Sir Robert Peel in mistake for the latter. The assassination was regarded by many persons as a political plot and there was indignation over M'Naghten's acquittal on the ground of insanity. Because of the public outcry, the House of Lords submitted, to a panel of judges, questions regarding the criminal responsibilities of persons afflicted with insane delusions. The judges' answers have been called the M'Naghten Rules.

These Rules state in essence, that in order to establish a defense of insanity, it must be shown that the accused was labouring under such a defect of reason from disease of the mind that (1) he did not know the nature and quality of the act he was doing, or (2) did not know that it was wrong. Ever since their introduction over a hundred years ago, the Rules have been criticized by both lawyers and psychiatrists. Lord Bramwell, for example, stated "nobody is hardly ever really mad enough to be within the definition of madman laid down in the Rules." Only the idiot, the grossly demented senile or the severely delirious patient can be said to have no knowledge of right or wrong and these persons are seldom seen in the criminal courts.

The Rules provide a purely intellectual criterion of responsibility and ignore completely the importance of emotional factors and instinctual drives in determining human behavior. As early as 1864 Maudsley wrote "The fundamental defect in the legal test of responsibility is that it is founded upon the consciousness of the individual . . . the most important part of our mental operations takes place unconsciously." The insane person who can distinguish right from wrong may not be free to choose between them. It is perhaps paradoxical that if M'Naghten had been tried under the Rules which bear his name, he might well have been found sane and sentenced to death.

In many jurisdictions the "right-wrong" test has been supplemented by a test of self-control. Even if the accused knew that murder was wrong, did he suffer from a mental disease that rendered him incapable of choosing the right and refraining from doing the wrong? Some of the new tests are so broad and vague that a successful plea of insanity became much easier than under the M'Naghten Rules. At one time all federal jurisdictions and about half the states were using a test based on the American Law Institute's Model Penal Code Test.

> "A person is not responsible for criminal conduct if at the time of such conduct as a result of mental disease or defect he lacks substantial capacity either to appreciate the criminality (wrongfulness) of his conduct or to conform his conduct to the requirements of law."

This was the test used in Washington, D.C. by the jury in the trial of John Hinckley who shot President Reagan, press secretary James Brady, a policeman and a Secret Service agent. Public outrage over the jury's finding that Hinckley was not guilty by reason of insanity prompted several states to adopt stricter tests of criminal responsibility. The insanity plea was already under attack. The public was concerned over the premature release of dangerous insane offenders after a short stay in a mental hospital. Some of these men killed again soon after their discharge from the hospital.

In the 1970s some courts made it much easier for persons found not guilty by reason of insanity to obtain their release. Previously a finding of insanity resulted in automatic indefinite commitment to a mental hospital, usually a special maximum security institution. Some courts however decided that a finding of insanity should be followed by another hearing to determine whether the legally insane person should be committed to a mental hospital under civil commitment statutes. Unless the hearing determined that the legally insane person was mentally ill and dangerous he would be released. Even if committed these persons had the same procedural rights as any civilly commited patient.

Critics of the insanity plea complain that defense attorneys always seem to be able to find psychiatrists who will testify favorably on behalf of their clients. In contested cases expert psychiatric witnesses almost invariably testify on both sides of the fence. A few states have abolished the insanity defense but whether such legislation will survive appeals to the United States Supreme Court remains to be seen. It has been suggested that instead of placing the burden on the district attorney to prove sanity beyond a reasonable doubt, the defense attorney should be required to prove his client's insanity either by a preponderance of the evidence or beyond reasonable doubt.

In those states which have provided an alternative verdict of guilty but mentally ill, the offender so convicted receives psychiatric treatment before serving his prison sentence. If this approach was intended to reduce the number of acquittals by reason of insanity, it does not seem to have accomplished its purpose. It has been suggested that persons found not guilty by reason of insanity should be committed to a state security institution for a specified term that takes into account the enormity of the crime. It has also been suggested that release decisions should be made by a parole board including representatives of the criminal justice system with authority to order conditions of release and to reconfine.

SIMULATED INSANITY

"Though this be madness, yet there is method in't."

Shakespeare, *Hamlet*

Psychiatric evaluation of the suspected murderer may be complicated by the suspect's attempts to fake insanity. Simulated insanity is as old as the history of medicine. In ancient literature the story is told that Ulysses feigned insanity in order to escape the Trojan War. He yoked a bull and a horse together, plowed the seashore and sowed salt instead of grain. Palamedes detected the deception by placing the infant son of the King of Ithaca in the line of the furrow. When Ulysses turned the plow aside to avoid the infant this act of discretion was considered sufficient proof that his madness was not real (2).

In the Bible there is a description in the First Book of Samuel of David's successful effort at feigning insanity in order to avoid punishment by the King of Gath. We are told that he scrabbled upon the gates and let the spittle fall from his beard. That Polonius' appraisal of Hamlet's sanity was correct is supported by Hamlet's comment, "I am but mad north, north west. When the wind is southerly I can tell a hawk from a handsaw."

The sane person who wishes to fake insanity usually has a very hazy idea of the behavior of an insane person. The jail library does not usually include a textbook of psychiatry and the ethical defense attorney provides no direct hints. The defense attorney's questions about voices and ideas of persecution may, however, have a suggestive effect, whether intended or not. The suspect has to fall back on his imagination, and his concept of psychotic behavior seldom resembles the true picture. The symptoms usually appear following the suspect's arrest and are seldom present prior to commission of the crime.

Jones and Llewellyn draw attention to the tendency of the malingerer to overact his part. "He sees less than the blind, he hears less than the deaf and he is more lame than the paralyzed. Obsessed with the idea that he must be a hopeless lunatic or imbecile 'un fou á grande orchestre' the pretender affects absolute rather than partial loss or perversion of the reasoning faculties. Determined that his insanity shall not lack multiple and obvious signs, he, so to speak, crowds the canvas, piles symptom upon symptom and so outstrips madness itself attaining to a but clumsy caricature of his assumed role."

Ossipov describes the extremes which the malingerer may exhibit. "If he is told to shut his eyes, he does not close the lids, but uses his fingers to bring the lids together. When someone shakes hands with him he uses his left hand instead of his right. Another malingerer when going to sleep, puts on his glasses and lights his pipe. Such conduct is due to the fact that the malingerer thinks that the stranger he behaves, the more psychotic he will be assumed to be."

Simulation is more frequent when a suspect faces the death sentence. Haines was about to report to the court that a certain patient was unable to cooperate with his counsel. However, the patient attempted to pass a letter to his wife but this was intercepted by a jail guard. In this twelve page letter, he explained his intent to appear insane. He gave a list of friends to call upon to testify that he gave the impression of being unstable, irrational and unsettled, that he would always lose interest in things he was doing; that he would begin a conversation and suddenly stop in the middle of it and start roaming; that he would sit and stare into space for long periods of time and would pay no attention to those about him.

He advised that all his friends be informed of this and then they be sub-poenaed to testify in court. Confronted with this letter, his behavior changed immediately and no overt signs of mental disease were elicited. Haines also quotes another case of malingering in which the suspect's sister, collapsing on the stand, was an excellent witness in his defense. Later it was learned that she had taken dramatic lessons to prepare for her court appearance.

The suspect may behave in an excited overactive manner, but it is difficult for a sane person to maintain this attitude for more than a few days. Often it is present only while the suspect is aware that he is being observed. The defendant who feigns a confused state may have a vacant expression and puzzled manner which disappears when he believes he is not under observation. The confusion does not extend to all subjects of conversation and he may show an inexplicable alertness in discussing certain topics.

One suspect appeared confused and disoriented. He was incoherent in his speech and seemed unable to grasp the meaning of even simple statements. When the first interview was concluded he thought the examination was completed. As he was sitting in the corridor outside my office waiting to be taken back to jail, he was heard complaining bitterly to his guards that he did not see how a psychiatrist could possibly complete his examination in one hour!

The suspect may assume a state of depression. Many suspects are in fact depressed. Their unfortunate plight in being charged with murder is a depressing situation. The suspect who feigns depression seldom exhibits the unrealistic self-reproachful ideas so often seen in the depressed patient. Instead of preoccupation with depressive thoughts, one may see an alert, vigilant attitude on the part of the suspect toward the physician. Concomitant symptoms of severe depression such as loss of appetite, weight loss, sleeplessness and constipation are difficult to simulate.

A suspect who entered a plea of insanity looked, on examination to be very depressed and appeared entirely oblivious of his surroundings. He made no spontaneous comments and did not reply to questions. Throughout the interviews, he sat slumped in a chair with his head drooped forward and his eyes downcast. One afternoon as he was being brought for interview, he was sitting dejectedly in the police car with a blank expression on his face. Out of the corner of his eye, he saw a girl adjusting her stocking in an alley. Before he realized what he was doing, he sat up quickly and turned his head sharply in order to get a better view of the girl before she disappeared from sight. In an unguarded moment, he had given himself away.

It is very difficult for a suspect to be consistent in his attempts to feign mental retardation. On intelligence tests the malingerer underestimates the difficulty of some tests and overestimates the difficulty of others. Thus, the malingerer may fail on easy items but pass more difficult ones.

The malingerer may claim that he hears voices or that he is being persecuted. He is usually somewhat ostentatious and eager to draw attention to such a complaint. He will refer to his voices at each interview. Yet he may become evasive when questioned at length about the voices. A schizophrenic patient may be willing or unwilling to talk about his hallucinations or delusions. However, the schizophrenic who is quick to draw the physician's attention to his delusional ideas is also willing to discuss these ideas at greater length, providing of course that the physician's attitude is not such as to discourage him.

The malingerer who thrusts forward his alleged psychotic symptoms may become very evasive if he thinks the questioning is for the purpose of testing the genuineness of these symptoms. Malingered hallucinations or delusions are often limited to one or two assertions which are repeatedly mentioned when listeners are at hand. They are not accompanied by the less dramatic but equally important signs and symptoms of the schizophrenic, depressive or other psychosis. When asked some simple question, he may give the appearance of profound concentration and then give an absurd answer, herein behaving differently from the schizophrenic. The total clinical picture presented by the malingerer fails to conform to the picture seen in a genuine psychosis.

A suspect charged with armed robbery volunteered, in a somewhat belligerent tone during the first interview, that he had committed the crime because he had been told to do so by voices from another planet. Clinical examination showed no evidence of psychosis apart from this one claim of "hearing voices." As the examination proceeded, he mellowed considerably and became very friendly toward the physician. In a further discussion of the crime, he was asked if he had ever pistol whipped or otherwise injured his holdup victims. He replied, in an offended tone of voice, "I'm a professional holdup man, I don't get nervous." In response to an inquiry regarding his use of leisure time he replied, "Drinking and thinking out ways of stealing money." He later agreed that he did not commit the crime in response to voices from another planet.

Malingering is not confined to the sane offender. The insane suspect ignorant of his true condition may feign insanity in order to avoid legal responsibility for his crime. Eissler points out that the act of malingering may constitute a defense against the approach of just that which the malingerer tries to enact as a conscious performance. Certainly, if a subject feels the threatening disintegration of his own personality, it may provide relief if he can convince himself "I am not submitting to it but performing it."

A confession of malingering does not by itself exclude psychosis. Persons known to have had a genuine psychosis may on recovery claim that they were malingering. For these persons a psychiatric illness is regarded as more humiliating than a jail sentence. The psychiatrist in examining the suspected murderer should combine sympathetic understanding with an attitude which is neither too skeptical nor too credulous. The story is told of a consulting physician who, walking into his ward one day with his intern remarked, "Well, how are they all this morning?" "All doing excellently," said the intern, "except the malingerer in the corner who died last night."

SIMULATED EPILEPSY

A man charged with murder succeeded in escaping the full penalty of the law by malingering epilepsy. The suspect, while in a prison hospital, occupied a bed next to an epileptic, and the latter coached him in the signs and symptoms of epilepsy (5). The convenience of a defense of epilepsy is obvious. The murderer will say that he has no memory for the period during which the crime was committed and will give a history of blackouts which appeared following a head injury at work or while in the armed services. That the head injury may have been slight, that the blackouts may have originated in alcohol and not epilepsy, and that the amnesia is simulated and not genuine is of little concern to some defense attorneys. To the ingredients of amnesia and blackouts add an abnormal brain wave tracing and you have the ideal setting for an insanity plea. Epilepsy is a frequent defense, especially when the defendant's guilt is not in doubt.

A suspect was arrested after armed robbery and claimed epilepsy as he could not recall his activities at the time of the crime. His attorney thought he might have had an epileptic attack as the crime seemed inexplicable. The suspect was from a good family, he had an excellent work record, he was not in financial need and also he was due to be married two days after the crime. In short, he did not seem to be the kind of person who would commit armed robbery.

On interview, certain additional information was obtained. He did appear to come from a respectable family, he assured me none of them had been in trouble. Inquiry revealed that by "in trouble" he meant getting a girl into trouble. More specific questioning revealed that his brother was in jail. His excellent work record was confirmed by casual inquiry, but detailed questioning revealed otherwise. His impending marriage was the result of an unwished for pregnancy and he was a somewhat reluctant bridegroom. He did appear to be the kind of person who would commit a crime. When questioned at length about his arrest he soon adopted a jocular attitude and showed no real concern about his predicament. He boasted about the manner of his arrest referring to the cop putting the jewelry on him — by this I took it to mean that he was handcuffed. Although no professional gunman would use such language he nevertheless showed a familiarity with criminal activities that suggested more than mere reading of true detective magazines. His explanation for having two guns in his possession when he set out to spend an evening with his girl friend was scarcely plausible. With a little persuasion, his account of his behavior changed sufficiently to exclude a diagnosis of epilepsy.

Popular belief suggests that assault and murder by epileptics are not uncommon. Statistical studies by neurologists who have treated large numbers of epileptics discount this popular belief. Hughlings Jackson who made the study of epileptics his life work could name seizures which were only potentially dangerous. Gowers who analyzed 3,000 cases mentions nothing more serious than a man who struck a bystander and a woman who threw her child downstairs. Muskens mentioned no instance of a crime committed by any of his 2,000 cases. Lennox and his colleagues reviewed the histories of perhaps 5,000 clinic and private patients. Several patients out of each thousand acted belligerently or caused minor injury to bystanders during or after a seizure.

THE GANSER SYNDROME

> *"As a rule disease as it stalks through the land cannot keep pace with the incurable vice of scribbling about it."*
>
> John Mayou, *de Rachitide, 1668*

"Depend upon it, sir, when a man knows he is to be hanged in a fortnight it concentrates his mind wonderfully." Samuel Johnson's words show that he was not familiar with the Ganser syndrome. Prisoners, waiting trial for murder or under sentence of death sometimes develop peculiar mental symptoms and behave in a very bizarre manner. The unconscious motivation is to avoid responsibility for the crime by appearing insane.

The Ganser patient may behave in a very grotesque fashion and give the appearance of having lost his memory for simple activities of everyday life. Thus, on entering the examining room he may stand on his head, a position which is rather difficult to maintain for any length of time. He may wear his clothes inside out, or peel a banana, throw away the banana and eat the skin. When asked to light a match he will rub the wrong end of the match on the inside of the folder. On being requested to unlock a door, he may try to put the handle of the key in the lock. Insane persons do not lose their memory for simple actions of everyday life, such as striking a match or unlocking a door.

A young man charged with attempted murder entered a plea of insanity. He claimed that during the trip to the hospital from jail he saw red horses, partially dressed in human clothing, sitting on the tops of lamp posts. Little men about twelve inches high ran ahead of the police car while it was traveling at high speed. While he was in the hospital, these little men came at night and took him to the moon where he saw American Air Force officers who were being held prisoners by cannibals. The total clinical picture was typical of the Ganser syndrome. During the course of the examination, he ventilated many feelings of resentment toward the police and court officials. Coincidentally, his bizarre symptoms disappeared, only to reappear in full force when the day came for his return to jail.

A young woman charged with murder denied memory of almost all the personal information which was requested. She said she did not know her first name, her age, the date of her birth, what grade she reached in school, where she was married and so on. To most questions she would respond immediately, "I don't know," but sometimes she would pause, then say, "That, I really don't know." She claimed that she could not recall the names of any makes of cars. When these names were read to her from the classified section of a telephone directory, she said she had never heard them before. Yet, she was able to recite the twenty-third Psalm.

A characteristic feature of the Ganser syndrome, which is an hysterical reaction, is the patient's failure to answer even simple questions correctly. Yet no matter how absurd an answer may be, it is usually clear that the question has been understood, and sometimes the error is so slight as to suggest that the patient is aware of the correct answer. Thus, the patient may say that $3+4=8$; $10-7=4$; $24 \div 6=5$; a dog has three legs, and there are 50 weeks in a year.

On the other hand the patient's response, while showing that he has understood the question, may not come near the correct answer. Thus $3 \times 4 = 100$; three days in a week; a dime is called a dollar; a watch showing the time of a quarter past three is read as 12 o'clock. When asked to count from 1 to 20, the patient may leave out certain numbers, yet when asked to repeat the same task, he may give the numbers which he omitted previously and leave out other numbers.

The patient may answer difficult questions correctly and fail in his answers to more simple inquiries. His performance on simple arithmetical or other tests may vary from one day to the next. Absurd remarks may be interspersed with thoughtful, intelligent and pertinent statements. Inconsistency is clearly a feature of the Ganser syndrome.

The disorder may last only a few hours or may continue over many weeks. As it appears almost invariably after the crime, its presence seldom affects the question of whether or not the patient was legally sane or insane at the time of the crime. The syndrome may occur in the setting of a genuine schizophrenic illness or other psychosis.

The following case is given as an illustrative example of the Ganser syndrome.

A thirty-three year old man was charged with the murder of his girl friend. At his first interview, he could hardly wait to sit down before volunteering that he had killed a girl and that God had told him to do this. "God told me to kill her, she's no good, she's full of sin. My father is next, I'm going to kill him, too. I'm going to kill lots of people, they are no good, they are full of sin. I like to shoot guns, I like to shoot guns. I like to hear them go off." He announced his intention of killing his wife, the judge and various other persons. He claimed he was a prophet who had been sent to the earth to destroy all sinners, after which he would take the remaining people on earth back to heaven with him. God and Jesus, according to his story, visited him regularly in the county jail. His victim also appeared wearing a long white gown and asked to be allowed to return to earth. The suspect told her he was unable to agree to this request.

When questioned further about his symptoms, he became very evasive but after much inquiry, he revealed that God had been speaking to him since he was five years of age. A chronic hallucinatory condition existing since the age of five was inconsistent with his past history and present mental status. At times, he was very suspicious in his attitude and in a theatrical manner would insist on seeing water being run out of a faucet before he would drink it. At other times, he was very friendly and in no way paranoid. He claimed extensive memory loss and he gave his year of birth variously as 1920, 1922, 1930, and 1952. Yet he was able to recall his eight figure Army serial number correctly. January, Monday and Wednesday were given as the months of the year. The next day, he gave the twelve months correctly in their proper order.

On physical examination, he was unable to touch his nose with his forefinger when his eyes were closed. Indeed, on one occasion, he touched his left shoulder instead of his nose, yet other tests showed no impairment of his sense of position or muscle coordination. He showed no facial or other reaction when a large spinal needle was inserted into a fold of skin in the back of his neck. The psychiatric diagnosis was sociopathic personality and Ganser syndrome.

Throughout interviews with the physician, he appeared alert and interested in his surroundings. During psychological testing, he appeared depressed and complained that his head hurt. He constantly held and rubbed his head displaying a marked tremor, first of one hand then the other. He gave the appearance initially of not hearing questions. After the same question had been put to him three or four times, he would mumble a response. On an intelligence test, his score gave him an IQ of 42 which was manifestly absurd in terms of his work record as a taxi driver. Of the twenty-five information items, he knew only the name of the president. He claimed that rubber came from water, that there were three pints in a quart and that he had no idea how many weeks there were in a year. On the vocabulary test, he responded to only three items and said he did not know the meaning of such words as "donkey, join, fur or cushion."

His responses on the arithmetical test are of interest. On three of the easier items his answers were 5, 17 and 9, whereas the correct answers were 4, 16 and 10 respectively. In each case, the error was one above or below the correct answer. He answered the following question incorrectly: "If a man buys six cents worth of stamps and gives the clerk ten cents, how much change should he get back?" Yet he was able to answer the following more difficult question correctly: "If a man buys seven two-cent stamps and gives the clerk a half dollar, how much change should he get back?" On the object assembly test he put the head of the human figure in the arm socket.

He was aware of the purpose of the psychiatric examination and also of the fact that he faced a possible death sentence in court. He was able to discuss the role of his attorney in defending him. Legal proceedings were prolonged due to Supreme Court reversal of his conviction at the first trial on legal technicalities, not connected with his psychiatric condition. At his final trial, in which he was sentenced to life imprisonment, he had new attorneys who were not familiar with his earlier behavior. These attorneys in their extensive dealings with the suspect were unable to detect any signs of mental disorder. The Ganser syndrome presumably disappeared while he was in jail prior to his final trial (9).

REFERENCES

1. Eissler, K.R.: Malingering. In Wilber, G.B. and Muensterberger, W. (Eds.): *Psychoanalysis and Culture.* New York, International Universities Press, 1951.
2. Glueck, Bernard: *Studies in Forensic Psychiatry.* London, Heinemann, 1916.
3. Guze, S.B., *et al.:* Criminality and psychiatric disorders. *Arch Gen Psychiat, 20*:583, 1969.
4. Haines, W.H.: The psychiatrist in court. *Dis Nerv System, 11*:273, 1950.
5. Hopwood, J.S. and Snell, H.K.: Amnesia in relation to crime. *J Ment Sci, 79*:27, 1933.
6. Jones, A.B. and Llewellyn, J.: *Malingering.* London, Heinemann, 1917.
7. Lennox, W.G.: Amnesia, real and feigned. *Amer J Psychiat, 99*:732, 1943.
8. Maudsley, Henry: *Insanity and Crime.* London, Churchill, 1864.
9. Macdonald, J.M.: *Psychiatry and the Criminal.* Springfield, Illinois, Charles C Thomas, 1976.
10. Mowatt, R.R.: *Morbid Jealousy and Murder.* London, Tavistock Publications, 1966.
11. Ossipov, V.P.: Malingering, the simulation of psychosis. *Bull Menninger Clin, 8*:39, 1944.
12. Taylor, P.J. and Gunn, J.: Violence and psychosis. *Brit Med J, 288*:1945, 1984.
13. World Health Organization: *Report of the International Pilot Study of Schizophrenia.* Geneva, World Health Organization, 1973.

CHAPTER 10

CHARACTER DISORDER AND MURDER

"Character is Destiny."

Heraclitus

I T IS OFTEN said, and with justification, that no two persons are alike. Nevertheless prominent character traits are shared by sufficiently large numbers of persons to permit descriptions of certain character types. Many unusual and abnormal people show throughout their lives striking patterns of behavior which make it possible to predict their likely reactions to varying situations. Murder is not confined to any one personality type but the sociopathic personality is disproportionately represented in the ranks of murderers.

THE SOCIOPATHIC MURDERER

"His intellect was in that most unfortunate of all states — too disordered for liberty and not sufficiently disordered for Bedlam."

Lord Macaulay

Sociopathic personalities (sometimes called psychopathic or antisocial personalities) are social misfits who from an early age prove a problem to themselves as well as to society. They are very plausible and often at first sight impressive persons, but they repeatedly disappoint their families and friends. They may form quick social relationships, but seem unable to maintain them. Sociopaths lack the capacity to **feel** with others and may be devoid of affection, callous and cynical. A review of

203

their life histories show that they fail to conform to accepted social customs. Lacking persistence of effort they go from one job to another in quick succession.

Their impulsivity and intolerance of frustration may lead to repeated antisocial acts. Egocentric and immature, they constitute an individualistic rebellious group, intolerant of discipline and of the legal and social restrictions of everyday life. As a rule they do not benefit from the type of treatment presently available in mental hospitals, and they seem unable to profit from experience or punishment. They are the living antithesis of the saying that a burnt child dreads the fire, since they repeat the same fiascos time and again in an impressively self-destructive fashion (3).

The manifestations of their lawlessness include alcoholism, drug dependence, sexual perversions, theft, assault and even homicide. In their criminal behavior as well as in other walks of life, they show a lack of judgment and foresight which is almost beyond belief, yet they may score well on intelligence tests. For example, a sociopath holds up a bank wearing a very distinctive sports shirt, without first checking the layout of the bank, and he fails to notice that the gas gauge of the getaway car is on empty.

Textbook descriptions mention the sociopath's ability to charm and impress others but tend to highlight the negative aspects of the sociopath. Bernard Shaw once said that we judge an artist by his highest moments and the criminal by his lowest. We tend to see sociopathic personalities as totally antisocial, yet the sociopath at times is capable of mature behavior.

Disregard for the truth is not seen in his every statement. His undoubted unreliability and irresponsibility do not show themselves in every situation. Not all his obligations are neglected, not all his promises remain unfulfilled and not all his checks bounce. Impulsivity does not preclude self-restraint. The sociopath with a long criminal record of impulsive assaultive behavior in response to trivial provocation may remain calm and apparently unmoved in the face of serious insult. He may be cruel, but he may also be compassionate.

Despite his apparent absence of guilt, the sociopath often commits his crime in such a manner as to ensure his detection. Thus one sociopathic murderer altered nine out of ten stolen articles so that they could not be recognized by the owner and then pawned only that article which he had not bothered to disguise. His conscience would appear to permit commission of the crime, yet demand punishment for the forbidden act. The apparent absence of guilt, or alternatively the inability of the individual to utilize such feelings in the control of his behavior, is one of the hallmarks of sociopathy.

The sociopath may commit crimes of great violence in a ruthless and callous manner. David F. Early, a prisoner at Leavenworth Penitentiary, informed the prison psychologist that he intended to commit murder as soon as he was released from the penitentiary. Three days after he was released he murdered a prominent Denver attorney, his wife and daughter.

Early's prediction of murder to the psychologist was made public at his trial: "I never think of the consequences, if I could say to myself, Early remember the consequences, then I could keep myself from doing it. I have a fear that I won't be able to control myself. I will get back at my landlady. I got a room in her place ten years ago. I guess she is a nasty hard-to-get-along with person. I get to thinking that the old one has been abusing people for many years. I'm just the one to go down there and give her a batch of trouble. I will get back there when I get out and I will stomp her over the head, tie her up and rape her and kill her finally.

"I will make it to death row yet. I have an uncle-in-law who is a corporation lawyer. I have a scheme for holding him up for ransom money and I would kidnap his family and threaten to kill his wife and children for ransom. Right now I am doing an illegal sentence and when I get out of this I am going to kill people to get money if necessary."

On his release from the penitentiary, Early travelled to Denver where he tried without success to buy a revolver. He did not seek out the landlady he had threatened to kill, but he did go to the home of K, the corporation lawyer and distant relative, with the intention of committing burglary. There was no one at home and entry was gained through an unlocked kitchen door. He found a rifle and pistol which he loaded. Mrs. K arrived home at 2 PM, followed at intervals of approximately one hour or more by her daughter, son and husband. Each in turn was bound hand and foot.

Early's intention was to wait in the house till nightfall and then leave with the money he had obtained. However when K attempted to get up off the bed: "I told him to lay down on the bed so he laid down on the bed and then he sat back up again and I told him to lay back down on the bed, and he said, 'No, you are going to shoot me,' and I said, 'No, I am not going to shoot you unless you start something.' So he says 'Yes, I know you are going to shoot me.' He says 'Don't shoot me.' I said 'All right, just lay down on the bed like I told you and I won't shoot you.' So he didn't lay down on the bed and I cocked the gun. When I cocked the gun he came up off the bed and came at me.

"I shot him. I wanted to stop him and I stopped him. I said, Well I guess I'll have to kill everybody else. There was never any doubt about it in my mind. Those peoples' lives weren't no value to me. They was all a danger. I realized that if I left them alive they could testify against me. If I killed all the witnesses, they'd have an awful hard time convicting me of murder."

After shooting the lawyer Early went to the bedroom where he had tied up Mrs. K and her seventeen year old stepson. He shot Mrs. K but, curiously, he did not shoot the youth. (His later rationalization for this oversight was that it was probably in his mind to shoot his victims in the order they returned home.) Instead he went to the room of the fifteen year old girl and shot her. In the meantime her brother succeeded in freeing his legs. He slipped out of the room and hid in the study. When Early went back to the bedroom, the young boy ran out of the house. Early fired at him but missed and the rifle jammed on the second shot.

My distress on hearing the detailed account of the triple slaying was evidently reflected in my facial expression as Early remonstrated with me saying, "You shouldn't let yourself be emotionally involved. You should be cool, detached and clinical. A good psychiatrist should culti-vate that ability." He then complained about the press reports of his crime which had not mentioned his acts of kindness, placing a pillow un-der Mrs. K's head and so on.

He reiterated that it was not his intention to kill when he visited the home. Throughout the psychiatric examination he was courteous and cooperative although he did say he would kill me if a chance to escape presented itself. When a nurse interrupted one interview to report that she had to awake the two police guards who had fallen asleep Early be-came very indignant at this shortcoming and expressed considerable so-licitude for my welfare.

Early was captured while driving away from the house. He showed no remorse whatever. "I killed three people. I killed them with no com-punction. It didn't mean any more for me to kill them than to turn off the lights. I wouldn't be backward about doing it again if it'd get me any gain. I don't get pleasure out of killing and it don't bother me neither. I feel it's alright for me to kill somebody if I feel it's necessary. If I got out today I'd probably be in trouble again, probably with a gun too, but I'd be more careful next time."

Ever since he was a child he had resented K. He envied K's excellent financial position and felt that K had looked down upon him. Although he had visited K's home many times he never felt at ease with him. He denied having told a policeman regarding the slaying of K's daughter, "She was his and he had everything and now he has nothing." However, he wondered whether he had in mind all the time killing K. Referring to his reason for shooting K he said, "Maybe it was just an excuse. I wanted to do it. I'm really glad that son of a bitch is dead. I was envious of that house it was real fine. All this trouble I've been in all my life I guess is a way of striking back — striking back at my parents. As bad as I am it ain't all my fault."

In reviewing his past life Early said he was not a model child, but a model of juvenile delinquency, and he recounted many delinquent acts in his youth such as theft, firesetting, flooding a basement and cruelty to animals including an attempt to electrocute a dog. He spoke in very bitter terms about his parents who separated when he was two weeks old. He complained that his mother was promiscuous, drank to excess and never really loved him. After his first sentence to a Federal prison his mother informed him that she never wanted to see him again or have anything to do with him. The stepfather was described as an unkind, vicious, overbearing, inconsistent alcoholic. He described many beatings at the hands of his mother and step-father.

His social adjustment was poor from an early age. On leaving school he changed jobs frequently. He was discharged from the Air Force when his mother complained that he was under age for enlistment. His naval career, which included brief service as a policeman, was terminated by an undesirable discharge. He tried to join the Marines but was drunk at the time of application.

His criminal record included sentences to a boys' industrial school, the Colorado State Penitentiary, El Reno Reformatory and the Federal penitentiaries at Lewisburg and Leavenworth for juvenile delinquency, check forgery, car theft and armed robbery. He estimated that he had committed thirty armed robberies. However, he described his murders as "straight killings, picayune crimes" compared with such offenses as cruelty to children, rape and dope peddling. "If I had my way the only penalty you could give them (dope peddlers) would be the death penalty, no ten to fifteen years but the straight death penalty." Early's prediction of making it to death row was fulfilled. He was executed in the gas chamber of the Colorado State Penitentiary.

PASSIVE-AGGRESSIVE PERSONALITY

The passive-aggressive personality has difficulty in expressing his hostile impulses and when aroused he will not openly express his anger. he does express his hostility indirectly in passive ways, for example by agreeing with his opponent yet not honoring his agreement by procrastination and obstructionism which are justified by specious explanations.

This character type includes the passive dependent person who lacks confidence and is unable to stand alone. He shows a childlike emotional dependency on others and has particular difficulty in expressing hostility. These are individuals who permit themselves to be pushed around with few if any protests, they fail to fight, they favor a policy of peace at any price (4). Rarely they may react with violence if pushed too far or if threatened with loss of dependency gratification as in the following case.

HCL, a forty-one year old Spanish-American male, walked into police headquarters late one night and informed the desk patrolman that he had stabbed to death his forty-five year old sister and that he had slashed her lover with a knife.

On psychiatric examination HCL, a compliant, swarthy man of medium height and muscular build, gave a detailed history of his past life. His mother died a month after his birth and he was raised by his elderly grandparents along with a cousin about his own age. Childhood was recalled with sadness and he bitterly resented favors shown to his cousin. His grandfather frequently beat him and once the beating was of such severity that the neighbors intervened. He felt unloved and unwanted.

School attendance was irregular because the family moved frequently and because he was required to spend long hours alone herding sheep. His clothes were so dilapidated that he was ashamed to go to school or to associate with other boys. He can only recall three occasions on which he saw his father and these visits were brief. His immediate response to the question of his earliest memory was an account of his first meeting with his sister Dora when he was ten years old. She clutched him to her and he felt the first thrill of love and warmth that he had ever experienced.

When he was twenty-three Dora came to live with him after she had been deserted by her second husband. They continued to live together for eighteen years and during this time Dora had three illegitimate children. HCL kept referring to these children as "my children" but denied paternity. He had little interest in women and his whole life was centered around his sister and her family. He was very dependent on Dora and showed a childlike devotion to her.

Although he worked steadily in a rubber factory he was unable to save money because of his readiness to satisfy his sister's extravagant whims. She used to complain because he was always ready to loan money to fellow workers. If repayment was not forthcoming he would rather overlook the debt than risk the possibility of unpleasant argument.

He avoided quarrels at any cost and until the tragedy he had never lost his temper and had never been involved in a fight. His foreman said nobody could get mad at him as he agreed with everybody on everything. A reliable and conscientious worker who was always ready to do a favor, he was well liked by all his associates. Once when his sister suggested separation because they were becoming too dependent on each other he attempted suicide by drinking Lysol.

Some years later she again talked of leaving him and again he became very distressed. He offered her his home and promised he would move out of the home but he did not fulfill his promise. One day he returned home to find that she had left with all the furniture. Resentful and angry he nevertheless continued to support her financially. Ten days after the separation he pleaded with her to return and despite her refusal he gave her a present of $100 and promised he would pay her department store bills. She told him that she was working but that evening while he was drinking with some friends in a tavern he learned that Dora was living with a Mr. Camarillo. His friends taunted him by telling him that his sister had made a fool of him all these years and did not really care for him. Shocked by this news he brooded for some hours before deciding to find out whether it was true.

On arriving at Camarillo's apartment he was refused admission. Enraged he obtained a hunting knife, broke down the door and searched the apartment. When he pulled open a closet door his sister jumped out and screamed. He stabbed her fatally and he then stabbed her lover. Later he claimed that his sister must have fallen on the knife.

"I just can't figure out how a man can be classed as a murderer when he doesn't have the heart to hurt a fly. If they hadn't told me my sister was with this man it wouldn't have happened. If I'd learned about it more slow we could have come to some agreement. When they said she'd got a man I didn't want to believe it. I felt like I'd been stabbed in the back. What I felt like was being left alone to face life by myself. Why did she suddenly leave me stranded, deserted in the world? My intention was to go out to this place and find out the truth. When he wouldn't open the door I began to get angry. This man he got me mad. I got uncontrollable. The first time in my life I've really been mad."

Following his arrest he was very remorseful and for several weeks he went without food each Thursday, the day of the killing, as an act of penitence. Three months after the tragedy while awaiting trial he became acutely depressed, refused food, slept poorly, and refused to talk to his lawyers. His behavior was very bizarre and on admission to a hospital he was found to be suffering from the Ganser state (Chapter 9). This disorder quickly responded to treatment. He later pleaded guilty to second degree murder and was sentenced to from twelve to thirty years imprisonment.

THE HYSTERICAL PERSONALITY

Threats to kill by hysterical personalities may give rise to considerable concern on the part of relatives, although the risk of homicide is negligible. The hysterical personality, usually seen in women, is characterized by immaturity, vanity and egocentricity; a remarkable tendency to display very vivid, if shallow, emotional outbursts, sexually provocative behavior often without actual promiscuity, together with demanding, dependent behavior. The following case is of interest.

A twenty-three year old musician was arrested after he had confided in a fellow university student that he intended to kill his girl friend's sister. The defendant was a short slim effeminate young man, dressed in a many colored sport shirt, jeans, and purple slippers. He was not at all concerned about his predicament and indeed seemed to relish the psychiatric examination which had been ordered by the court.

During the interview he paced up and down the room, pausing from time to time to tap the ashes from the cigarette in his long ivory cigarette holder. With a wealth of dramatic gestures, he recounted the story of his life interspersed with his views on politics, music, modern art, philosophy and religion.

His girl friend was an attractive, but poorly educated shop assistant whom he had planned to transform into a society girl after the manner described in Bernard Shaw's famous play **Pygmalion.** The plan was wrecked when the girl's older sister intervened and the musician in his anger told a number of his fellow students of his plans to murder his girl friend's sister. These threats were taken seriously despite their melodramatic nature.

"I want to be cured, but I am not sure how. My problem is that I feel driven to commit a murder. I have this compulsion. I'm afraid I might commit a murder by reflex. I justified this intellectually and emotionally and every way I knew how. I made no physical attempts to kill, but I was desperately afraid I would. I have grown up in an intellectual community, then I went to an emotional community. I felt myself forced into a mechanical world worked by clocks. I prefer to be rational rather than instinctive. I'm not ashamed of my emotions, but the intellect must rule. The impulse to kill is like a cancerous growth inside of me—it's destroying me—I'm trying to stamp it out with my intellect, with the emotions of love within me.

"The picture I draw of her would be different from that drawn by a camera, by an IBM machine. I think my attitude toward her is one of hate. She tries to be just, but she does not understand. I noticed my hands moving forward to strangle her. I don't know enough about the mechanics of strangulation to know whether I could have killed her or not, before I was pulled off. They couldn't have stopped me if I had gone ahead with it. They couldn't have stopped me if my drive had been strong enough.

"I set myself aside from society, my norms, my goals are so different. I am a good person, not normal. Some have called me a beatnik but this is not quite applicable. What I fear so much is that this impulse to kill is becoming a part of me. I want to destroy it before it destroys me. It will not be easy to destroy. I cannot set it on a table and say you have not a place in me. There's no intellectual reason for it—there may be emotional reasons, but they are in the past now and should be dead. These impulses are so much a part of me, I can't just dismiss them, that's why I'm here."

This young man suffered from a hysterical personality disorder and despite his expressed wish to kill there was no danger that he would act on his homicidal impulses.

MULTIPLE PERSONALITY

> "*Every man has three characters: that which he exhibits, that which he has, and that which he thinks he has.*"
>
> Alphonse Karr

Robert Louis Stevenson's story of Dr. Jekyll and Mr. Hyde is an example in fiction of a man with two personalities, the one good and the other evil. Stevenson described Henry Jekyll as having "every mark of capacity and kindness," whereas Edward Hyde was "shaken with inordinate anger, strung to the pitch of murder, and lusting to inflict pain." The multiple personality has two or more personalities that may differ in age, sex, sexual orientation (heterosexual or homosexual), race, cultural background, social class, outlook on life, ethical standards, sociability and other patterns of behavior. Thus one personality may be friendly, optimistic and law abiding and another personality may be gruff, cynical and frankly antisocial.

In one example the primary personality, "the square," is shy, sensitive, polite, passive and highly conventional. The second personality, "the lawyer," is purely intellectual, rational and without emotion. He enjoys twisting words, engaging in debate, talking his way out of difficulties, and getting what he wants by legal means. The third personality, "the lover," is pleasure oriented, a glib talker and quite a ladies' man. He smiles frequently and radiates a certain warmth and charm. The fourth personality, "the warrior," is a cold, belligerent, angry, sullen person, occasionally sarcastic, and quick to respond to any threat in an intimidating manner (5).

The original, birth or primary personality usually has no knowledge of the secondary, alternate, or subpersonalities, but is aware of lost periods of time. Subpersonalities may be aware of each other. Change from one personality to another may be preceded by stress or headache and is often sudden and dramatic. It can also occur under hypnosis. Claims have been made that the original personality and subpersonalities have different brain wave (EEG) patterns but Spanos, et al. point out that the results are far from clear or consistent, furthermore in one study a patient who simulated different personalities produced even more marked between personality EEG differences than did patients with multiple personality (8).

The disorder has been attributed to childhood physical or sexual abuse and onset is usually in childhood or adolescence. Multiple personality was formerly regarded as a rare disorder but many cases have been reported recently and psychiatrists in a University Department of Psychiatry have claimed a 10 percent incidence among psychiatric inpatients and outpatients (2). Thigpen and Cleckley, authors of **The Three Faces of Eve,** a book on a multiple personality, have expressed concern about the recent claims of a high incidence of this disorder. After publication of their book many persons called them on the telephone, each personality identifying itself in a different voice. In letters each personality would write a section in its own unique handwriting.

In the twenty-five years since publication of the book, the authors have examined hundreds of patients who were thought to have this disorder, either by therapists or by the patients themselves, yet they found only one patient with a genuine multiple personality. They pointed out that many people who claim to have a multiple personality appear to be motivated (either consciously or unconsciously) by a desire to draw attention to themselves or to avoid responsibility for certain actions. They expressed concern about the use of multiple personality as a defense against prosecution for major crimes.

If a murder is committed by a subpersonality, should the primary personality, who claims no knowledge of the murder, be held responsible for the crime? An English judge told a defendant, who claimed that he had two personalities, that both personalities would have to go to jail. Such robust common sense is unlikely to be found in every courtroom. It is easy to fake multiple personality. An accused murderer can conceal the fact that he has read **The Three Faces of Eve** or other books on the subject, deny any knowledge of the murder, and later tell a psychiatrist, perhaps under hypnosis, that he has several personalities, one of whom raped and killed twelve women.

Kenneth Bianchi, the Hillside Strangler, provides an example of the simulation of multiple personality to avoid punishment. In 1977 and 1978 the nude bodies of ten women who had been raped, bound or handcuffed and strangled, were found on various hillsides in Los Angeles County. In 1979 two young women were raped and strangled in Bellingham, Washington. Bianchi was arrested and at first said he had alibis for the Bellingham murders, but these alibis could not be confirmed. The defense attorney, requesting an examination by Dr. John Watkins, raised the possibility that there might be another "part" of Mr. Bianchi.

Under hypnosis Bianchi responded to Dr. Watkins' request to speak to another "part," of Ken by revealing "Steve" who took credit for the two Bellingham killings and also implicated himself, and his adoptive cousin, Angelo Buono, in the Hillside Strangler killings. He was able to provide details which only the guilty person would have known. After hypnosis Bianchi continued to claim innocence and disclaimed knowledge of Steve. Dr. Watkins diagnosed multiple personality and one week later the defense entered a plea of not guilty by reason of insanity (6).

Five experts found Bianchi insane. Watkins, Allison and Markman diagnosed multiple personality and Lunde diagnosed extremely severe dissociative reaction bordering on psychosis. (Multiple personality is one of the dissociative disorders.) Two experts found Bianchi sane. Faerstein diagnosed sociopathic personality and Orne diagnosed antisocial personality (10).

A search of Bianchi's apartment revealed fourteen books on psychology including a book on hypnosis. Bianchi had seen the film **Three Faces of Eve** and may have seen the film **Sybil** in his cell shortly before the interview with Dr. Watkins. These films provided information on amnesia and the sudden shifts in behavior in multiple personality.

Furthermore police investigators on learning that Bianchi had used the name Steve Walker under hypnosis, wondered whether Bianchi knew a Steve Walker. He did indeed. Bianchi misrepresenting himself as a psychologist, had placed an advertisement in the **Los Angeles Times** requesting psychologists seeking employment to send him their college transcripts. Steven Walker did so and Bianchi, using the name Steve Walker, wrote to the college requesting new diplomas except for his name. He explained that he had retained a calligrapher to print his name in a fancy script of his choice. He requested that the diplomas should be sent to Thomas Steven Walker, c/o Mrs. K. Bianchi. After obtaining the blank diplomas, he had a calligrapher affix "Kenneth A. Bianchi" to them (6).

Bianchi's credibility is surely further damaged by the fact that he requested his mother and another woman to provide alibis for him. A young woman who had become interested in him and visited him in prison attempted the murder of another woman in the style of the Hillside Strangler. After her arrest she admitted that this had been discussed with Bianchi and was an attempt to show that the killer was still at large (6).

Psychological tests were administered to Kenneth Bianchi and to "Steve" in an attempt to authenticate the presence of different autonomous personalities. Psychologists interpreted the test results to both support and refute the claim of multiple personality. Orne believes that the data did not support this diagnosis. Spanos, et al. in 1985 asked college students to play the role of Harry who had been accused of brutally killing three women. Despite much evidence of guilt, a not guilty plea had been entered and a psychiatric evaluation had been requested. The students were asked to role play Harry throughout the psychiatric interview that might involve hypnosis.

Some students were "hypnotized" through a fake hypnotic induction and were asked almost the identical questions which were put to Bianchi in the interview in which "Steve" confessed to the murders. "I've talked a bit to Harry but I think there might be another part of Harry that I haven't talked to." Most of these students adopted a different name, had post-hypnotic amnesia and displayed other major signs of multiple personality. The two different personalities performed very differently on psychological tests. Students who were not "hypnotized" did not claim another personality (8).

Orne, et al. have provided a long review of the evidence that Bianchi was simulating multiple personality and that the correct diagnosis was sociopathic personality. Bianchi who was working as a security guard planned the murders in Washington, he told another guard that he would patrol the area that included the house where the murders occurred, he called one of the victims and told her he would pay her $100 to watch the house for two hours while a burglar alarm was being repaired but to tell no one about this for security reasons, he called on the telephone to say that he would not be attending a meeting of the sheriff's reserve that night, and he made other preparations for the murder. One of the victims told her boyfriend about the $100 payment and when she disappeared Bianchi became a suspect.

Bianchi entered a plea of guilty to the two murders in Bellingham, Washington and to five of the murders in Los Angeles. As part of a plea bargain to escape the death penalty he agreed to testify against his cousin, Angelo Buono. After a trial that took 345 days during two years, Buono was found guilty of nine murders. Both were sentenced to life imprisonment. In Los Angeles posing as police officers, they stopped women in the street, handcuffed them, raped them in the back of their car, strangled them and then dumped the bodies on hillsides.

Bianchi was adopted at the age of three months. Urinary incontinence was a problem in childhood and his mother took him to numerous urologists in search of a physical cause. Psychotherapy was recommended but was rejected by his mother. When she went to work a neighbor took care of him and the urinary problems disappeared. His mother was a domineering woman and a University of Rochester psychiatrist reported "The impression is gained that this mother is herself a seriously disturbed person, and her discussion about the handling of the child by various medical men indicates some apparent paranoid trends. It is apparent that she has been strongly controlling toward this boy, keeping him out of school very frequently, particularly in the last several months because of her fear that he would develop a sore throat and begin to wet" (7). His father died when he was thirteen.

There were reports that he was an habitual liar and that he killed a cat and dog. His wish was to become a police officer but he was only able to obtain work as a security guard. Criminal activity included shoplifting, use of stolen credit cards, sale of drugs, pimping of juvenile prostitutes and impersonating a California Highway Patrolman.

The murders began during his common-law wife's pregnancy during which he did not have sexual relations with her. His first wife commented regarding their sexual relations, "And after we did have sex I always think he looked at me as a little soiled, you know. I don't think he got any pleasure out of it at all. It was more of a once in a while duty."

THE SCHIZOID PERSONALITY

The schizoid personality is a shy, aloof, distant person who often lives alone, avoids social relationships and is preoccupied with his private world of daydreams and fantasies. He is very sensitive and is quick to interpret commonplace comments or actions of others as evidence of rejection or criticism. Yet people see him as "cold," lacking in tender feelings and indifferent to praise or criticism. Some schizoid personalities may become schizophrenic and before the appearance of the psychotic illness their behavior may be odd or bizarre.

The male schizoid personality is uncomfortable in the presence of women, seldom goes out with girls and rarely marries. Yet he may collect pornographic magazines and have great curiosity about women's bodies. The schizoid murderer will remove the underclothing of his female victim and possibly place some object in her vagina, but is unlikely to have sexual relations with her. He may also stab his victim repeatedly and mutilate her body. Following the crime he may leave his job and move to another city. Ultimately his remorse over the murder may lead him to confess to the police as in the following example.

An unknown man telephoned the Denver Police radio dispatcher to report that he had killed a woman in her downtown hotel room. Police officers found that an eighty-five year old woman had been strangled with an electrical appliance cord, which was looped tightly around her neck. Her pajama top had been pulled up above her breasts and a pair of scissors had been forced up to the hinge in her chest. Numerous pills were scattered on her chest and on the floor. Her pajama bottoms had been removed and were wrapped around her right foot. A peeled banana was on the floor between her thighs near her crotch. She had not been raped. There were no signs of forcible entry into her room.

Three days later a twenty-nine year old single laborer, who lived at the same hotel as the victim, appeared at the police building and confessed that he had committed the crime. Following his plea of insanity I examined him. He said that most of the people in the hotel were senior citizens without a family and he wanted to do something nice for them. "I took a rose, knocked on the door, she opened the door, I think she smiled, said something, I don't know what it was. She took the chain off the lock and I went in. I said something, I don't know what I said, I think we talked for a couple of seconds or so. Something was said and she started screaming.

"I put my hand over her mouth, told her I didn't want to hurt her, if she was quiet I'd let her go. I think she struggled and fell on the floor. My hand was still on her mouth and she was making more noise. I think I started choking her. She kept making more noise, I think I kept choking her . . . I dumped something in the bathtub I don't know what it was . . . I think I found some pills in a bottle. I think I dumped them out but I can't remember. There were some bananas . . . I thought about eating but I changed my mind and I threw them on her legs. I'm not sure if I was sick before or after. I was real sick."

He took the key to her room and left but returned later, put a cord around her neck and stabbed her because he was afraid she would wake up and tell the police who choked her. In addition to telephoning the police department he also called the fire department and a local television station. He left Denver and stayed in a city about thirty miles away. "I thought about leaving the state but I knew eventually it would catch up to me. I thought it was better if I gave up."

Lady Macbeth tortured by guilt over the murder of King Duncan complained "What will these hands ne'er be clean . . . Here's the smell of blood still. All the perfumes of Arabia will not sweeten this little hand" (**Macbeth** Act V Scene 1 Shakespeare). In like manner this man told me "My hands had the smell of death. I'd wash my hands, it didn't make any difference. You could smell the death on my hands, sometimes you could taste it too."

It is perhaps significant that after his arrest he did not hear from his mother or his stepfather. His father visited him once briefly in the jail and his stepmother visited him only long enough to obtain the name of his attorney. His parents, prior to their separation, did not get along well together and his father, a long distance truck driver, was frequently away from home for three to four days at a time. He was whipped three times by his stepfather, but one whipping with a two by four left bruises on his legs for many weeks. There was other violence in the home and he commented "The way I was raised had a lot to do with (my) being a loner."

As a child he was afraid of the dark and used to stutter. Because of a learning difficulty he was placed in a special school which he attended until he left school in the ninth grade. He also had difficulty studying during his basic training in the Navy and he needed an extra two months to complete the course. After his discharge from the Navy he worked in laboring jobs in restaurants, on oil fields and ranches. Usually he would leave a job after two or three months.

A shy lonely person, he had few close friends. he never went with women because he never knew what to say to them. Occasionally, as on the day of the murder, he would drink a lot of beer. His only prior offense was stealing a truck and some rifles while working on a sheep ranch, because he was angry at his employer over the working conditions and poor pay. He pleaded guilty to second degree murder and was sentenced to twenty years in the penitentiary.

REFERENCES

1. Allison, R.B.: Difficulties diagnosing the multiple personality syndrome in a death penalty case. *Int J Clin Exp Hypnosis, 32*:102, 1984.
2. Bliss, E.L. and Jeppsen, E.A.: Prevalence of multiple personality among inpatients and outpatients. *Amer J Psychiat, 142*:250, 1985.
3. Greenacre, P.: Conscience in the psychopath. *Am J Ortho Psychiat, 15*:495, 1945,
4. Guttmacher, M.S.: *The Mind of the Murderer.* New York, Farrar, Strauss and Cudahy, 1960.
5. Ludwig, A.M., *et al.*: The objective study of a multiple personality. *Arch Gen Psychiat, 26*:298, 1972.
6. Orne, M.T., *et al.*: On the differential diagnosis of multiple personality in the forensic context. *Int J Clin Exp Hypnosis, 32*:118, 1984.
7. Schwarz, Ted: *The Hillside Strangler: A Murderer's Mind.* New York, Doubleday and Company, 1981.
8. Spanos, N.P., *et al.*: Multiple personality: a social psychological perspective. *J Abnorm Psychol, 94*:362, 1985.
9. Thigpen, C.H. and Cleckley, H.M.: On the incidence of multiple personality disorder. *Int J Clin Exp Hypnosis, 32*:63, 1984.
10. Watkins, J.G.: The Bianchi case, sociopath or multiple personality: *Int J Clin Exp Hypnosis, 32*:67, 1984.

CHAPTER 11

CHILDREN AND ADOLESCENTS WHO KILL

"The unloved cannot love."

William Blake

A CURLY-HEADED youngster aged two years and a half was the petted darling of his parents until a second arrival appeared on the scene to dispute his way. After forebearing for a month the partial loss of attention and affection that ensued, he resolved to put an end to a state of affairs which was to him unendurable. Left alone with the baby girl one day, he seized a bronze statuette and battered it in her face, causing a fracture of the skull and immediate death. A verdict to this effect was returned by the jury, and it is worthy of notice that the boy — his troubles being over — has regained his customary cheerfulness and exhibits no remorse whatever. Indeed, he constantly expresses gladness that the baby has gone.

Cases of this kind, as Ernest Jones points out, are by no means as rare as a casual newspaper reader is apt to suppose. He also cites the case of a little girl, aged two, being very jealous of her baby brother, four months old, got a large knife and cut his throat with it. The first infant murderer lived in New York, the second in Finestere, France.

A seven year old boy drowned another boy in order to obtain possession of a cheap toy. The death was at first attributed to an accident but later the boy confessed the deed and this was confirmed by another boy who had been present during the act.

Adults find it difficult to believe that a child would commit murder and painstaking criminal investigation may be neglected when the assailant is a child. There are many cases on record where deaths from drowning or shooting were falsely attributed to accidental causes. A young boy becomes enraged with his playmate and shoots him to death. He tearfully explains that he was playing cops and robbers and did not know the gun was loaded. The explanation is accepted without question and the truth only comes to light if the boy spontaneously confesses the truth.

Burt quotes the case of a country girl of five, having one day with great interest watched her father slaughtering a sheep; said to her younger brother afterwards, "Let's play killing baa lambs," and making him lie on the floor, proceeded to slash his throat from ear to ear, so that he died.

The **Petit Parisien** reports the case of a boy of nine who lured a little girl of six to the river bank and deliberately pushed her in. She was rescued and the boy was confined to his room for three or four days as punishment. When, however, the first opportunity for escape occurred, he did precisely the same thing with a baby girl of three, and was seen from a distance enjoying himself by gloating over his drowning victim and repulsing her feeble attempts at regaining the bank. This time he was sentenced to a reformatory, to remain there until the age of sixteen.

Havelock Ellis described a girl of twelve condemned to eight years imprisonment for the murder of a playmate by pushing her out of a window in order to take her earrings and sell them for cakes. Previously, she would torture her school fellows, stick forks in the eyes of rabbits and afterward slit open their bellies. She showed and expressed no remorse.

The following three children who committed murder were examined by the author. The victims included a mother, father and brother of the slayers.

AB, an eleven year old farm boy, on waking at a quarter to five one morning, carried out a plan which he had confided the previous day to a younger brother. He armed himself with his father's rifle, opened the door of his parent's bedroom and from a distance of eight to ten feet he aimed the rifle at his father's head, held his breath and pulled the trigger. After replacing the rifle he returned to bed and calmly informed his brothers "I shot daddy." His father died without regaining consciousness before the arrival of the ambulance.

The family was questioned at length about the shooting and it was not until his third interview with the police that AB confessed. His mother had a "hunch" that AB had shot his father because he seemed so unconcerned about his father's death. In explanation of the killing he said that he was angry because his father had mistreated him.

"He wouldn't help us with the chores. He'd say he might be down pretty soon but he'd just stay inside and listen to the radio. He wouldn't let me go anywhere, wouldn't let me go to town with him after I worked real hard. He hurt my feelings a lot. I said to myself I had enough beatings. I walked in and shot him."

AB complained that his father would not let him have a young calf which had been offered to him by a 4-H club. Money earned by working for neighbors was taken from him and his only allowance was twenty-five to fifty cents a year. There were few toys and he had to forego school lunches to save enough money to buy himself a pocketknife. He expressed no remorse for his action and mentioned without apparent concern that he might go to the electric chair.

On the poverty stricken farm AB had been expected to do the work of a man. A very self-possessed boy, who kept the hospital staff at a distance, he seemed to have a need to demonstrate that he could do anything expected of a man. He answered questions in an impersonal fashion and he revealed his thoughts and feelings only to a very limited extent. Of dull intelligence he had a poor vocabulary for his age. Brain wave tracings revealed abnormalities in both temporal areas.

After his transfer to an unlocked ward in the hospital he slipped two table knives under the door of the locked ward to a federal prisoner. The latter sharpened one of the knives and held it against the throat of an attendant while he made good his escape from custody. It was later learned that before coming to the hospital AB had while in jail helped another inmate to escape.

The court was informed that AB was unable to distinguish between good and evil with respect to the homicide. This opinion led to his acquittal and he was placed on a boys ranch. It is significant that his mother insisted on giving up all custody rights as his parent, despite advice that this action might hamper successful rehabilitation.

CD, a thirteen year old boy, played hooky from school for the first time on the day that he killed his mother. When his truancy was discovered his parents were informed and he was told to return home immediately. When he arrived home his mother scolded him and told him she would take away his rifle and make him quit his job as a shoe shine boy. The rifle, which was his prize possession, had been given to him by his grandparents. CD became very upset and rushed to the closet where his rifle was hanging. He loaded it with one of three shells he had in his pocket.

As he was running out of the house to hide his rifle, he was startled by the sudden appearance of his mother from the bathroom. Impulsively he attempted to frighten her by pointing the gun at her. It was not his intention to shoot her, however he fired at her from a distance of about twelve feet. He was unable to give an explanation for pulling the trigger. She screamed and fell mortally wounded to the floor. Although she was unconscious, if not already dead, CD reloaded the rifle and shot his mother at close range in the head below the right ear "so that she could not do anything to me." After reloading the rifle he locked his six year old brother and four year old sister in a room and left the house. He rang a school friend asking him to go to a hotel with his .22 caliber pistol.

This friend in his statement to the police said, "On the way to the hotel CD told me he had shot his mother and we had to leave town fast. We had made plans about two months ago about how we might leave town in the event of any trouble with the police. We planned to go to a hotel and watch for a salesman and when he got in his car I would slide in the front seat and CB in the back. I would point a gun at him and force him to drive to Albuquerque, then knock him out and throw him out of the car."

CD was arrested in the hotel. He showed very little emotion over the death of his mother, apart from a short period of tears and, refusing to sign a statement, he asked to see a lawyer. On admission to the hospital for psychiatric examination, he was at first rather quiet and reserved but later he became much more outgoing. He continued to show little emotion over the death of his mother.

His school record was excellent. His teacher reported that he always sat right in front of her desk and was one of her best pupils. At school he preferred to play with boys several years younger than himself. Despite his reputation as a well-behaved obedient child, he had been shoplifting for two years and had stolen a radio from an appliance store. One of the reasons for his stealing was the need to prove to his friend that he was not a coward. He admitted to fantasies of becoming a big time gangster. Several times after reading gangster stories he had thoughts of killing his parents, but he quickly dispelled these thoughts from his mind.

In talking about his home life CD said that his father was very strict and complained that he was usually blamed, often unjustly, for things his younger brother had done. He described his mother as being fussy and over-protective; for example, she would drive him to school although it was only a couple of blocks from his home. She made him bake cakes and do other chores usually reserved for girls. He was ashamed of these duties and deeply resented them. The sleeping arrangements were unusual in that the parents took turns to sleep in the boys' room.

The year before the tragedy his tonsils were removed and he was circumcised. The latter operation was done at the request of his mother who had not permitted the operation when he was an infant because she thought it was cruel. CD was afraid before the operation that the surgeon might "goof" and cut his throat. After the operation his mother applied ointment three times a day to his genitals. CD particularly resented his mother doing this and after she hurt him on one occasion he insisted on taking care of himself.

This boy wished to be dependent upon and close to his mother, but coexisting wishes to be independent aroused conflict and great anger toward his mother. Her unwitting seductive behavior and her encouragement of a passive feminine role in her son added to his hostility. Her threat to deprive him of his rifle and job, and all that they stood for, converted his fantasies of homicide into action.

On being informed that CD was unable to distinguish between good and evil, the court arranged for the boy to be sent to a charitable institution for boys.

EF, an eleven year old boy, walked stealthily into the living room of his home where his fifteen year old brother was watching television. He pointed the rifle at the back of his brother's head and shot him. Then he enlisted the aid of an older and a younger stepbrother in cleaning up the blood and dressing the victim. All three put the dead brother on a sled with the intention of dumping him in a nearby river. However they noticed a man was following them so they dumped the body in some weeds and covered it over with weeds.

EF expressed no grief at having killed his brother, rather he boasted about his deed and said he would do it again if he had the chance. The shooting occurred while both parents were out of the house, after the victim had slapped his younger brother for not bringing him his clothes when ordered to do so. EF went outside to get his brother's shoes. On the porch he noticed the .22 caliber rifle and he decided to "get" his brother, who had been picking on him and bullying him for some time.

The boy's mother died two months after his birth and for a time he was looked after by an aunt. His father thought that he was neglected and a physician told the father that the boy was undernourished. When his father remarried the boy went back to live with him. About two years before the tragedy EF began getting into trouble at school and was suspended on two occasions. He was arrested by the police after he had broken into a grocery store to steal some candy. The father worked on the railroad and was frequently absent from home for five to six days at a time. The mother also worked and the children saw comparatively little of their parents.

While in the hospital EF had many angry outbursts. On one occasion when he got into an argument with an older patient, he proclaimed to the whole ward that he was in the hospital on a charge of first degree murder, and he was going to kill this particular patient when he got out. A brain wave tracing showed abnormal waves (14 per second).

Although EF spoke without remorse about the killing, it was considered that he was attempting to defend himself against great fear and anxiety by adopting a callous indifferent attitude. A very striking painting which he made while in the hospital showed a murderer standing alongside the body of his victim. The murderer, in the form of the devil, is strikingly portrayed in vivid colors: red, yellow and black. His hands, or rather claws, are dripping with blood, and red lines entering the body indicate the trajectory of cannon shells fired from two black jet planes in the sky overhead.

This boy was committed to a state mental hospital by the court after psychiatric testimony was presented that he could not be held responsible for his behavior.

ADOLESCENTS WHO KILL

Thirteen to sixteen year old homicide offenders include antisocial youths who kill in the course of an armed robbery or other felony. Resistance to armed robbery through fight, flight, cries for help or refusal to hand over money may have fatal consequences for the victim. Adolescents who murder strangers are significantly more likely to have a history of poor impulse control, aggressive behavior, previous arrests and sentences to training schools than adolescents who kill their parents (5). Antisocial youths may also kill members of rival street gangs to gain status within their gang, in defense of their own lives in a street fight, or in revenge for theft, prior injury or loss of face.

Adolescents without a prior history of antisocial or delinquent behavior may kill parents who have physically abused them. Often these offenders are unusually well behaved and appear to be mature beyond their years. They anticipate the needs of adults, show a respect for authority and can be relied upon to complete tasks assigned to them. They do well in school despite adverse conditions in the home, work regularly in part-time jobs outside school hours, in addition to performing household chores and taking care of younger brothers and sisters. They may kill in order to protect their mother or a sibling from physical or sexual assault by father. The mother they protect may also be physically abusive.

There is a pseudo-maturity in these adolescents. Their compliant behavior is designed to protect themselves from further beatings. They are committed to "looking good" and their helpful actions are not spontaneous and heartfelt. Their lack of empathy and their arrogant holier than thou attitude contribute to the difficulty they have in forming close relationships with others. After killing father they assume even more of a paternal role in the family and tend to show the same irritable impatience, and expectation of immediate obedience as the dead tyrant. For example one youth shared his dead father's fear that his sister might be sexually molested by male students at her high school. He tried to impose quite unreasonable limits on her relationships and activities and became very angry with her when she did not observe his rules.

The situation is not made easier by the failure of mother, brothers, and sisters to show gratitude for his getting rid of father. Indeed there may even be criticism and expression of regret that father is no longer with them. Treatment may be further complicated if there is an incestuous attachment to mother, even though there may not have been any frank sexual activity. One father encouraged his fifteen year old son, who was later to kill him, to sleep with his mother, saying that he wanted no other female to take his son's virginity. Once when his wife said she was going to leave him he told her "Take your dirty son with you" and he told his son "You want to sleep with Mommy all by yourself?"

Parental sexual abuse of an adolescent may also lead to murder. The love that kills is incestuous love (9). A fourteen year old youth who killed his mother eventually revealed that he had sexual relations with her on her initiative about once a month. She was separated from her husband. The killing was unusually brutal and prolonged. Patricide by a daughter is rare. Antony and Rizzo reported the case of a fifteen year old girl who shot and killed her violent and seductive father.

He had sexual relations with three of his four daughters as well as his son "from behind." Two daughters, including the one who killed her father, had been made pregnant. He terminated one pregnancy with a television antenna. The other pregnancy resulted in a full-term baby that father drowned two hours after birth. Mother helped bury this baby in a field near the home. Father was killed after he accused his daughters of having sexual relations with men at a drive-in theater. He took them home and following an argument he started to strangle one daughter and another daughter shot him (1).

Killing of mother may occur when a sexually immature but homosexually oriented son, is trapped in a dependent but hostile relationship with a possessive mother (4).

A parent may encourage a child to kill the other parent. Malmquist gives the example of a fifteen year old youth who shot and killed his stepfather. The youth had seen his mother beaten many times when his father was intoxicated. On the occasion of the homicide, the father had gone outside mumbling he wanted a piece of wood with which to beat his wife. During his brief absence, the boy's mother sat down next to him on a couch and, laying a pistol down between them, stated: "I know you're big enough to protect me now" (8).

A man, divorced from his wife, had the delusion that he was Jesus Christ. He had the fixed idea that he would die at the hands of his children when he was thirty-three and a half years old, the age at which he believed Jesus was crucified. One of his sons shot and fatally wounded him on the day he became thirty-three and a half years of age. Sargent suggested that the father, in order to fulfill the requirements of his religious delusion, managed to commit suicide by provoking his son to kill him. Sargent also suggested that the boy's mother planted the idea in his mind that she would not be unhappy if his father were dead.

Bender has personally examined thirty-one boys and two girls who have been responsible, or have been considered by themselves or others to be responsible for the death of another person. Fifteen of these thirty-three children had psychiatric examinations, before the death occurred. These examinations pointed out severe abnormality and forecast dangerous behavior. In the majority of these cases there had been recommendations which had not been followed.

Danger signs consisted of some combination of the following: 1) Organic brain damage with an impulse disorder, and abnormal brain waves and epilepsy. 2) Childhood schizophrenia with preoccupations with death and killing or sociopathic behavior. 3) Compulsive firesetting. 4) Reading disability. 5) Extremely unfavorable home conditions and life experiences. 6) A personal experience with violent death.

Six children caused death by fires. Among the twenty-seven children who caused death by some means other than fire, there were eight who were compulsive firesetters, including all five who were associated with a death by drowning. The group examined by Bender included three mental defectives, three epileptics and twelve schizophrenics.

REFERENCES

1. Antony, E.J. and Rizzo, A.: Adolescent girls who kill or try to kill their fathers. In Antony, E.J. and Koupernik, C. (Eds.): *The Child in His Family*. New York, John Wiley and Sons, 1973.
2. Bender, Lauretta: Children and adolescents who have killed. *Amer J Psychiat, 116*:510, 1960.
3. Burt, C.: *The Young Delinquent*. London, Univ. of London Press, 1944.
4. Chiswick, Derek: Matricide. *Brit Med J, 283*:1279, 1981.
5. Corder, B.F., *et al.*: Adolescent parricide: a comparison with other adolescent murder. *Amer J Psychiat, 133*:957, 1976.
6. Ellis, Havelock: *Studies in the Psychology of Sex*. Philadelphia, F.A. Davis Company, 1927.
7. Jones, Ernest: Infant murderers. *Brit J Dis Children, 1*:510, 1904.
8. Malmquist, C.P.: Premonitory signs of homicidal aggression in juveniles. *Amer J Psychiat, 128*:461, 1971.
9. Rubinstein, L.H.: The theme of Electra and Orestes. *Brit J Med Psychol, 42*:99, 1969.
10. Sadoff, R.L.: Children who kill. In Danto, B.L., *et al.* (Eds.): *The Human Side of Homicide*. New York, Univ. of Columbia Press, 1982.
11. Sargent, Douglas: Children who kill—a family conspiracy. *Social Work, 7*:35, 1962.

CHAPTER 12

SELF-MURDER

*"We have long known, that no neurotic is preoccupied
with suicide, who has not turned back towards
himself, a murderous impulse against others."*

Freud, *Mourning and Melancholia*

MEN FEAR death as children fear to go in the dark (Bacon). It is the greatest fear which besets the life of man yet some persons actively seek death. One can commit suicide in order not to be tortured by the fear of death. Suicide is not often the subject of inquiry. One reason for the relative dearth of research is that "dead men tell no tales." Another reason is that there is a strong unconscious resistance to consideration of this subject. Many well-known psychiatrists have committed suicide. Thus, it is given to these men to direct the lives of others, yet they have failed in the direction of their own lives.

The problem is a serious one, suicide in the United States stands tenth among the leading causes of death, and accounts for more than 27,000 deaths each year. Few persons are not touched in their lifetime by this phenomenon. If it does not occur among one's family or friends it is heard of through acquaintances or their families (4). Karl Menninger in **Man Against Himself** states that in the end each man kills himself in his own selected way, fast or slow, soon or late. This is an extreme viewpoint, but it serves to focus attention on such forms of chronic suicide as asceticism and martyrdom, alcohol addiction and unconsciously purposive accidents.

"Historically suicide has been known in all eras of written history, though the practice has been far more common in some cultures than in others. In primitive society suicide was unknown in some groups but fairly common in others. In one group among the Caroline Islanders the thought of suicide had simply never occurred to the group, and when it was explained to them they responded in effect, 'Ridiculous!' Among American Indians certain tribes had a high rate of suicide—in others it was unknown. Among the Navajo Indians, a war-like tribe, the practice was frequent, while among the Zunis, a peace-loving tribe which lived in an adjacent valley, the practice was unknown. Some primitives were indifferent to suicide while others considered it a serious sin. Among the Dakota Indians it was believed that a woman who committed suicide by hanging, which was the common method of suicide, would have to drag the tree on which she hanged herself through the lands of the Spirits forever. It therefore became a common practice for Dakota women to choose the smallest possible tree that would support them in their suicide attempts. Among the Eskimos suicide has a utilitarian factor. In old age suicide is common in order to decrease the burden of support on the younger members of the group.

"In the Orient suicide is condoned by most religions. Among the Hindus widows commonly were expected to commit suicide, a practice known as Suttee. In both India and China the practice of widows committing suicide was most prevalent among the wealthy class possibly because the practice prevented women from inheriting wealth. In India Suttee was outlawed in the nineteenth century. The Mohammedans are violently opposed to suicide, and the practice is proscribed in the Koran although it is not condemned in the Bible. In Jewish history suicide was rare until very recent times. The Old Testament theme of sacredness of life possibly played so strong an emphasis on the positive aspect of living that no thought was given to suicide. In fact there are only four instances of suicide mentioned in the Old Testament. The first was that of Samson when he pulled down the temple. The second was that of Saul and his armor bearer when he saw that he was about to be defeated and pled with his armor bearer to kill him, without success. The third was the case of Abimelech, who when hit on the head by a stone thrown by a woman during an attack, killed himself so that it could not be said that he was slain by a woman. And finally that of Ahithophel who, when Absalom rejected his counsel to march on King David, set his house in order and hanged himself. All of the examples were apparently pardonable suicides as no reprimand is set down in the Bible, and each received a ritual burial.

"The early Christian Church did not condemn suicide, for many early Christians committed suicide to avoid torture, and this was condoned as martyrdom. It was not until the time of St. Augustine that suicide was denounced as a sin under all circumstances, and by the fifth century suicide was condemned by ecclesiastical law. In St. Thomas Acquinas' time suicide became a crime as well as a sin. During the Middle Ages the practice of suicide was considered so reprehensible that barbaric practices were carried out on the corpses of suicides" (Robert D. Wright).

In England until abolished by statute in 1823 it was customary to bury suicides at four crossroads with a stake driven through the body. Instead it was ordered that the body be buried privately in a churchyard or other burial ground, without any stake being driven through the body, between nine and twelve at night and without religious rites. This act was repealed in 1880. Suicide and attempted suicide ceased to be criminal acts in England in 1961.

Some nations have much higher suicide rates than others. Thus the suicide rate in Denmark is over five times that of the Republic of Ireland. The present rate in the United States is about twelve suicides per 100,000 population each year. More men than women commit suicide but more women than men attempt suicide. Suicide is more than three times as frequent in men than it is in women. It has been estimated that about 10 percent of persons who attempt suicide eventually kill themselves. Suicide rates are higher in persons over fifty-five years of age.

In recent years there has been an increase in the number of suicides among adolescents and young adults. Younger children from four to eight years of age usually run into traffic, hang themselves or jump from high places. They seldom leave notes. Older children take drugs or poison, slash their wrists, shoot themselves or use other methods.

The greatest number of suicides occur not in winter as might be expected, but in the spring and early summer. Suicides are most common in May and least common in December. People are most likely to take their own lives on Monday and least likely on Saturday. Within each month, except February, suicides are most frequent around the fifth of the month and least frequent in the last days of the month. MacMahon found these patterns in a review of suicides reported in the United States for the years 1972 to 1978. There was no relationship between the number of suicides and the phases of the moon. The suicide rate falls during time of war and usually rises sharply when the war is over, after which the rate returns to the prewar level. The figures may be misleading as suicide in battle is likely to pass unnoticed. The suicide rate among white persons is twice that found among Blacks.

Professional men and businessmen have a higher suicide rate than men in lower socio-economic groups. Gainsburg believes that poverty becomes an important factor in suicide according to its context. The indigenous poor, to whom poverty is an accepted feature of their position in society tolerate it with equanimity. This attitude does not foster suicide. A change from comparative affluence to poverty, or loss of employment, is however, more disruptive, since the person affected often fails to adjust himself to his altered circumstances.

High density of population, employment in industry and residence in large towns contribute to a higher rate of suicide. Zorbaugh studied those living in furnished rooms. He describes how the entire population of these rooming-house areas changes every few months. The population includes a disproportionate number of single males, and few children, and is largely made up of "white collar" workers, students and shopgirls. He stresses the anonymity and loneliness of these people; their cursory relationships and the way in which this isolated, unsupervised mode of life leads to irresponsible and egregious behavior. He quotes from the biographies of some of these people poignant extracts which emphasize the forlornness and dejection of their existence; their thwarted emotional outlets, compensating fantasies and, ultimately, the trend of their thoughts toward suicide. In Chicago, suicides are more common in these districts than anywhere else. In fact, the desperate authorities demolished a bridge adjoining one "rooming house" district, so regularly was it used for the purpose through which it acquired its name—"Suicide Bridge."

Loneliness and enforced idleness contribute to suicide. Elderly single women are however less prone to suicide than childless widows. Permanent emotional ties, the married state and a large number of children reduce the risk. Divorced persons commit suicide much more frequently than either married, widowed or single persons.

There is a common misconception that psychosis is one of the most frequent causes of suicide. Only about one in five suicides is the result of psychosis. A Metropolitan Life Insurance Company study of 2,000 suicides attributed 18 percent to the presence of psychosis. Several psychiatric studies give a figure of approximately 20 percent.

Robins in his study of 134 deaths from suicide in St. Louis, Missouri found that 94 percent of the suicides had a mental illness. Almost 50 percent were depressed in the months before their deaths and 25 percent suffered from alcoholism. Four percent had organic brain disorder and 2 percent were schizophrenic. Four subjects (3 percent) committed homicides and 3 subjects (2 percent) attempted to murder someone, before taking their own lives.

Awareness of physical and mental decline is an important factor. Persons commit suicide more frequently on account of anticipated suffering than because of actual suffering, however severe. Thus man seems to be more capable of adjusting to physical pain than to anticipating dread of it. In malignant or incurable illness, the two most critical periods with regard to suicide seem to be that of uncertainty, while diagnosis and prognosis are still at issue, and that of shock following the first realization of the upheavals and suffering, true or fancied, that are to follow. Once the patient has settled into the routine of chronic illness, suicidal thoughts tend to disappear from the picture. The suicide rate is lowest in men of normal weight. Persons who are under or overweight show excessive suicide mortality, that of the overweights being one-third above those of normal weight.

Many coroners' statistics bear out possible relationship between menstruation and suicide. One study reported thirty-nine suicides in women, with eleven occurring just before and eleven during the menstrual period, making a proportion of more than 50 percent coincidental with the event.

There is an intimate relationship between suicide and murder. This is not surprising as both are manifestations of hate and aggression. One-third of all murderers in England commit suicide. In the United States four percent of all homicide offenders kill themselves shortly after the offense (6). It has been stated that countries with a high suicide rate have a low homicide rate; countries with a low suicide rate have a high homicide rate. This relationship is not constant.

The more popular methods of suicide include hanging, shooting, drowning, poisoning and jumping in front of moving vehicles. The use of sedative or narcotic drugs has increased in popularity in recent years. I have seen a number of patients admitted to a hospital following automobile accidents who have confided that they deliberately wrecked their cars in the hope of taking their own lives. Bizarre methods are sometimes employed, particularly by psychotic patients. Persons have taken their lives by swallowing strong acids, or red hot coals, by diving into the flames of a furnace or into vats of molten iron, by throwing themselves upon revolving circular saws, by exploding dynamite in their mouths and by decapitation with homemade guillotines. In Los Angeles, a man, feeling despondent, clamped a .38 caliber automatic pistol to an ironing board, ran ten yards of gauze from the trigger to an electric mixer, suspended a heavy sash weight over his head by a thread and poured gasoline all around. He set fire to the gasoline, started the mixer, winding up the gauze and sat down before the gun under the sash weight. The sash weight failed to fall down, the bullet merely wounded him and a neighbor put out the fire. Police took him to the hospital.

A twenty-seven year old New Zealand electrician used a foolproof suicide machine to kill himself with six bullets in the heart. He was found on a platform in his home surrounded by devices that gave him no chance of survival.

Suspended above his body was an automatic .22 caliber rifle with its trigger connected to a solenoid which in turn was wired to two time clocks, two doors and an electromagnet. Police believe the machine took weeks to manufacture and gave the following reconstruction of the man's death:

The man built the platform complete with snaplocks on chains and wooden crossbars so that once he was on it he could not escape, even if he changed his mind at the last minute. Intricate and carefully installed wiring and electronic devices assured that after a lapse of time the rifle would fire six shots through a hole carefully drilled in a board above the man's heart. Two time clocks assured that, if one of the clocks failed, the other would work. Anyone entering the room also could have set off the mechanism by opening either of the two doors. If there was a power failure an electromagnet would switch off and pull the trigger.

Probably the most remarkable case on record, is described by Dublin, of the Italian shoemaker who attempted to crucify himself. He nailed two pices of wood together in the form of a cross, placed a bracket in position to hold his feet, sat down upon the lengthwise beam, nailed his feet to the bracket, and transfixed his left hand completely by a nail which had previously been driven through the arm of the cross. The right hand he could not manage to fasten, and so it hung at his side. He stripped himself with the exception of a loin cloth, put a crown of thorns upon his head, and wounded himself on the side with one of his shoe-making tools. Then by means of a pulley arrangement he managed to drag this whole contrivance out of the low windowsill of his room in such a fashion that the populace of Venice soon discovered the crucifix with its living burden suspended against the wall of the house. Since this happened at eight o'clock in the morning, it was only a few minutes before he was taken down and removed to a hospital where he slowly recovered. When asked the reason for this action by a physician who was much interested in the case and who has written it up in great detail, his only explanation was that: "The pride of man must be mortified, it must expire on the cross."

The reasons which are usually proffered to account for suicide or suicidal attempts seldom provide an adequate explanation of the self-destructive act. All too often the act is attributed to a series of family or business misfortunes and the fact that other persons exposed to similar or more severe trials and tribulations do not take their lives, is not taken into account. Karl Menninger in **Man Against Himself** suggests further investigation of the popular attitude that suicide is an escape from an intolerable life situation.

Menninger points out that the individual always, in a measure, creates his own environment, and thus the suicidal person must in some way help to create the very thing from which, in suicide, he takes flight. he adds that this is very well brought out by many novelists who have described the way in which the man who ultimately commits suicide begins his self-destruction long beforehand. The illustration given is derived from O'Hara's version of a famous legend. "A servant ran to his master in fright, saying that he had been jostled and threatened by Death in the market place and wished, therefore, to go as rapidly as possible to Samarra where Death would not find him. His master let him go and himself went to the market place and seeing Death there asked him why he had threatened the servant. To this Death replied it was not a threat but a gesture of surprise that he should see in Bagdad the man with whom he had an appointment that night in Samarra." That a person may inexorably keep a rendezvous with death even while ostensibly fleeing from it is intuitively recognized by novelists (3).

All of us harbor negative as well as positive feelings for family members and friends. The combination of a harsh conscience and marked ambivalent feelings toward a loved person may result in strong feelings of guilt upon the death of the loved person. The conscience may demand death as punishment for the forbidden hostile feelings or actions; however, the person may be unaware of the intensity of his forbidden feelings and attribute his suicidal impulses to feelings of grief.

Menninger draws attention to the fact that some persons take their lives following, not misfortune, but some sudden good fortune. "I have known men and women to become overwhelmed with depression and attempt or commit suicide immediately following a promotion, an increase in income, or a sudden realization of their importance and prestige in their community. I remember one man, who, owing in part to his good judgment and in part to some good luck, was able to make a considerable success of his bank at the same time that his competitor's bank and many other banks were failing, and he no sooner realized this fully than he became depressed and ultimately shot himself. I remember another man whose business sagacity had enabled him to succeed in a number of enterprises during the same period of economic distress who reacted the same way.

"How shall we explain this? . . . why should they become depressed and suicidal in reaction to success? Freud was the first to point out that this was the reaction to the disapproval of an overgrown 'hypertrophied' conscience. Such a man lives his entire life under the dictates of a conscience which says 'You must work; you must renounce; you must sacrifice; you must earn; you must give; you must achieve; you must deny your expectation to be blessed with gifts, with love, with an easy life. This is what you want, to be sure, but you may not have it. For you to have it means the robbing or displacing of someone else, the failure of someone else, the usurpation by you of the position once occupied by your envied baby brother or someone else in the family. This you may not have on pain of death.' "

The element of spite and punishment of others is sometimes a contributing factor. "When I'm dead they'll be sorry." Hysterical personalities make suicidal gestures to gain attention, to arouse sympathy, to frighten others into submission, or to dramatize themselves; however fatal accidents are apt to occur: leaning too far out of a window, overdosing with drugs believed to be harmless, or miscalculating the arrival of someone to shut off the gas jets may lead to a fatal outcome. Here death is an accident in a dramatic setting.

The existence of rational suicide is disputed. Sociologists regard suicide as the outcome of social forces against which the individual is powerless. The cultural attitude toward suicide no doubt influences the suicide rate. Suicide is approved in some countries and condemned in others. In some cultures suicide is demanded when the moral code is broken or under other circumstances, as for example in Japan where hara-kiri is regarded with honor.

REFERENCES

1. Dublin, L.I. and Bunzel, B.: *To Be or Not To Be.* New York, Smith and Haas, 1933.
2. MacMahon, Kathleen: Short-term temporal cycles in the frequency of suicide. *Amer J Epidem, 117:*744, 1983.

3. Menninger, K.A.: *Man Against Himself.* New York, Harcourt Brace, 1938.
4. Murphy, G.E.: Problems in studying suicide. *Psychiatric Developments,* 4:339, 1983.
5. O'Hara, John: *Appointment in Samarra.* New York, Harcourt, Brace and Company, 1934.
6. Robins, Eli: *The Final Months.* New York, Oxford University Press, 1981.
7. Wright, R.D.: Suicide—a problem in social medicine. *Neuropsychiat,* 1:4, 1951.
8. Zorbaugh, H.W.: *Gold Coast and Slum.* Chicago, University of Chicago Press, 1929.

CHAPTER 13

CRIMINAL INVESTIGATION

"It has long been an axiom of mine that the little
things are infinitely the most important."

Conan Doyle, *The Adventures of Sherlock Holmes*

THE IDEAL homicide team includes two detectives who are both expert crime scene investigators and talented interviewers. The crime scene is vital because it tells what happened and may provide the only clues. Yet these clues may be subtle and escape the notice of someone who is not a skillful, experienced detective. He has to be alert and have a quick mind because his first visit to the scene, perhaps late at night, may be his only opportunity to recognize and seize evidence. The recent trend of courts to suppress confessions, sometimes for dubious reasons, and the reluctance of juries to believe witnesses who are themselves crooks, have increased the importance of crime scene evidence in securing conviction of the guilty.

Witnesses to a homicide are not always willing informants. When the witness is related to the murderer, family loyalties may seal his mouth. In high crime areas residents often withhold information from the police. There were thirty-five persons in the **Outlaw Bar** when a woman's boyfriend shot and killed her husband. Couples were dancing alongside the body when the police arrived. Everyone in the small bar heard the shots but no one saw the shooting. Each person in the bar explained that he was in the john. The two toilets each measured five feet by five feet. Homicide suspects have compelling reasons for remaining silent. Yet all these handicaps may be overcome by a homicide detective, who has a way with words and with people.

Other members of the homicide team include the crime laboratory detectives who take photographs, look for fingerprints and collect shell casings, bullets, hairs (animal hairs can be identified as coming from a dog, cat, deer and so on; human hairs can be identified by race, body area, and whether bleached or dyed), fibers, glass, paint scrapings, cigarette butts, traces of soil and samples of blood, saliva, urine and semen for analysis and identification. The forensic pathologist estimates the time of death (some would say it is often no more than an educated guess) and through his autopsy provides evidence on the cause of death. The Behavioral Science Unit of the FBI Academy after assessment of the murder scene may be able to provide a psychological profile of the unknown suspect.

While all these experts are at work the homicide detectives are busy checking the background of the victim to determine who might benefit from his death. They also follow up information obtained from many sources including anonymous informants. Psychics are ever ready to volunteer their assistance in any unsolved killing that attracts national attention, but not every detective welcomes their clues, which are often as nebulous as their sources.

THE CRIME SCENE

"You see but you do not observe."

Conan Doyle, *The Memoirs of Sherlock Holmes*

The first police officer to arrive at the scene will check to see whether the victim is still alive and whether there are other victims or suspects in the immediate area. It is his responsibility to protect the crime scene. If the area is not immediately secured, whether by a protective tape at waist level or other barrier, the crime scene will be destroyed, altered, or contaminated by curious onlookers, police officers eager to see what is to be seen, or the criminal himself if by mischance he is brought back to the scene.

Often a fire department rescue team or paramedics arrive before the police. In their efforts to save the victim's life they may move crucial evidence. This might not be such a problem if they informed the detectives, but they depart as quickly as they arrived, without telling anyone what they found and what they did. Occasionally the good intentions of citizens serve no useful purpose, for example providing cardiopulmonary resuscitation on a victim stiff with rigor mortis.

One homicide offender claimed that he fired his pistol in self-defense after the victim attacked him with a claw hammer. But there was no claw hammer at the scene. Fortunately a police officer had noticed a fireman pick up a claw hammer and place it in the victim's truck, which was parked nearby.

A drunk, who apparently fell in an alley and suffered a fractured skull, was dead upon admission to a hospital. It was observed there that his pockets had been turned inside out. This first led the investigators to believe he had been assaulted and robbed. Later, it was discovered that the first officer at the scene had turned the subject's pockets inside out seeking identification and then failed to notify anybody about what he had done (2).

The unnecessary intrusion of police officers, not directly involved in the homicide investigation, can lead to the trampling underfoot of a bullet and the displacement or crushing of a shell casing, in both examples ruining the items for the purpose of comparison in the laboratory. The suspect's shoe prints in dust or snow may be obliterated or shoe prints that suggest the route of the suspect may be those of an officer. The fingerprints on the telephone are those of the patrol sergeant, who called his wife to say that he would be late for dinner.

Officers should try to avoid touching anything and should not move items. They should not use the telephone nor the toilet. They should not open or close curtains or windows, turn on or off lights, radio or television set and should not adjust the thermostat. If they have to open a closet to make sure that no one is inside, they should leave the closet door in the position in which they found it. If they alter the crime scene they should write a note to this effect to the homicide detective.

Many officers seem compelled to handle any firearms they see and if they change the position of the hammer or turn the cylinder of a revolver, they will be afraid to admit it later. They may say that they picked up a shotgun to see if it was loaded, or they took possession of a revolver because they were afraid a paramedic would pick it up. Firearms and other evidence should be left in place until a crime scene has been videotaped, photographed, measured and sketched. Officers stand alongside small items to protect them, or place their hats over them.

Whenever an officer confiscates an electric clock he should note in his report the exact time appearing on the clock, or preserve a record of the time by photographing the clock. In an arson-murder case the time on the clock was critical to placing the defendant on the premises at the time of the fire. Because the officer did not make a record of the time on the clock it was not possible to prove that the time on the clock was the same as when it was originally confiscated.

Officers use their experience and their eyes and are quick to notice something that seems unnatural or out of place. At an apparent burglary homicide with ransacking of the home detectives noted that a living room window had been broken in the middle, but the glass had not been removed from the lower section. Burglars do not like to climb over jagged glass. A plant had been thrown over in the living room, but it must have been tipped over gently because the earth around it was only slightly displaced. Greeting cards on a TV set were standing upright yet they fell over when the TV set was slightly jostled by the detective. Clothes in one room had been taken out of the closet and then laid on a sofa still in their hangers. It was believed that the homicide was committed by an associate of a family member who lived in the home.

Offenders who have a proprietary interest in the scene of a crime betray themselves by taking care to avoid destruction or loss of items. For example, a female tenant in an apartment house was stabbed twenty-seven times. There was no weapon near the body, but a laboratory check of a knife in the kitchen drawer tested positive for blood stains. It had been washed and replaced in the drawer after the homicide. Questioning of the apartment house manager resulted in a confession of murder.

A homicide offender may take just one item from the victim's apartment and this theft may not be apparent to the detectives. It is a good practice to ask a friend of the victim to look over the apartment to see if anything is missing. In one homicide a small radio was missing. It was a gift from a former boyfriend, who regained possession of his gift after killing his victim. The radio was found in his apartment.

The crime scene includes the suspect, the victim, the location where the body is found and the site of the homicide which may be in the next room or several miles away. After death the blood settles by gravitation in the lower parts of the body. If the victim is lying on his back there will be a purple discoloration of the skin on his back, with white patches on pressure points over the shoulder blades and buttocks. This is referred to as postmortem lividity. If the victim is found lying on his face but his back is discolored, then the body may have been moved some hours after death.

In carbon monoxide poisoning and in death due to asphyxia there may be relatively little clotting of the blood so that if the body is turned over up to twenty-four hours after death, the post-mortem lividity will slowly shift to the new dependent position. In carbon monoxide poisoning there is a cherry red discoloration of the skin.

The hardening of muscle fibers after death is one of the least reliable indicators of the time of death. Rigor mortis begins two to four hours after death and reaches a peak within four to twelve hours, but it can disappear within nine hours in a very hot environment. In cold conditions rigor mortis may persist for up to sixty hours. Once rigidity has been broken by forcible manipulation it will not reappear unless the manipulation occurred very shortly after death.

Bite Marks

Bite marks, whether on the victim or on evidence left at the scene, can lead to identification of the suspect. In a rape-murder bite marks, on a cucumber forced in the elderly victim's vagina, were used as evidence to convict her murderer. In child-battering homicides there may be both old and recent bite marks. As only a limited number of persons may have the opportunity to assault the child over a period of weeks or months, they can be asked to make bite marks in wax for a forensic odontologist to compare with pictures of the bite marks on the child.

Bite marks on victims are also found in sex-related murders (on breasts, around the vagina and on thighs in rape murders; especially on back and shoulders in homosexual murders) and in the killing of one child by another child (the assault may begin with a bite on the face). Saliva left at the location of the bite can be tested to determine the suspect's blood group. About 80 percent of the population are secretors who have in their saliva, semen or vaginal fluid, detectable amounts of the same ABO group characteristics as in their blood.

Tape Recorders

In this electronic age it is important to check all tape recorders found at the scene of the murder. The victim may have on him a tape recorder that records his own murder. Construction foreman Billy Stanton concealed a microcassette recorder under his shirt when he went to pick up his daughter on a visit to his ex-wife and her new husband near Brownsville, Texas. There had been trouble over visitation rights and he wanted to record evidence of animosity toward him. He was beaten with a baseball bat and shot and his fiance was shot. Their bodies were taken to an isolated area in the trunk of a car and dumped. Investigators discovered the recorder. After a brief conversation there were the sounds of the beating with the baseball bat. The murderers were convicted and sent to prison.

In Florida, Michael Phillips was shot and killed in his office. A detective noticed a wire leading from a tape recorder in a desk drawer to a microphone in a pencil holder. Phillips stated on the tape that he was about to have a meeting with Antony Inciarrano, who said "We have a deal, yes or no." This statement was followed by an argument, five shots and the protracted moans of the dying Phillips.

Inciarrano pleaded no contest to a charge of murder and was sentenced to life imprisonment. Florida has a state law against tape recording private conversations unless all parties consent and Inciarrano appealed his conviction because the tape recording violated his right to privacy. A lower appellate court ruling that the tape should not have been admitted at trial has been appealed to a higher court.

Drag Marks

"A search for drag marks must be made. This applies to both outdoor and indoor scenes. In outdoor scenes, the drag marks may lead to tire tracks of a vehicle used to transport the body. Disarranged clothing or scuffing of the shoes confirm the necessity to find drag marks. Drag marks are characteristically a double, roughly parallel set of marks that are produced by the heels or toes of a body while being dragged by the shoulders. However, be alert for a wide "swath" of disturbed foliage, rug nap, or dust which may be produced when a body is dragged by the feet. In rare instances a body may be dragged first by the feet and then by the shoulders, or vice versa. This makes for a very confusing set of patterns, which can only be sorted out with patience.

"Dragging of the body will produce changes in the clothing and body which can be very confusing if the investigator does not realize their cause. Assuming that a body is dragged by the feet, the primary pressure area will be the thorax, and the clothes around the thorax will be pushed upward. In addition to possible exposure of the breasts in females, numerous parallel superficial abrasions or scratches will be inflicted on the surface which is lower. In the case of dragging by the shoulders, the clothes of the lower body may be pushed downward and similarly expose genitalia and inflict abrasions.

"Should the surface be extremely rough or contain sharp stones, these abrasions can be deep. Confusion can be severe if the body is dragged by both shoulders and legs, thus exposing the breasts and genitalia and causing multiple abrasions. This situation must be distinguished from a rape murder. Clothes that are pushed out of place by dragging usually are rolled rather than folded, and bits of earth, stone, or lint may be caught in the rolled clothes, giving the clue that dragging took place. They will rarely be torn as they usually are in rapes" (1).

Dying Declaration

If the victim is still alive an officer should go with him in the ambulance to the hospital, and recover his clothing. It has been suggested that if the victim is dying he should be told this, and then asked to make a dying declaration which can be introduced in evidence. How many officers would be willing to tell a man that he is dying during an ambulance trip to the hospital? The situation is different when a victim has been treated and returned to a hospital room. Under these circumstances a homicide detective can do a videotaped interview.

SCIENTIFIC EVIDENCE

"A little monograph on the ashes of
one hundred and forty different varieties
of pipe, cigar, and cigarette tobacco."

Conan Doyle, *The Adventures of Sherlock Holmes*

Fibers and Hairs

The interchange of fibers and hairs at the crime scene, especially between the murderer and his victim, may provide crucial evidence. For example a man suspected of stomping his victim to death had very small specks of material in one heel of his cowboy boots. These were identified under the microscope as consisting of four different colored acrylic orlon fibers that matched similar fibers in the victim's jacket. Fiber and hair evidence played a vital role in the conviction of the serial killer Wayne Williams who strangled most of his victims.

Thirty children and young men were murdered or reported missing in Atlanta, Georgia between July 1979 and May 1981. In February 1981, an Atlanta newspaper article revealed that several different types of fibers had been found on two murder victims. Following publication of this article, bodies recovered from rivers in the Atlanta metropolitan area were either nude or clothed only in undershorts. On May 22, 1981, Atlanta police and FBI agents on surveillance duty at a bridge over the Chattahooche River heard a loud splash and stopped an automobile being driven off the bridge by twenty-three year old Wayne Bertram Williams.

Two days later the body of Nathanial Cater was pulled from the river approximately one mile downstream from the bridge. A yellowish-green nylon carpet fiber recovered from the hair on Cater's head matched fibers recovered from nine other murder victims in Atlanta. Search warrants were obtained for Williams' home and automobile. The yellowish-green carpet fibers matched fibers from a green carpet in Williams' bedroom. An estimation, based on sales records of the carpet manufacturer, showed that there was one chance in 7,792 of finding a carpet like Williams' carpet by randomly selecting occupied residences in the Atlanta area (3).

Williams was charged with the murders of Nathanial Cater and Jimmy Payne. During the trial evidence was introduced linking Williams to these two murders and to similar murders of ten other young men or boys. On the bodies of all these twelve victims were fibers matching fibers from a violet and green bedspread in Williams' room. There were dog hairs on eleven victims similar to dog hairs from Williams' dog. The Williams family had access to a large number of automobiles including rental cars. Nine victims were linked to automobiles used by the Williams family.

Of the nine victims who were killed during the period when Williams had access to a 1970 Chevrolet station wagon, fibers consistent with having originated from both the station wagon carpet and the bedroom carpet were recovered from six of the victims. The probability in 1981 of randomly selecting an automobile having carpet like that in the 1970 Chevrolet station wagon from the 2,373,512 cars registered in the Atlanta metropolitan area is one chance in 3,828, a very low probability representing a significant association (3).

Transferred fibers are usually lost rapidly as people go about their daily routine, therefore foreign fibers on a person are most often from recent surroundings. Seven types of fiber linked Payne's body to the Williams' environment (Williams' home, automobile or person) and six types on Cater's body. The fiber evidence shows that these victims' bodies were apparently associated with Williams shortly before or after their deaths. Furthermore the locations of the fibers—on Payne's shorts and in Cater's head and pubic hairs—were not those where one would expect to find fibers transferred from an automobile or house to victims who had been fully clothed (3).

Williams denied knowing any of the victims but the FBI forensic expert provides convincing evidence of Williams' association with the bodies of the murder victims, however he points out that evidence dealing with Williams' character and behavior, eyewitness accounts of his association with several victims, and his link to a victim recovered from the Chatahooche River, were also essential to the case. One witness testified that Williams had offered him money to perform oral sex, and another described how, after he had accepted a lift, Williams had fondled him through his trousers, then stopped the car in secluded woods; the teenager had jumped out and ran away (9).

THE AUTOPSY

"The Doctor said that Death was but a scientific fact."

The Ballad of Reading Gaol, Oscar Wilde

The forensic pathologist's autopsy may aid in determining whether the victim's death was the result of an accident, suicide or homicide. The suicidal person may make superficial cuts on his skin ("hesitation marks") before making a deep fatal cut, or he may fire his weapon away from himself ("test shots") before shooting himself. Furthermore he will often push aside clothing to uncover his skin before cutting or shooting himself. Homicide offenders do not push aside clothing before stabbing or shooting their victims. A suicidal right-handed person usually will shoot himself in the right temple or cut the left side of his throat obliquely. There may be scars on the wrist or elbow from previous suicide attempts. Victims of homicide may have "defense wounds" on their forearms or hands from trying to protect themselves.

Most persons who commit suicide with handguns shoot themselves in the head. The most common site is in the temple, followed by the mouth, under the chin and the forehead. About 18 percent shoot themselves in the chest and about 1 or 2 percent shoot themselves in the abdomen with handguns. Women seldom shoot themselves in the face.

As Di Maio points out there are people who will be different and shoot themselves on the top of the head, in the eye, in the back or even in the back of the head. The fact that a wound is in an unusual location does not necessarily mean that it cannot be self-inflicted, but one must always start with the assumption that such a wound is a homicide. In rare unquestioned instances, individuals have committed suicide by shooting themselves in the back of the head (4).

Suicidal persons sometimes shoot themselves several times. Di Maio quotes the case of a man who shot himself nine times in the chest with a nine-shot .22 caliber revolver. Even after bullet wounds penetrate the heart, a person may do extraordinary things. Snyder recalls the case of a police officer who was shot by a gangster through the heart with a bullet from a .38 special. He was not knocked off his feet and after receiving the wound, took out his own revolver, fired all six loads, put it back in its holster, walked across a wide street and climbed into his automobile where he died.

Contact wounds occur when the muzzle of the firearm is held directly against the body. Soot and powder are deposited inside the wound. When the muzzle is held a short distance from the body there is "powder tattooing" of the skin. This results from unburned powder grains that are blown into the skin. The distance at which powder tattooing occurs depends on the caliber of the gun, the length of the barrel, and the type of ammunition. A .38 caliber revolver, with a four inch barrel, and cartridges with flake powder produced powder tattooing out to eighteen to twenty-four inches (4).

In distant gunshot wounds the only mark on the skin is a reddish-brown abrasion ring which is usually present in most entrance wounds. Exit wounds are usually larger than entrance wounds and the skin edges are usually ragged or irregular, but they can be round or oval. Contact wounds of the skull, where there is only a thin layer of flesh over the bone, have an irregular stellate appearance unlike the usual small round or oval entrance wounds.

Knight points out that medical evidence can sometimes confirm or exclude possible motives for a shooting, but extraordinary events occur in medicolegal practice and a careful evaluation must always be made to ensure that dogmatic statements by doctors do not mislead detectives. He gives the example of a fatal shooting with an entrance wound in the chest and an exit wound on the back. There was another entrance wound on the back and inside the thorax was a deformed revolver bullet. The natural assumption was that the victim had been shot twice from two different directions, but this was inconsistent with the circumstances, and on careful investigation it was discovered that the deceased had been standing against a brick wall. A single projectile had entered the front of the chest, passed through the back, richocheted from the wall and reentered the back (6).

Accidental Death or Child Battering?

Autopsy findings which suggest child battering include: bruises of varying ages, "fingertip" bruises from a parent gripping the child around the elbows and knees, black eyes, lacerations of the mouth, especially tearing of the inside of the upper lip, bite marks, cigarette burns, burns from boiling water or from sitting in a bath of very hot water, malnutrition and poor skin hygiene. X-rays of the entire skeleton may show fractures in varying stages of healing. Ruptured liver, bruising of the intestines and subdural hemorrhage may also be found.

INTERVIEWING WITNESSES

> *"The chief of police of a Southern city once gave me*
> *a description of a man, complete even to a mole*
> *on his neck, but neglected to mention*
> *that he had only one arm."*

Dashiell Hammett, *Memoirs of a Private Detective*

"Never, **never** ask for names and addresses until **after** the person has told you, in the form of general discussion and comment, conducted in friendly conversational tones, what he has seen. Then get **every** address and telephone number he has; work, home and close relatives — even a neighbor's telephone number, where appropriate. Scan the crowds and look for persons who are explaining the incident to others." This advice of Powis to fellow police officers is especially important in homicide investigations.

It is not always easy to identify quickly those persons at a homicide scene who either witnessed the homicide or have important information. These witnesses should be taken to the detective's office for further questioning, possibly on videotape. This is essential in those high crime areas where many citizens do not like to be seen talking to the police. Even in low crime neighborhoods citizens who know the suspect may be reluctant to talk because they have seen crime dramas on television about a criminal who stalks and kills the witness.

When there are many persons at the crime scene patrolmen will speak to them and write down their comments on relevant issues. This is more likely to be productive than simply handing each person a witness statement form and asking him to write his statement. Patrolmen will visit homes and businesses in the vicinity in a search for additional witnesses. Someone may have seen the suspect's car yet not volunteer that he wrote down the license number, so it is necessary to ask direct as well as indirect questions.

CRIMINAL PROFILES

"Singularity is almost invariably a clue."
Conan Doyle, *The Adventures of Sherlock Holmes*

Agents at the Behavioral Sciences Unit (BSU) of the FBI Academy developed a technique for classifying murderers into one of two categories — organized or disorganized. In a scientific study it was found that there were significant differences in the crime scenes of organized and disorganized offenders. Certain background differences were also found. Agents interviewed thirty-six convicted sexual murderers, twenty-five were serial murderers (the murder of separate victims with time breaks between victims ranging from two days to weeks or months) and eleven had committed either a single homicide, double homicide or spree murder. Twenty-four were organized murderers and twelve were disorganized murderers. The following account is based in part, not exclusively, on the report of the study (7).

The Organized Murderer

He plans his crime carefully and takes steps to avoid detection. Victims, although strangers, are carefully selected at a location far from the offender's home or place of employment. Often the victims of serial murderers resemble one another in age, appearance, hairstyle, occupation or lifestyle. The victims may be adolescent youths, hitchhiking college coeds, nurses, women frequenting bars, women sitting in cars with male companions or women alone in cars. The victim is approached in a friendly manner and may be asked for directions or for assistance. There may be an attempt to establish a friendly relationship.

The organized murderer may claim to be a police officer or other official. Whether dressed in a suit or casual clothing he presents a good appearance and is unlikely to arouse suspicion. Friendly persuasion is

Table I

CRIME SCENE DIFFERENCES BETWEEN ORGANIZED AND DISORGANIZED MURDERERS

Organized	Disorganized
Planned offense	Spontaneous offense
Victim a targeted stranger	Victim/location known
Personalizes victim	Depersonalizes victim
Controlled conversation	Minimal conversation
Crime scene reflects overall control	Crime scene random and sloppy
Demands submissive victim	Sudden violence to victim
Restraints used	Minimal use of restraints
Aggressive acts prior to death	Sexual acts after death
Body hidden	Body left in view
Weapon/evidence absent	Evidence/weapon often present
Transports victim or body	Body left at death scene

From *FBI Law Enforcement Bulletin* 54(8), August 1985.

replaced by direct orders or the use of force after he persuades the victim to get in his car or after he gets in the victim's car. The murder takes place at another location.

Victims are often handcuffed or tied with a rope. They may also be gagged and blindfolded. Torture precedes rape and murder. The offender brings his own weapon to the crime scene. Care is taken not to leave the weapon or other evidence at the scene. The body may be concealed or displayed naked in a posture likely to offend citizens. Some personal possessions of the victim or a body part such as an ear, finger or nipple may be taken as a souvenir or trophy.

The organized murderer may return to the crime scene. If the body has not been discovered he may move it so that the police will find it. He may volunteer to join a search party for his missing victim and inject himself in the police investigation, perhaps providing misleading information. If the body has been discovered and buried he may visit the grave. He may contact the victim's family on some pretence and may return his souvenir anonymously. There is no remorse and no change in his everyday behavior.

The organized murderer has an average or higher than average IQ, has graduated from high school and may have attended college. Although socially adept with a high IQ, his work record may be unsatisfactory because his persistence of effort is not equal to his ambition.

Furthermore he may have been fired from jobs because he does not relate well to persons in authority. He may work at jobs below his abilities, for example as a laborer, truck driver, or oil rig worker. Military service may have been in the Marine Corps, Rangers or Green Berets.

He may have worked as a reserve police officer or deputy sheriff. Failure to obtain employment as a police officer may lead him to become a security guard. He likes to carry weapons, handcuffs and some type of badge resembling that of a police officer. There may have been arrests for carrying a concealed weapon, assault, assault with a deadly weapon, arson, theft and impersonation of a police officer. If sentenced to an institution, he is a model prisoner and secures early release because he knows how to manipulate the system to his advantage.

He has a succession of girl friends because they tire of his selfish, self-centered behavior but there may be a submissive long-suffering wife who remains loyal to him. His friends may say that he is a great guy and fun to be around because of his friendly facade. He drives a car in keeping with his macho image, perhaps a four wheel drive pickup or a late model sports car that is well maintained.

"Precipitating situational stress, such as problems with finances, marriages, employment, and relationships with females, is often present prior to the murder . . . The organized offender may report an angry frame of mind at the time of the murder or state he was depressed. However, while committing the crime, he admits being calm and relaxed. Alcohol may have been consumed prior to the crime . . . Newspaper clippings of the crimes are often found during searches of the subject's residence, indicating the offender followed the criminal investigation in the newspaper" (7). John Gacy, Albert DeSalvo and Ted Bundy are examples of organized murderers.

The Disorganized Murderer

"The overall imprint of the disorganized crime scene is that the crime is committed suddenly and with no set plan of action for deterring detection. The crime scene shows great disarray. There is a spontaneous, symbolic, unplanned quality to the crime scene. The victim may be known to the offender, but age and sex of the victim do not necessarily matter.

"If the offender is selecting a victim by randomly knocking on doors in a neighborhood, the first person to open a door becomes the victim. The offender kills instantly to have control; he cannot risk that the victim will get the upper hand.

"The offender uses a blitz style of attack for confronting the victim, who is caught completely off guard. He either approaches the victim from behind, unexpectedly overpowering her, or he kills suddenly, as with a gun. The attack is a violent surprise, occurring spontaneously and in a location where the victim is going about his or her usual activities.

"The offender depersonalizes the victim, targeting specific areas of the body for extreme brutality. Overkill or excessive assault to the face often is an attempt to dehumanize the victim. Such facial destruction may indicate knowledge of the victim or that the victim resembles or represents a person who has caused the offender psychological distress. The offender may wear a mask or gloves, use a blindfold on the victim, or cover the victim's face as he attacks. There is minimal verbal interaction except for orders and threats. Restraints are not necessary, as the victim is killed quickly.

"Any sexually sadistic acts, often in the form of mutilation, are usually performed after death. Offenders have attempted a variety of sexual acts, including ejaculating into an open stab wound in the victim's abdomen. Evidence of urination, defecation, and masturbation has been found on the victim's clothing and in the home. Mutilation to the face, genitals, and breast, disembowelment, amputation, and vampirism may also be noted on the body.

"Disorganized offenders might keep the dead body. One murderer killed two women and kept their body parts in his home for eight years. He made masks from their heads and drums and seat covers from their skins. Earlier, he had exhumed the bodies of eight elderly women from their graves and performed similar mutilative acts.

"The death scene and crime scene are usually the same in murders committed by the disorganized offender, with the victim being left in the position in which she or he was killed. If the offender has mutilated the body, it may be positioned in a special way that has significance to the offender.

"No attempt is made to conceal the body. Fingerprints and footprints may be found, and the police have a great deal of evidence to use in their investigation. Usually, the murder weapon is one obtained at the scene and is left there, providing investigators with evidence" (7).

The disorganized offender may return to the scene of the crime and further mutilate the body or he may replace a souvenir that he had taken. If the victim has been buried he may go to the gravesite, leave flowers, and speak aloud to her, especially on the anniversary of the

Table II

PROFILE CHARACTERISTICS OF ORGANIZED AND DISORGANIZED MURDERS

Organized	Disorganized
Average to above-average intelligence	Below-average intelligence
Socially competent	Socially inadequate
Skilled work preferred	Unskilled work
Sexually competent	Sexually incompetent
High birth order status	Low birth order status
Father's work stable	Father's work unstable
Inconsistent childhood discipline	Harsh discipline as child
Controlled mood during crime	Anxious mood during crime
Use of alcohol with crime	Minimal use of alcohol
Precipitating situational stress	Minimal situational stress
Living with partner	Living alone
Mobility with car in good condition	Lives/works near crime scene
Follows crime in news media	Minimal interest in news media
May change jobs or leave town	Significant behavior change (drug/alcohol abuse, religiosity, etc.)

From *FBI Law Enforcement Bulletin* 54(8), August 1985.

murder. A hidden microphone near the grave can record his statement. Following the murder acquaintances may note a change in his behavior. He becomes more withdrawn, increases his use of alcohol or drugs, or he may become very remorseful and fanatically religious. He may quit his job and leave the area.

The disorganized murderer is likely to be of below average intelligence and a high school dropout. If he served in the armed services he was probably discharged within a few months. He has a menial job and a poor work record because of frequent failure to appear at work. He does not own a car and may be unable to drive so that he rides a bicycle or is dependent on public transportation. Unlike the organized murderer he is not athletic and he is a sloppy dresser. A loner with solitary interests such as watching television or reading comic books, he lives alone or with his parents. He may have a physical handicap such as acne, a hair lip, or stuttering and he has a poor self-image. His prior crimes are non-violent and may include window peeping or petty firesetting not involving the use of accelerants. Crimes are usually in his own neighborhood.

Case Example of a Disorganized Murderer

A young woman was found shot to death in her home. Her sweater had been pulled above her breasts and her pants had been pulled down. She had been disembowelled. There were slash wounds on her breasts but there was no evidence of sexual assault. Animal feces were in her mouth. There were indications that he drank her blood from a cup. Garbage was strewn about the house. Human tissue and steak knives were taken from her home.

On the same day a burglar broke into another house, urinated on female clothing and defecated in the house. Garbage was strewn throughout the home. Two days later a dog was shot with the same weapon used in the murders, and disembowelled. Four days after the first murder an older man, a woman and her young son were shot to death in the woman's home. Her twenty-two month old baby was missing from the home but a bullet hole was found in the pillow and there was brain tissue in the baby bed. This woman had also been disembowelled and her body had been slashed and mutilated. A knife had been forced up her anus. There were indications that a container had been used to collect her blood. The man's station wagon was stolen.

The Behavioral Science Unit profile of the offender included the following information: "Suspect description: White male aged twenty five to twenty-seven; thin, undernourished appearance; single, living alone in a location within one mile of the abandoned station wagon owned by one of the victims. Residence will be extremely slovenly and unkempt, and evidence of the crimes will be found at the residence. Suspect will have a history of mental illness and use of drugs. Suspect will be an unemployed loner who does not associate with either males or females and will probably spend a great deal of time in his own residence. If he resides with anyone, it will be with his parents. However, this is unlikely. Subject will have no prior military history; will be a high school or college dropout; probably suffers from one or more forms of paranoid psychosis" (7).

The police made a search within a one mile radius of the stolen vehicle. Their inquiries revealed that there was indeed a strange man who fit the profile. He had been asking for puppies. Pets had started disappearing after he moved into an apartment complex. He was a twenty-seven year old man who lived in an apartment in the same block as the abandoned car. He was in possession of a gun that matched the murder weapon. In his apartment were blenders containing animal and possibly human tissue. Steak knives taken from the first victim's home were also found.

"The man had previously been diagnosed as a paranoid schizo-phrenic and had been committed to a mental facility after he was found sucking blood from a dead bird. After he had been released, he was found in the desert bloodstained and wearing a loincloth. He told police he was sacrificing to flying saucers. He was released by police; however, later a child's body was found in the same vicinity" (7). He had delusions that rays projected on him from outer space were drying up his body fluids and he believed that the only way to replace these fluids was to drink the blood of squirrels, rabbits, cats, dogs, and human beings. He was found guilty of first degree murder but he committed suicide in jail.

One Murder—Two Profiles

The crime scene in a mutilation sex murder suggested a disorganized murderer but there were puzzling features. Death was from severe head injuries with excessive trauma to the face. The mutilations, which included removal of the breasts and a large abdominal incision, occurred after death. The fact that the murder did not occur at the garbage dump where the nude body was found and the presence of sperm in her vagina suggested an organized offender. FBI profilers decided there were two suspects.

The murderer was probably a high school dropout with a learning disability, brief military service and social problems. He would have evidence of the crime in his home and at night would visit his victim's grave. The suspect who raped the victim and provided the vehicle to move her body would be close to both the murderer and the victim. He would have a history of assaultive behavior and recent stress such as a divorce or pregnant wife.

The profile of the murderer ruled out five of six suspects, including a good prospect who discovered the body, had a few minor skirmishes with the law and secured an attorney after questioning by the police (5). The profile fit the remaining suspect, the victim's live-in boyfriend. Only recently on the request of his very controlling mother, she had sexual relations with him. She was very critical of his sexual performance and compared him unfavorably with her other lovers. He was seen at her grave at night. His brother, whose wife delivered a baby on the night of the murder, fit the profile of the other suspect and he confessed his involvement in the crime.

THE HOMICIDE DETECTIVE

"Our day begins when yours ends."

The homicide detective has to keep careful notes so that he can answer the defense attorney's questions "Who was at the scene; what were the weather conditions; were the neighbor's garage lights on or off?" He has to make sure that everyone involved in the investigation does a thorough job. Otherwise he may be embarrassed when the defense attorney asks the crime laboratory detective "Did you look for fingerprints under the toilet seat, did you do a gunshot residue test on the victim, did you get her fingernail scrapings?"

He has to make sure that a new inexperienced pathologist swabs the nasopharynx and anus for semen especially in those brutal murders that seem to be a hallmark of the homosexual assailant. He should check the tapes of all emergency calls for help to the 911 telephone operator about the time of the slaying. So many crank calls for help are received that a call which does not include name, address or telephone number and is not completed may not be passed on to the homicide detail. The detective may be surprised to hear a call for help that suddenly ends "No Terry don't shoot, don't shoot" and Terry is the name of the homicide victim's former boyfriend.

Telephone answering devices in the victim's home and office should also be checked. A man who was thought to have committed suicide by setting his car on fire had the following message on the telephone answering machine at his home "You better pay up or you won't believe what happens to you, when it happens."

In unsolved homicides review of the case with another detective may provide fresh leads. Further interviews with witnesses and neighbors may provide information that was previously concealed or not reported. A background check of the victim may point to his involvement in drug smuggling and his punishment for suspected betrayal or failure to pay debts.

A review of television tapes of the crime scene may show the presence of a suspect or witness who claimed that he was several miles away at the time of the murder. Often the person who finds the body is the killer. Has this person found any other bodies in the past or has he previously suggested where to look to searchers for a missing person? Above all who stands to benefit from the victim's death? This is one of the first questions that a homicide detective asks. It may deserve further consideration.

REFERENCES

1. Aronson, M.E.: Onsite investigation. In Gottschalk, L.A., *et al.* (Eds.): *Guide to the Investigation and Reporting of Drug Abuse Deaths.* Washington, D.C., U.S. Government Printing Office, 1977.
2. Bruhns, John: Police and homicides. In Danto, B.L., Bruhns, J. and Kutscher, A.H. (Eds.): *The Human Side of Homicide.* New York, Columbia University Press, 1982.
3. Deadman, H.A.: Fiber evidence and the Wayne Williams trial. *FBI Law Enforcement Bull, 53*(3):13, 1984.
4. Di Maio, V.J.M.: *Gunshot Wounds.* New York, Elsevier, 1985.
5. Geberth, V.J.: *Practical Homicide Investigation.* New York, Elsevier, 1983.
6. Knight, Bernard: Firearm injuries. In Tedeschi, C.G., Eckert, W.G. and Tedeschi, L.G. (Eds.): *Forensic Medicine.* Philadelphia, W.B. Saunders Company, 1977.
7. Ressler, R.K., Burgess, A.W., Depue, R.L., Douglas, J.E., Hazelwood, R.R. and Lanning, K.V., *et al.*: Crime scene and profile characteristics of organized and disorganized murderers. *FBI Law Enforcement Bull, 54*(8):18, August 1985.
8. Snyder, LeMoyne: *Homicide Investigation.* Second edition. Springfield, Illinois, Charles C Thomas, 1967.
9. Wilson, Colin and Seaman, Donald: *The Encyclopedia of Modern Murder, 1962-1982.* New York, G.P. Putnam's Sons, 1983.

CHAPTER 14

THE DEATH PENALTY

"A deep reverence for human life is worth more than a thousand executions in the prevention of murder; it is in fact, the great security of human life. The law of capital punishment, whilst pretending to support this reverence, does in fact tend to destroy it."

John Bright

THE EARLIEST known record of a death sentence for murder dates back to 1850 BC. Inscriptions on a clay tablet unearthed by archeologists in Iraq record the trial and punishment of three men who killed a temple official. The case was brought before King Ur-Ninurta, who turned it over for trial to a citizens' assembly which acted as a court of justice. The three men were sentenced by the assembly to be executed in front of the chair of the murdered man.

In Biblical times the Jews, despite their respect for the **lex talionis** of Moses were reluctant to inflict capital punishment. In the "Mishnah" it is stated that the Sanhedrin were themselves called murderers if the death penalty was inflicted more than once in seven years, and some Rabbis affirmed that once in seventy years was far too frequent. There is no doubt that the extreme rarity of Jewish judicial executions is to be explained by the almost insurmountable difficulties imposed by Rabbinic regulations as conditions precedent to a conviction leading to a capital sentence. At least two witnesses were required who should have seen the crime from the same place, or have been visible to each other, and who had actually warned the malefactor of the nature and consequences of the act he was about to commit (3). Today Israel has abolished capital punishment for murder other than genocide, which is the systematic extermination of a racial, political or cultural group.

Through the centuries various methods of capital punishment have been employed. Crucifixion, stoning, burning, drowning, burial alive, poisoning, boiling to death, mutilation, pressing to death and various other unpleasant procedures are recorded. Many crimes besides murder were punishable by death. At the beginning of the nineteenth century the criminal law of England was commonly known as the Bloody Code. It was unique in the world inasmuch as it listed between 220 and 230 offenses to be punished by death, from the stealing of turnips to associating with gypsies; to damaging a fishpond; to writing threatening letters; to impersonating out pensioners at Greenwich Hospital; to being found armed or disguised in a forest, park or rabbit warren; to cutting down a tree; to poaching, forging, picking pockets, shoplifting and so on through 220 odd items. The exact number of capital offenses was not known even to the best legal authorities (6).

In 1808, a boy and his sister, aged seven and eleven respectively, were hanged; in 1814, a man was hanged for cutting down a tree; in 1831, a boy of nine was hanged for setting fire to a house; and in 1833, a boy of nine was condemned to death at the Old Bailey for stealing two pennyworth of children's paints. Efforts to eliminate the death penalty for crimes other than murder and treason were long resisted on the grounds of the deterrent effect. Public executions were thought to add to the deterrent effect and "hanging days" were public holidays. Yet, evidence before the Royal Commission of 1866 revealed that of 167 persons who had been under the sentence of death, in one town, during a number of years, 164 had themselves witnessed a public execution.

Advocates of the death penalty claim that it has a valuable deterrent effect which if removed would result in an increase in the number of murders. They are quick to draw attention to the Old Testament teaching of "an eye for an eye and a tooth for a tooth." They are seldom aware of the later Old Testament teaching (Ezekiel 33:11), "As I live, saith the Lord God, I have no pleasure in the death of the wicked, but that the wicked should turn from his way and live." New Testament teachings forbid the taking of life by way of retribution.

The deterrent effect of the death penalty has been questioned. The Royal Commission on Capital Punishment (1949-1953) after studying statistics from many countries including the United States, concluded that there is no clear evidence that the abolition of capital punishment has led to an increase in the homicide rate or that its reintroduction has led to a fall. "Whether the death penalty is used or not, and whether executions are frequent or not, both death penalty states and abolition states show rates which suggest that these rates are conditioned by other factors than the death penalty."

Opponents of capital punishment claim that its use lowers rather than increases respect for the sanctity of human life. Capital punishment may act as a positive incentive to murder for the suicidal and the exhibitionist. Maudsley quotes the case of Burton, an eighteen year old youth, who made up his mind to murder somebody because he wanted to be hanged. He said he had an impulse to kill someone so he sharpened his knife, then followed a boy, the first person he saw, to a convenient place where he killed him. During the trial he was the least concerned person in court. When sentenced to death, with a smile, he thanked the judge.

As an example of the exhibitionist, for whom the existence of capital punishment may act as an incentive, Gardiner quotes the case of the English murderer Marjeram. In 1930 this young man stabbed a girl to death on Dartford Common. He had never seen her before and there was no attempt at any sexual assault. When the police could not find the knife, Marjeram obligingly showed them the place on the Common where he had thrown it. The Recorder, when charging the Grand Jury, described the crime as "inexplicable." At Marjeram's trial it was suggested that the cause was a desire to be in the limelight.

The suggestion would seem to have been well merited. While still at the Police Station Marjeram asked for the newspapers, saying, "I wish to read the account of the murder and all that has been said in the newspapers about me. There must be a lot about me as a job like this has not been done for a long time." He dressed himself with care for his trial and kept asking the police whether he looked all right. He smiled throughout his trial, which he appeared to enjoy very much. While the jury were out considering their verdict he sat laughing and joking with the warders at the top of the steps leading to the cells. It would appear from the letters he wrote from the condemned cell to his mother that he retained the same attitude there until he was hanged. All the doctors agreed that he was sane. But he was clearly of a highly abnormal mentality.

At the age of five he had had an abscess on the brain and had had to be strapped down because the pain was such that he said that he wanted to die, and it was feared that he might do some injury to himself. When grown up he had attempted suicide, but from what he himself later said it would seem probable that the real object of the attempted suicide was to draw attention to himself. He subsequently gave himself up for a murder in a shop at Reading which he had not committed, but the police were quick to appreciate that in fact he had had nothing to do with it. He was then sentenced to six months imprisonment for stealing a handbag at a time when the condemned cell in his prison — Maidstone — was occupied by a young man named Fox, who was waiting to be hanged, and who was duly hanged.

Any ordinary person would also think that if the death penalty was ever peculiarly deterrent, it would be so to a young man, like Marjeram, who had lived in close proximity to another young man who was waiting to be hanged in the condemned cell. In fact, however, his experience appears to have had precisely the opposite effect. Marjeram appears to have been aware that while the warders treated him with contempt, they spoke respectfully to the young man in the condemned cell.

Even the Prison Governor — himself — treated Fox with respect. It seems clear that Marjeram simply decided that this was the place which he wanted to occupy. According to his mother he came out of Maidstone prison on the 5th of April; on the 9th Fox was hanged there; and on the 11th having referred to Fox as a "hero" to his mother, he murdered this girl on Dartford Common. It would be difficult for any rational man, applying his mind to the facts, to come to any other conclusion but that to this type of disordered mind the hanging process, with all its attendant publicity and sensationalism, in fact operates not as a deterrent, but as an incentive, and that but for the existence of capital punishment, the girl on Dartford Common would be alive today (3).

Capital punishment involves the risk of execution of innocent persons. Juries are not infallible and tragic mistakes have been made. Stephen Tonka, a Hungarian landowner who was hanged in 1913 for the murder of his daughter, was subsequently proved to be innocent of the crime. A farewell letter from the daughter, announcing her intention to commit suicide, had come to light fourteen years too late to save her father's life. Leopold Hilsner of Austria spent eighteen years in prison before he was released because the charge against him was found to have been false. In this case it was possible to reverse the verdict as there was no death penalty in Austria.

Relatively few convicted murderers are executed. Between 1900 and 1950 only one in twelve murderers in England and one in twenty-five murderers in Scotland, was hanged. A study of 588 cases of criminal homicide in Philadelphia showed that only seven offenders were sentenced to death. One-third of English murderers take their own lives. About four percent of the offenders in the Philadelphia study commited suicide.

METHODS OF EXECUTION

Hanging

"Execution by hanging is a practice of great antiquity and obscure origin. It may be presumed to have been invented rather for its advertisement value than as a more effective way of taking life than other early methods of execution, such as beheading, drowning, stoning, impaling, and precipitation from a height. Hanging inflicted a signal indignity on the victim in a uniquely conspicuous fashion. It displayed him to the onlookers in the most ignominious and abject of postures, and would thus be likely to enhance the deterrent effect of his punishment on anyone who might be tempted to do what he had done. Moreover until comparatively recent times, execution by hanging caused a slow and distressing death by suffocation; the victim's last agonies would be a warning not soon forgotten by the crowds that watched them. Thus hanging came to be regarded as a peculiarly grim and degrading form of punishment" (12).

The task of hanging is sometimes bungled. Untoward incidents were not uncommon in earlier years. Often much confusion was caused by faulty tying or breaking of the rope. Thus, when Captain Kidd was hanged in 1701, the rope broke and he had to be raised from the ground and hanged again (11). In 1789, in England three men were executed. One of them, William Snow, had hung but a few seconds when the rope slipped from the gallows and he fell to the ground. Snow heard the sorrowful exclamations of the spectators, and said with an air of compassion, "Good people, be not hurried, I am not hurried, I can wait a little." And the executioner wishing to lengthen the rope, Snow calmly waited till his companion was dead, when the rope was taken from the deceased's arms, in order to complete the execution of Snow (7).

Laurence gives the following description of the execution of David Evans. The rope broke, and the unhappy man fell down beneath the gallows, unhurt, but completely unnerved. There were loud cries immediately from the crowd who were watching: Shame! Let him go! The half hanged man, staggering to his feet, exclaimed, "I claim my liberty. You have hanged me once, and you have no authority to hang me again." . . . "You are greatly mistaken," replied Calcraft (the hangman) firmly. "There is no such law as that—to let a man go if there is an accident and he is not properly hanged. My warrant and my order are to hang you by the neck until you are dead. So up you go and hang you must until you are dead." Evans was forced up the scaffold by Calcraft and two wardens and duly hanged, with protests still on his lips.

The English executioner, James Berry, had some unfortunate experiences. His biographer, Justin Atholl, comments that the craftsman aims at perfection, but in the nature of things sometimes falls short of it and even the most skilled and conscientious worker with his hands has his mishaps. Berry operated at a period when hanging was still to be perfected and the confidence of those concerned in carrying it out exceeded their knowledge and experience.

Atholl's account of Berry's attempts to hang John Lee in 1885 deserve mention. "Berry put Lee on the trap, pinioned his legs, drew the white cap over his head and adjusted the noose. This took only a few seconds and Lee said nothing. Then Berry stepped back and drew the lever. There was a grinding noise, but no movement of the doors. For a few seconds Berry was frozen in astonishment. He pulled the lever again, but it was fully drawn. Then he put a foot forward and stamped on the doors. They remained immovable. When Berry's stamping proved ineffectual, warders joined him in trying to force down the trap. All this time — and it seems that about six minutes were spent in this first attempt — Lee remained immovable on the drop. The chaplain had continued to read the burial services. At last Berry removed the noose from Lee's neck and took off the white cap. Lee's face was ashen, but no whiter than that of some of the witnesses, and he seemed still cool and collected. Lee was taken into a room nearby and Berry, helped by the warders, tested the trap all over again. Berry even climbed down into the pit to examine the drawbolt, which seemed to be in order. He pulled the lever and the trap doors fell. No one seems to have considered the effect on the condemned man nearby of the crashing doors, but the fact was that by this time everyone was really past caring about anything except getting it over somehow."

"Lee was brought back and once more Berry went through the ritual of pinioning his legs, putting on the white cap, adjusting the noose. This time Berry, acting under great emotion, pulled the lever with such force that he bent it. The trap doors remained immovable. There was more stamping. It had no effect. Lee was again taken off the trap. The officials, like Berry, were by this time controlling themselves with extreme difficulty. According to Berry more than one fortified himself with brandy which was offered to Lee but refused, but it is possible that Berry's memory was faulty in this respect as it was in believing that he made only two attempts to hang Lee.

"In fact, Lee was led away a second time with the chaplain to a room in the prison. Berry and a prison tradesman tried to put things right. A plane was brought into use and bits of wood hacked off with a saw and axe. The accompaniment to this business was the sound of the crowd outside who had at first thought the fact that the black flag was not hoisted at the expected time was due to a reprieve and then, by some mysterious prison grapevine, learned of the truth.

"At every test the trap doors fell perfectly naturally. John Lee was brought back for the third time. For the third time the Rev. John Pitkin began the burial service. And for the third time when Lee was stood on the trap, capped and noosed, the doors refused to open in response to the lever. The chaplain reeled and would have fallen if one of the prison officers had not held him up. He recovered. The prison surgeon urged him to ask for the execution to be stopped. The prison governor seems to have been in a poor state but in consultation with Mr. Henry M. James, the Under-Sheriff, agreed that the attempts to hang Lee should be ended and that a messenger should be sent immediately by the express about to leave to report to the Home Secretary . . . Later in the day Berry learned that the Home Secretary, immediately on hearing the facts had ordered John Lee to be respited and his sentence was commuted to one of penal servitude for life.

"No official explanation was offered . . . The mistake according to the most plausible theory lay in using a warped board in the platform in front of the trap. This board curved downwards slightly towards its ends so that when a weight was placed on it, it is flattened and lengthened, one end moving under the edge of the trap doors. The weight on this board during the execution was the chaplain standing in front of the condemned man. Of course as soon as Lee was removed, the chaplain moved away and the trap worked perfectly. But each time Lee was brought back, the chaplain moved back into position to take up the service for the burial of the dead again and ensured that the doors did not work.

"Three months later Berry executed a Moses Shrimpton and the execution appeared to have passed off without incident. When Berry went down to the pit to inspect the body he discovered that the nine foot drop had half pulled the victim's head from his body and the walls were running with blood. A few months later Berry executed a Robert Goodale. Goodale was incapable of standing alone and was held up by warders. Berry signalled to them to let go and pulled the lever. Goodale dropped out of sight and one of the warders with his foot on the drop also fell, only saving himself by catching the edge of the opening. But no one had eyes for the warder. They were hypnotized by the sight of the rope rebounding through the opening. For a moment Berry thought the noose had slipped or the rope had broken, but the truth was soon apparent. The rope had cut through Goodale's neck as cleanly as a knife. A glance into the pit showed the head still in its white bag lying beside a body covered in blood under the rope now swinging freely.

"The execution of Goodale led, in due course, to the official inquiry into the methods of hanging used in England already described. The effect on Berry was undoubtedly to make him much more 'conservative' in deciding on the drop and a consequent number of cases in which death was not produced by dislocation of the neck and was by no means instantaneous. When he hanged Henry Delvin at Duke Street Prison, Glasgow, the drop was underestimated and as a result Delvin was slowly strangled, although the fact was not made public at the time. George Horton, executed for poisoning his young daughter, 'did not die until two or three minutes after he had been dropped.' When Arthur Delaney stood on the scaffold Berry said that he had a feeling the drop had been underestimated but that it was too late to alter it. The medical aspects of hanging were at this time arousing considerable interest and there were no less than three doctors present at this execution. With Berry they remained gazing into the pit some time after the prisoner had dropped, watching him dying slowly.

"When he came to execute David Robert at Cardiff Gaol, Berry found a very heavy man like Goodale. He was determined there should be no repetition of that horror and gave him a drop of only three feet seven inches, although the stretching of the rope, in fact, resulted in a fall of four feet. The spectators, who included reporters, noticed that there was a hardly perceptible thud when the body fell. Owing to the short drop, the wretched man's head remained visible above the opening and spectators saw his convulsive twitching and breathing. There was a horrified silence for a minute after which Berry said, 'I think he's dead now,' but the body continued to move and take convulsive breaths. Berry walked over to the Governor and requested him to order the Press to leave, which they did. The man had been struggling for three minutes at this point and how much longer elapsed before death became apparent was not therefore recorded. Another man named Hayes lived for five minutes on the end of the rope. Berry himself was sensitive about these strangulations, but curiously not upset by them in the same way as by shedding blood.

"He would 'steady the rope' with his hand so that if it went on vibrating the spectators should not have their feelings harrowed by the thought that the movement was due to struggles by the man suspended on it. He was upset by criticism in the Press when a victim was seen to breathe or convulse after the drop. When Upton was hanged at Oxford the drop was too long and his neck was severely lacerated so that there was much blood. Berry, as I have described, was very irritated at the inquest and at one point burst out, 'If I had given the man two feet six instead of five feet and he had fidgited, the Press would have been down on me' " (1).

The present technique of hanging is designed to cause death by fracture dislocation of cervical vertebrae with laceration or crushing of the spinal cord. Some skill is needed otherwise slow death from strangulation will result. Mr. Albert Pierrepoint, the English executioner, gave evidence on this point to the Royal Commission on Capital Punishment (1949-1953).

Question: The knot as you showed us this morning, must always be under the angle of the left jaw? **Answer:** Yes.

Question: That is very important, is it? **Answer:** Very important.

Question: Why is it very important? **Answer:** If you had the same knot on the right-hand side it comes back behind the neck, and throws the neck forward, which would make a strangulation. If you put it on the left-hand side it finishes up in front and throws the chin back and breaks the spinal cord.

Question: It depends on where he is standing on the trap? **Answer:** No, I do not think so. The knot is the secret of it, really. We have to put it on the left lower jaw and if we have it on that side, when he falls it finishes under the chin and throws the chin back; but if the knot is on the right-hand side, it would finish up behind his neck and throw his neck forward, which would be strangulation. He might live on the rope for a quarter of an hour then.

"In most of the English prisons equipped for execution the execution chamber adjoins the condemned cell. The chamber itself is a small room and the trap occupies a large part of the floor. The trap is formed of two hinged leaves held in position from below by bolts which are withdrawn when the lever is pulled, allowing the leaves to drop on their hinges. Above the trap a rope of a standard length is attached to a strong chain, which is fitted to the overhead beam in such a way that it can be raised and lowered and secured at any desired height by means of a cotter slipped into one of the links and a bracket fixed on the beam. This enables the length of chain to be adjusted to make the drop accord with the height and weight of the prisoner.

"The executioner and his assistant arrive at the prison on the afternoon before the execution. They are told the height and weight of the prisoner and are given an opportunity to see him from a position where they themselves cannot be seen. While the prisoner is out of his cell they test the apparatus to ensure that it is working satisfactorily. For this purpose they use a sack of approximately the same weight as the prisoner, having ascertained the proper drop from a table which gives the length appropriate to a prisoner's weight. Some adjustments in the length given in the table may be necessary to allow for other physical characteristics of the prisoner, such as age and build.

"On the morning of the execution a final check of the equipment is carried out. The rope is coiled, fitted to the chain, and secured in position by a piece of pack-thread which will be broken by the weight of the prisoner when he drops. Just before the time of execution the executioner and his assistant join the Under-Sheriff and the prison officials outside the door of the condemned cell. The Under-Sheriff gives the signal; the executioner enters the cell and pinions the prisoner's arms behind his back, and two officers lead him to the scaffold and place him directly across the division of the trap on a spot previously marked with chalk. The assistant executioner pinions his legs, while the executioner puts a white cap over his head and fits the noose round his neck with the knot drawn tight on the left lower jaw, where it is held in position by a sliding ring. The executioner then pulls the lever. The medical officer carries out an immediate inspection to assure himself that life is extinct and the body is then left to hang for an hour before being taken down. Mr. Pierrepoint said that the time which elapses between the entry of the executioner into the cell and the pulling of the lever is normally between nine and twelve seconds but may be twenty to twenty-five seconds in a few prisons where the condemned cell does not adjoin the execution chamber" (12).

The brief period of time which elapses between entry of the executioner into the prisoner's cell and his death by hanging is one of the arguments advanced in favor of this method of execution. Although a greater period of time is usually taken when execution is by lethal gas or electrocution this is not invariably true. Thus the time interval between entry into the prisoner's cell and unconsciousness varies between forty seconds and seven minutes. Disfiguration of the body in hanging (stretching of the neck) was not a problem in England where the body was not returned to the relatives, but buried within the prison.

Electrocution

New York was the first state to adopt electrocution as a means of capital punishment. "The first criminal to be executed by electricity was a man named Kemmler, who had killed his mistress in a fit of jealousy. He was condemned to death on June 24, 1889. An appeal was entered on the ground that the new method of execution was against the Federal Constitution, which stipulated that executions should not be 'cruel or unusual.' As the new law had abolished hanging in New York, there was no method of executing Kemmler until the point which had been raised was settled. It was not until August 6, 1890, over a year after he had been sentenced to death, that Kemmler was executed in Auburn Prison. Drying of one of the electrical conductors at the point of contact caused a burning of the flesh.

"One or two succeeding electrocutions passed off without incident, but on July 27, 1893, the execution of William Taylor, at Auburn, once again caused an outcry against the new method of capital punishment. With the first passing of the current, the chair broke and the unhappy man fell forward semi-conscious. He was removed to a bed and given chloroform and injections of morphia to keep him unconscious while the apparatus was being repaired. It was sixty-nine minutes before the current was restored and the execution completed" (7).

No similar mishap has occurred since but in some states there have been occasions when the current failed to reach the chair when the switch was engaged. Emergency generators are usually provided in case there is a power failure. The procedure in Washington, D.C. is as follows:

"The execution takes place at 10 AM. At midnight on the preceding night the condemned man is taken from the condemned cell block to a cell adjoining the electrocution chamber. About 5:30 AM the top of his head and the calf of one leg are shaved to afford direct contact with the electrodes. (The prisoner is usually handcuffed during this operation to prevent him from seizing the razor.) At 7:15 AM the death warrant is read to him and about 10 o'clock he is taken to the electrocution chamber. Five witnesses are present (including representatives of the Press) and two doctors — the prison medical officer and the city coroner. The witnesses watch the execution through a grille or dark glass and cannot be seen by the prisoner. Three officers strap the condemned man to the chair, tying him around the waist, legs and wrists. A mask is placed over his face and the electrodes are attached to his head and legs. As soon as this operation is completed (about two minutes after he has left the cell) the signal is given and the switch is pulled by the electrician; the current is left on for two minutes, during which there is alternation of two or more different voltages. When it is switched off, the body slumps forward in the chair. The prisoner does not make any sound when the current is turned on, and unconsciousness is apparently instantaneous. He is not, however, pronounced dead for some minutes after the current is disconnected. The leg is sometimes slightly burned, but the body is not otherwise marked or mutilated (12).

Lethal Gas

The gas chamber is still used for execution in several states. The following description of the method and equipment employed in North Carolina is typical of the procedure in other states:

"A chamber or room, when the doors are closed, is hermetically sealed to prevent leakage of cyanide gas. This room contains two observation windows. One window is for observation by the required witnesses and the other for officials required to be present at the execution. The doors leading to the chamber are connected with the electrically controlled panel. This is a safety measure, and unless the doors are properly closed the trap, allowing the cyanide pellets to drop into the acid, cannot be thrown. In this room is a wooden chair with leather straps for strapping the prisoner's arms, legs and across the abdomen to the chair. In the seat of his chair is a trap door electrically controlled which releases the cyanide pellets.

"Prior to the execution all equipment is double checked and a pound of sodium cyanide pellets is placed in the trap in the seat of the chair. Twenty minutes before execution three pints of USP sulphuric acid and six pints of water are carefully mixed in a lead container. The container is covered with a lid of similar material and is placed under the chair in a position to receive the pellets when dropped.

"There are two copper pipes adjacent to the chair which lead under the floor outside the physician's stand. At the end of the pipe in the chamber is a rubber hose which is to be connected to the head of a Bowles stethoscope strapped to the prisoner's chest. Attached to the other end of the copper pipes at the physician's stand are the earpieces of a stethoscope for determining the time of the prisoner's death.

"The prisoner has been previously prepared in his cell in this manner;

clothing removed, with the exception of shorts; the head of a Bowles stethoscope strapped over the apex of the heart with broad strips of adhesive.

"After the above preparations the prisoner walks to the execution chamber preceded by the chaplain and followed by the warden or one of his deputies. He is then strapped in the chair under the supervision of the warden or deputy; a leather mask applied to the face; the stethoscope head connected with aforementioned tube; the chaplain's prayers completed and all officials leave the chamber. The last person leaving the chamber quickly removes the cover from the acid container. The doors to the chamber and ante-room are quickly closed and the pellets dropped in the acid by the electrically controlled switch.

"After the prisoner is pronounced dead by the attending physician, ammonia gas is forced into the chamber until indicators within the chamber show that all cyanide gas has been neutralized. Ammonia gas is then removed by a specially constructed exhaust fan" (12).

Shooting

Shooting is the method of execution used in many countries during war time for offenses against the Military Code. There are many cases on record of executions which have been bungled by a nervous firing squad. The execution in World War II of the U.S. Army deserter Eddie Slovik is a case in point. The twelve men in the firing squad were picked on the basis of being expert riflemen. Yet Slovik struggled up twice after he had been shot. Huie quotes an Army physician who was present as follows:

"The shooting had been very poor and reflected the nervousness of the riflemen. Not one of the bullets had struck the heart. The bullets ranged from high in the neck region out to the left shoulder over the left chest, and under the heart. His body was quivering slightly; his breathing was extremely shallow; the heartbeat, faint, rapid and irregular. The firing squad had almost finished reloading for a second volley when Slovik was reported dead."

When Utah gave the condemned murderer the choice between shooting and hanging, shooting was preferred by almost all the condemned prisoners. The first hanging in Utah since 1912 occurred in 1958 when Barton Kirkham was executed for killing two persons in a $50 holdup in 1956. He refused to appeal for clemency. "I want to die, man, I'm fed up with it. I don't want life. My parents are the ones

who want me commuted. They think you can be rehabilitated in prison
. . . but rehabilitation comes from within. I chose hanging instead of the
firing squad because of the publicity . . . the novelty . . . to put the state
to more inconvenience."

Lethal Injection

The hypodermic needle may well replace the noose, the electric chair
and the gas chamber. Oklahoma, the first state to adopt lethal injection
in May 1977, coupled humanitarian with economic arguments: the
rusted electric coils and rotting wood in the state's old electric chair—last
used in 1966—required repairs costing $62,000. An alternative plan to
build a gas chamber would have cost more than $200,000. Death by in-
jection, law makers were advised, would cost only $10 to $15 "per event"
(8).

A barbiturate drug to render the person unconscious, a muscle relax-
ant, and potassium chloride to stop the heart are administered intrave-
nously. Usually there is rapid loss of consciousness. On November 2,
1984, fifty-two year old Margie Barfield was the first woman to be executed by the injection of drugs. She had herself, on different occasions,
poisoned her boyfriend, her mother and two elderly persons for whom
she had worked as a live-in housekeeper.

Three bottles of saline hung from the gurney to which she was
strapped. Two of them fed needles in her arms for about twenty minutes
to keep her veins open, while the third dripped into a bucket. Three
technicians behind a plastic curtain administered the drugs, but only
two of the technicians' injections went in her arms. As the drugs were injected into her arms, her mouth was moving quickly as if she were saying something. One witness said "It was almost as if she was praying."
There were no signs of a struggle or pain.

It took James Autry fifteen minutes to die on March 14, 1984. At
12:25 AM the prison warden asked Autry if he had any last words. Autry
answered no and the warden said "Let it begin." At 12:30 AM he grunted,
sighed and winced. He began breathing more deeply and said "Oh, it's
hurting." At 12:33 AM he raised his head, looked around at the warden
behind him, then at his pen pal, Shirley Tadlock, whom he had asked to
be a witness. "I love you" he said. At 12:35 AM his legs moved. Five
minutes later a doctor pronounced that Autry was dead (10).

Difficulty in locating a suitable vein may delay the execution. This is
particularly likely to happen when the person has been injecting heroin

into his veins with the result that many of the veins become blocked with scar tissue. This was the problem when the time came in March 1985 to execute the serial murderer and drug abuser Stephen Morin. It took technicians more than forty minutes to begin the lethal injections. After unsuccessful attempts on both arms and one leg a technician finally slipped the needle into a vein in his right arm.

The Guillotine

The guillotine, an instrument for beheading, was named after a French physician who advocated its use in 1789 on humanitarian grounds. The condemned prisoner is placed face downward on a platform, with his neck resting between semicircular depressions in two boards, which are held in position by two upright posts. When a lever is released, the guillotine blade, set into an eighty pound metal weight, slides down between the grooved upright posts. In order to prevent excessive mutilation an assistant executioner is responsible for preventing the victim from drawing his head into his shoulders. Because it is his duty to position the victim correctly, he is known in criminal slang as "the photographer."

Today France is the only country which uses this form of execution. "The prisoner is not informed of the date of his execution and he learns that his appeal for clemency has been rejected only when he is awakened by the officials charged to hand him over to the executioner. Nightly, he must go to sleep wondering if the guillotine is even then being silently mounted in the courtyard for the removal of his head a few hours later. Only on Saturday nights and the nights preceding religious or national fete days can he sleep without apprehension, knowing that Article 25 of the **Code Penal** prohibits the carrying out of death sentences on those days.

"A little before dawn, two wardens approach the condemned man's cell. They are in stockinged feet: nothing must disturb the prisoner's last few seconds' sleep. Suddenly they open the door, cross rapidly to the condemned man and seize him before he has had time to realize that this is no mere continuation of his dreams. The chaplain, the officials who have waited outside in the corridor, enter the cell. The prison director speaks the traditional words: 'Your appeal has been rejected. Be brave.' There is no hurry. The victim may smoke a final cigarette, drink a final glass of rum, write a letter, receive—if he wants it—such consolation as the chaplain can provide" (5).

THE EXECUTIONER

It is tempting to speculate on the motives and psychopathology of persons who seek employment as executioners. In England the number of applications for the post was very great and the applicants have included clergymen, lawyers, undertakers and doctors. In earlier times many hangmen were themselves criminals and their conduct on the gallows was often heartless and unseemly. The **Daily Mercury** for April 6, 1738, gives the following description of a public execution: "This day Will Summers and Tipping were executed here for housebreaking. At the tree, the hangman was intoxicated with liquor, and supposing that there were three for execution, was going to put one of the ropes round the parson's neck as they stood in the cart, and was with much difficulty prevented by the goaler from so doing."

Not a few executioners (Cratwell, Price, Rose, Thrift and others) have themselves died on the gallows or have suffered lesser punishment for murder. Others committed or attempted suicide. The English hangman, Ellis, resigned after executing a woman (Edith Thompson) and shortly after attempted to hang himself. Eight years later he committed suicide. Laurence describes two hangmen who executed relatives. Roger Gray, a seventeenth century executioner, hanged his own brother. He wrote the following letter to his nephew, "I am much afflicted to be the conveyancer of such news unto you as cannot be very welcome. Your father died eight days since, but the most generously I ever saw man, I will say this of him everywhere; for I myself trussed him up."

In the days of Charles II a father and his two sons were tried at Derby assizes for horse stealing. All were found guilty, and the bench of judges in a cruel whim, said they would pardon any one of the criminals who would consent to hang the other two. This barbarous offer was first made to the father, who indignantly refused it.

"What!" said he, "a father hang his two sons? Can I consent to take away the life I gave? Shall I put to a cruel death the boys I have cherished, and who to me have been dearer than life itself? No, No! Let me suffer a hundred deaths first!" . . . The elder son likewise refused, but the younger son accepted the offer and was later appointed hangman for Derby and neighboring counties.

The post of executioner is sometimes passed on from father to son and grandson. Between 1685 and 1847, seven generations of the Samson family were represented in the ranks of French public executioners. At one period seven Samson brothers were all engaged in the unusual profession. For over 200 years the male and even a few female members of eleven families, in effect held hereditary office as officials of the guillotine. These families tended to intermarry—a practice which was facilitated by the reluctance of most families to include among their relatives an executioner.

The post is seldom a popular one and even the most enthusiastic supporters of capital punishment hold the executioner in doubtful regard. The executioners of Spain were for a time compelled to have their houses painted red, and were not allowed to walk in the streets except in a garment which had a gallows embroidered on it (7). Following public executions strong forces of police were sometimes necessary to protect the hangman from assault by the crowd.

THE INTERVAL BETWEEN SENTENCE AND EXECUTION

In England the condemned murderer was executed within several weeks of his sentence. In 1950 when there were nineteen executions in England and Wales, the average period was about five weeks; in the twelve cases in which there was an appeal the average was slightly over six weeks, and in seven where there was not, it was just under three. The interval between sentence and execution is much longer in the United States.

In 1951, Frank Wojculewicz killed two persons, a police officer and a bystander in a packing house robbery and was himself paralyzed from a police bullet in his spine. He was convicted and sentenced to death in 1952. Several appeals were made based upon his injury and resulting mental condition. The State countered that his condition was of his own making and that the crime was not committed while he was ill. After waiting seven years in a Connecticut prison he was taken in 1959 to the execution chamber in a wheelchair. His wasted body was lifted into an electric chair which had been specially modified because his knees could not bend.

The first eight years of his second child's life (she was born shortly after the slaying) were spent while her father was under sentence of death.

Caryl Chessman, convicted of kidnapping for robbery with bodily harm—a capital offense in California in 1948—spent almost twelve years in death row before his execution in 1960. He fought off eight scheduled executions through court appeals. The thirty-eight year old man spent almost a third of his life under sentence of death.

While on death row he wrote four books, including a best seller **Cell 2455 Death Row.** The royalties financed his appeals. Before his execution Chessman described his nearness to death as terrifying. "It's almost as though you are walled off from the living. There is an awareness, hard to describe, that pours in on you like waves pounding against a beach. If you ask me how I feel about my approaching execution, let me say I do not believe I can project my feelings to anyone. I have been through this so many times that I just can't say how I feel. You die with the pungent odour of peach blossoms in your nostrils, strapped down, gagging, stared at." Chessman died with dignity, mouthing words to the witnesses, who could not hear him through the soundproof walls of the gas chamber.

Melvin Leroy Sullivan was only nineteen years old when he was sentenced to death with another man for the October, 1949 slaying of a youthful Utah service station attendant. Six and a half years later he was executed at dawn by a firing squad.

The attorneys for a condemned man should be given adequate time in which to prepare an appeal; but the practice, so common in the United States, of prolonging the period between sentence and execution for several years is surely undesirable.

GALLOWS HUMOR

"Nothing they did in life became them so well
as their manner of leaving it."

Grierson Dickson, *Murder by Numbers*

The last remarks of prisoners before execution are often given considerable publicity. Even the most banal comments are carefully noted and repeated for the benefit of a curious public. When the multiple murderer Crawford Goldsby, alias Cherokee Bill, was asked if he wanted to say anything to the crowd, he replied "No, I came here to die not to make a speech." Such reticence is not common. In earlier times in England condemned prisoners would often make speeches on the gallows, sometimes for as long as fifteen minutes or more. Last minute confessions or denial of guilt and religious comments commonly comprise the final comments of the doomed man.

Many anecdotes are told of humorous or insulting remarks by departing murderers and doubtless a significant percentage are apocryphal, as for example the statement attributed to the English poisoner, Dr. William Palmer. When offered a glass of champagne, just before the entrance of the hangman, he blew off the bubbles remarking: "They always give me indigestion the next morning if I drink in a hurry." Another prisoner waved aside a proffered glass of rum with the comment, "I lose all sense of direction when I'm drunk." Neville Heath's last words were a request for a whiskey, to which he added "You might make that a double." The mass murderer, Landru, adhering to his teetotal principles refused a glass of rum with the words, "Thank you, but I do not require it, I shall die bravely." Later he interrupted the chaplain, "I am very sorry" he murmured courteously, nodding toward the waiting executioners, "but I must not keep these gentlemen waiting" (2).

Peace, who had been worried by a cough for some days, wondered after a fit of coughing, whether the executioner "can cure this cough of mine." The plane bomber, Graham, extended an invitation to the Denver Post reporter, Zeke Scher, who had covered his trial, to sit on his lap—in the gas chamber. Commonly quoted comments are, "This will teach me a lesson I'll never forget" and the response to an impatient warder, "What's the hurry, they can't start without us." One offender when advised before entering the gas chamber that it would be easier to take deep breaths asked indignantly, "How would you know?"

The last words of one condemned man to the prison warden, prior to electrocution were, "Tell me, is it direct or alternating current, I've often wondered." A man, who had murdered his parents, complained to the executioner, "What! Would you execute an orphan?" Another who had killed his son complained that it was unjust to execute the father of a family. Christie, the multiple murderer, was opposed in principle to capital punishment.

John Sellhurst, while awaiting execution for the murder of his wife, penned this rhyme:

"With her a fearful life I led,
The drink it did so fly to her head;
On the devil's tipple she used to dote,
But I cured her with a cut on the throat,
I wish I could the deed undo,
And so, dear people all, must you."

James W. Rodgers, before his execution by the firing squad in Utah, spent his last few moments joking with a chaplain and prison officials.

When asked for his last request, he replied, "I done told you my last request, a bulletproof vest."

Kenneth Neu prior to his execution composed a song entitled, "I'm fit as a fiddle and ready to hang." He sang a verse of "Love in Bloom" to the accompaniment of a tap dance on the gallows. When the hangman approached, black cap in hand, Neu asked, "Has that thing been laundered since the last time you used it?" His last words were, "Don't muss my hair."

When the judge was reviewing the crime of Potts Harris, the prisoner, prior to pronouncing sentence of death, he made a slight error in a date and was corrected by the prisoner. The judge replied brusquely that it was a matter of slight importance. "I beg your Honor's pardon," Harris retorted, "you see, I have never been sentenced to death before and am not as familiar with the procedure as might be."

Not all men go to their death with a jest on their lips. In Columbia, South Dakota, a condemned rapist fought fiercely for twenty minutes before seven penitentiary guards could strap him into the chair. One guard suffered a deep bite on his wrists. The guard captain remarked: "I was so exhausted that for the first time in eighteen years I failed to ask a condemned man if he had any final word."

Pablo Vargas, sentenced to death for the rape murder of a sixteen year old girl, fought with guards for the last moments of his life. His composure collapsed as he approached the death chamber, and he struggled with guards, screaming, "Don't, please don't." The guards finally managed to drag him to the electric chair. It was the first time in the last 600 executions at the Sing Sing penitentiary that guards could recall a prisoner struggling. It is not unusual for a doomed man to comment adversely on the absence of the prosecutor and judge at the execution.

The great majority of condemned men and women show surprising fortitude and die bravely on the scaffold. Nothing so well becomes the murderer as his bearing on departing this world. The psychopath, who cannot live like a man, can die like one. The great majority of cases show a substantial gain in weight between the date of arrest and execution. Hobson found that only two out of fifty consecutive murderers awaiting trial at Brixton prison lost weight. The remaining forty-eight men all gained weight, and one or two of them gained as much as fourteen pounds. There may be considerable anxiety or depression so long as the murderer's fate is in doubt. Yet these symptoms may disappear as soon as the prisoner learns that his final appeal has been rejected.

The traditional last meal is often refused, which is perhaps not surprising. Some men, however, take full advantage of their privilege to request a special delicacy. For his last meal Kurten ordered Wienerschnitzel with fried potatoes and white wine, enjoying it so much that he asked for it again and ate a second meal (2).

The murderer, Morris Mason, who was electrocuted for raping an elderly woman, nailing her hand to a chair and then setting her house on fire, ordered a final meal from a McDonald's restaurant of four Big Macs (hamburgers), two large orders of french fries, two hot fudge sundaes, a piece of hot apple pie and two large soft drinks.

The final indignity of capital punishment is the autopsy. It's purpose is not clear as the cause of death is surely not in doubt. The argument that it is kinder to execute a man than to imprison him for life probably has few supporters among those best qualified to judge — the inhabitants of death row.

REFERENCES

1. Atholl, Justin: *The Reluctant Hangman.* London, John Long Ltd., 1956.
2. Dickson, Grierson: *Murder by Numbers.* London, Robert Hale Ltd., 1958.
3. Gardiner, Gerald: *Capital Punishment as a Deterrent and the Alternative.* London, Victor Gollancz Ltd., 1956.
4. Hobson, J.A.: Personal communication.
5. Kershaw, Alister: *A History of the Guillotine.* London, John Calder, 1958.
6. Koestler, Arthur: *Reflections on Hanging.* London, Victor Gollancz Ltd., 1956.
7. Laurence, John: *History of Capital Punishment.* London, Samson Low, 1932.
8. Malone, Patrick: Death row and the medical model. *Hastings Center Report,* 9(5):5, 1979.
9. Maudsley, Henry: *Insanity and Crime.* John Churchill and Sons, 1864.
10. *Medical Tribune,* February 6, 1985.
11. Radzinowicz, Leon: *A History of English Criminal Law.* New York, Macmillan and Company, 1948.
12. Royal Commission on Capital Punishment Report. London, H.M. Stationery Office, 1953.

CHAPTER 15

PREVENTION OF CRIMINAL HOMICIDE

"Any man's death diminishes me,
because I am involved in Mankind.
And therefore never send to know
for whom the bell tolls. It tolls
for thee."

John Donne, *Devotions*

IMPERFECT KNOWLEDGE of the origins of criminal homicide handicaps formulation of suitable preventive measures. Those who see criminals as victims of their social environment advocate social measures such as elimination of discrimination against minority groups, assurance of employment and clearance of slums. Many social reforms are needed independent of their possible influence on crime rates.

Sociologists emphasize the importance of delinquency areas, those crucibles of crime which contribute significantly to the incidence of delinquency and adult criminal behavior. Slum clearance is recommended but rehousing by itself is not sufficient. Various British studies have shown that as the slum areas have been cleared and their inhabitants transferred to new municipal housing estates, the centers of delinquency have shifted with them. The new estates have begun to surpass even the old central areas in the number of crimes committed by those who live in them (3).

Those who see crime as the product of warped personality development and mental disorder focus on the need for child guidance centers and the psychological treatment of offenders. Other solutions include better law enforcement, a prompt efficient judicial system with greater concern for the rights of victims and less emphasis on the rights of criminal suspects, stringent gun controls, research to enable recognition of the potential murder, longer prison sentences and more frequent use of the death penalty. Many of these proposals have two things in common: great expense and no clear evidence of their effectiveness in reducing the rates of criminal homicide.

It has been said that a country has the criminals it deserves. Crime prevention cannot be left to the police, the courts and the prisons. Citizens need to become involved in anti-crime crusades, in groups which promote campaigns against drunk drivers, child molesters and other offenders. Court watchers have contributed to more efficient operation of the courts and have drawn public attention to judges who give dangerous offenders, including murderers, short prison sentences, or place them on work-release programs so that they stay in jail only at night.

CITIZEN AWARENESS

Those persons who because of their occupation, age, sex or lifestyle are more likely to become victims of homicide should take steps to lessen this risk. Women who work alone at night in donut shops and convenience stores that are not located in busy shopping centers place their lives at risk. Hitchhikers and drivers who pick up hitchhikers place themselves in danger. Elderly persons who cash large checks at supermarkets may be observed by muggers in need of money. Prostitutes are ready victims for serial killers.

The increase in violent crime and political terrorism may have unpleasant consequences for any citizen. Radzinowicz and King warn that even in the most law-abiding countries, we have to come to terms with the fact that we had tended to develop expectations of security for ourselves and our property which are no longer realistic. "We have lost a measure of our freedom. We have been compelled to face the need for greater caution in our dealings with others. The possibility of falling a victim to crime, in its traditional sense, has increasingly to be taken into account in our daily lives" (8).

Some of the preventive measures against becoming a victim of crime have dismal implications that we are regressing to a paranoid lifestyle in which persons are afraid to open their doors to strangers, banks conduct their business by television screens and pneumatic tubes, and cities plan long narrow parks as protection against assault and robbery. Home owners should have entrance lights and a strong front door with a peephole. Large shrubs should not be located near the door. Even if a caller is in police uniform, check to see whether there is a police car parked in the street before opening the door. Call utility and telephone companies to confirm the identity of employees when they make surprise visits. Do not allow strangers inside to use the telephone.

In the United States 10 percent of all criminal homicides occur during armed robberies. If approached by an armed robber in the street it is wise to hand over your wallet or purse without argument or discussion. It is not wise to give up a weapon, allow the robber to take you to another location or permit him to tie you up. If you are taken to an isolated area there is no one there to help you. If you are tied up you are completely helpless. It is the writer's impression that criminals who tie up victims are more likely to kill or inflict physical injury. Resistance to these demands gives you a sporting chance of survival by calling for help or fighting your assailant.

The reader may say that it is easier to give this advice than to follow it. I was seized as a hostage in a county jail by a man charged with two counts of murder and three counts of armed robbery and assault. He seized me from behind and started choking me. No attempt was made to reason with him. Instead I shouted for help at the top of my voice and repeatedly kicked him in the shin. He responded by biting my ear and he did not let go. Two deputy sheriffs responded to the interviewing room and despite his threat "Get out of here or I'll cut his throat" immediately seized the prisoner and released me. He was armed with a razor blade but he did not cut my throat.

Keep your car doors locked at all times. A young couple were sitting in their car on a Denver street when a man jerked a door open and at gunpoint told the driver, "Just drive me where I tell you and no one will get hurt." Near a farmhouse he ordered the couple out of the car, robbed them, then shot the man in the back killing him. He attempted to rape the woman but she struggled with him and despite a bullet wound in the shoulder was able to escape.

Before getting into your car, check your back seat to make sure that no one is hiding there. Before getting out of your car check for suspicious persons outside your home or apartment house. Do not get out of your car to help someone requesting assistance. Drive to the nearest pay telephone and notify the police that someone needs help. If your car breaks down, raise the hood, turn on your flasher lights, and ask anyone who stops to help you to call the police or a garage. You will make exceptions to these rules, for example when a car with a family stops to help you. The serial murderers, Sherman McCrary and Carl Taylor, travelled across the United States with their wives. Taylor's wife was McCrary's daughter. At least one victim, after being abducted from a Denver donut shop, was taken in the family car to a lonely spot, raped and murdered.

Businesses should take steps to reduce the likelihood of armed robbery. Store owners should keep their store windows as uncluttered as possible. Large signs and advertising displays make it difficult for officers driving by in police cruisers to see inside the store. Robbers prefer to conduct their business in privacy and often avoid stores where the cash register and safe are close to a large front plate glass window. Invite the police to check your security measures. Check the identification, arrest records and backgrounds of new employees. An employee who shows no identification and gives a false address may be planning to set up a robbery.

Handle money with care. Never advertise possession of large sums of money nor discuss payroll or other money matters in public places. Keep as little money as possible in cash registers. A criminal who purchased a carton of milk in a supermarket was impressed by the amount of money in the cash register. Two weeks later he robbed the store. Following his arrest he told police, "I wouldn't have hijacked them if they hadn't been so careless with their money."

Money not needed for making change should be placed in a locked safe. "Drop safes" permit employees to place money in the safe without having to open the safe. If they do not have the key, they cannot be forced to open the safe. Money can also be kept or hidden in some place other than the cash register. Care should be taken not to betray the location of this money. Make bank deposits in daylight whenever possible. Vary the time and route of trips to the bank. Failure to take this elementary precaution may have fatal consequences as in the following example.

A store manager went to the bank at the same time every day, and drove the same car over the same route to and from the bank. He was watched, timed and checked each day by four men who knew every move he made. The store manager had a habit of locking the door on the passenger's side of his automobile and leaving the driver's door unlocked at the bank. This was known by the robbers and on the day of the robbery, while the victim was in the bank, one robber entered the victim's car and unlocked the door on the passenger side. He wiped off all his fingerprints inside the car to prevent his identification.

The store manager left the bank, entered his car, locked the door on the driver's side and placed the money sack containing $7,600 on the front seat beside him. He sat there for a few minutes, then backed from the parking space. As he started to drive from the lot, his car was blocked in front and rear. Two men from the car in front walked up to the manager's car, opened the passenger door, shot him twice, removed the money bag, and drove away (4).

BUILDING DESIGN

Buildings, especially apartment houses are now being designed to make them as crime proof as possible. High-rise apartment houses are most susceptible to crime. Apartment houses with more than thirteen floors have twice as much crime as blocks with the same number of apartments but on only three floors. The safest shape for an apartment house is not a tall, square building but an "L" shape in which the ends of the "L" touch the street and the entrance way lies in the angle between the two arms. This creates a private triangular zone between the street and the apartments which the residents come to know and in which the activity of strangers can be quickly spotted. The entrance is easy to light at night and because it is the only one in the block it remains busy.

The most important factor in the design of entrance ways, elevators and staircases (where up to half the crimes of violence take place) is their visibility from and proximity to the street. Many architects like to design housing precincts with the entrances facing inward, for the sake of privacy. But these are not safe. Robberies from people in entrance ways (where the mailboxes are often situated) are twice as common when the entrances face away from the street.

Newman notes the safety of areas densely and regularly enough populated to provide a number of possible witnesses, who might choose to come to the aid of a victim. He suggests that entries to residential buildings should be planned in juxtaposition to these "safe" areas such as high schools, hamburger joints and shopping centers. Fire doors to fire escapes should open only from the inside.

GUN CONTROL

"How oft the sight of means to do ill deeds
Makes ill deeds done!"

Shakespeare, *King John*

A person who is determined to commit murder will do so with any available weapon, a knife, a piece of wood, or with his bare hands. Some persons who would not hesitate to shoot their victim on an impulse might flinch from hand to hand combat or might be unable to accomplish their purpose without the advantage of a firearm. It is tempting to think of gun control as a means of reducing the homicide rate, but prohibition of the sale of alcohol in the United States did not eliminate the sale of alcohol, and gun control will not eliminate the sale of guns.

Advocates of gun control recommend that the private possession of handguns should be prohibited for all persons other than law enforcement and military personnel. In support of this measure reference is often made to the lower incidence of armed crime in England where gun control laws sharply restrict the possession of handguns. Yet figures from that country suggest that guns were less used in crime when there were no controls whatever. Furthermore fifty years of control have not deprived the criminal of access to a vast pool of illegal weapons.

Legislators would do well to study **Firearms Control** by Colin Greenwood, a Chief Inspector of the West Yorkshire Constabulary. His book is based on considerable research conducted while he was a Fellow of the Cambridge University Institute of Criminology. He shows that about half a million firearms have been surrendered to the police since 1946 — half of these were pistols most of which were illegally held. Unfortunately criminals are not likely to take their handguns to the police and despite fifty years of very strict controls on pistols, there is far greater use of this class of weapon in crime than ever before.

THE POTENTIAL SLAYER

It is often stated that a considerable percentage of homicide offenders are not persons of criminal tendencies, that slaying another person is their first offense against the law. Wolfgang's study of homicide in Philadelphia suggests otherwise. Sixty-four percent of the offenders in this study had previous arrest records, largely for offenses against the person, including aggravated assault. Wolfgang believes that if sufficient attention, supervision and follow-up by appropriate authorities were applied to the person who commits aggravated assault, assault with intent to kill, or a series of less serious personal assaults, society would be able to exercise some control over the offense of homicide, and the number of killings accordingly might decrease.

It is surely a matter for concern that persons convicted of serious, or potentially serious bodily assault are not infrequently fined a small sum of money, sentenced to a few days in jail or given a prison sentence, which is suspended providing the defendant leaves town. (If you must shoot someone, please do so in another town or state.) Doubtless there are cases of bodily assault, where a prison sentence is not indicated.

Nevertheless, there are many cases on record of criminal offenders, who, despite a history of dangerous propensities, have been fined or given short prison sentences for serious bodily assault. In other cases there was either no pre-sentence investigation or an inadequate investigation.

THREATS TO KILL

Threats to kill, like threats to commit suicide, should not be taken lightly. Homicidal threats may be made seriously or in jest, in the heat of anger or in deceptive calm. A young soldier decided to kill his NCO. The next morning he informed a fellow soldier of his intended homicide, naming the victim. That day he shot the NCO and then returned to his barracks, where he related the full story to the other soldier after opening with the remark, "Mission accomplished, mind at ease." He told one soldier to notify his commanding officer and asked another to play the tune, "In the Jailhouse Now."

Another soldier when informed that he was to be transferred to Camp Hale, Colorado, announced that he would kill himself or someone else first. He stated that he did not care about the consequences of such an action. Arrangements were being made to discharge him from the Army, but he shot and killed a man while stealing a car in which he had planned to go absent without leave. In both these examples, the calm statement of intended murder was deceptive.

Conditional threats may have lethal consequences. "If you ever leave me, I'll kill you" may lead to "If I can't have you, I'll make sure no one else does." As promiscuous wives tend to remain promiscuous, the threat, "If you ever step out on me agian..." may foreshadow tragedy. The husband who can live neither with his wife nor without her may resolve his dilemma through homicide.

A five to six year follow-up study of 100 patients admitted to a psychiatric hospital because of homicidal threats showed that seven had either taken their own lives or those of others. Four committed suicide and three committed homicide. The incidence of homicide or suicide may be more than 7 percent as twenty-three patients could not be traced (5).

The threat which is expressed in gesture, the hand drawn across the throat or clasped to some weapon, has a melodramatic quality which may be misleading. A change in facial expressions, "if looks could kill," sometimes conveys greater menace than the spoken word. The threat may be made in writing, stated clearly in an extortion note or perhaps disguised in the fantasy of a classroom essay. When a teacher asked the class to write a theme on a book, a fifteen year old student wrote the following:

> This book does not have a title, but it is the story of a boy who was fed up of living. His name, that doesn't matter. It's what he will do will shock you. One night when his parents went to bed, he got up from his bed, took his shotgun, loaded it and went quietly into their bedroom.
>
> His mother and father were sleeping, he took aim, shot his father first, his mother screamed, he shot her. His smaller brother came running out of his room to see what was the matter, he fired again. What was the reason for this gruesome murder? What made him to do it? He hated them. His life ambition was to get a car. They promised him one, but always fell down on their promises. This story is not fiction, although it sounds fantastic, it happened in my family.

That night the student went to his parent's room and wounded both with two blasts from a shotgun.

Symbolic expression of the homicidal threat include burning, firing bullets at, or sticking a pin in a picture of the intended victim. The husband who rips or burns clothing belonging to his wife or stabs her pillow repeatedly with a knife may be warning her of his homicidal anger toward her. A mother who stabbed a favorite childhood doll later attempted to kill her infant daughter. False confessions of murder may also betray homicidal inclinations. Clifford Allen pointed out the need for psychiatric examination after a young man made such a confession. His warning was disregarded. A few days later, the young man stabbed a girl to death on Dartford Heath (1).

It is not easy to provide protection for wives who have been threatened by their husbands. Mrs. LS was warned that her former husband intended to come to Denver to kill her. She tried to get help from the authorities, but was told that nothing could be done until S actually came to Denver and started bothering her. S arrived by plane from New York at 4 PM on a Monday afternoon. Early Tuesday morning he called at his ex-wife's home and, in the presence of their son, he killed her before shooting himself. Four months earlier S had been released from a Colorado mental hospital to the care of his mother in New York. She had promised to keep him under close supervision and to place him under private psychiatric care.

MENTAL ILLNESS AND HOMICIDE

Each year there are a number of tragic killings by psychotic persons. The tragedy is compounded by the fact that often there is a clear indication, for weeks or even months before the act of homicide, that the offender was suffering from severe mental illness. Families often procrastinate and avoid taking action to secure psychiatric treatment until some major untoward event occurs. It is perhaps understandable why relatives of a sick person delay taking the necessary steps to seek help. It is not so clear why physicians so often acquiesce in this delay. Expectations of a spontaneous improvement in the patient's condition; failure to recognize the serious nature of the disorder and reluctance to antagonize the patient are possible explanations. Delay is especially likely to occur when the patient is a prominent or wealthy member of the community.

The severely depressed person who complains that he can see no hope for the future may take his own life or the lives of his family. The paranoid person who believes that he is being persecuted may seek help from a lawyer or from the police. When he fails to obtain the help he expects, namely protection from his alleged persecutors, he may feel justified in taking the law into his own hands. The writer during a period of three years saw two paranoid persons accused of murder under these circumstances.

A middle-aged woman had delusions that her husband was having sexual relations with their teenage daughter. The police department, on receipt of her complaint, arranged for physical examination of the daughter. The woman did not believe the results of the examination, which refuted her accusation, and she later shot and killed her husband. A railroad worker complained to a sheriff's office that officials of the railroad union were doping him. The complaint was recognized as being absurd, but no attempt was made to obtain psychiatric examination and the man subsequently murdered one of his imagined persecutors.

The sociopathic personality, who figures so prominently among those who threaten homicide, is not usually welcome in psychiatric hospitals because of his disruptive influence on patients and staff. Involuntary commitment to a mental hospital often provides only brief protection for society. It may further undermine his self-respect as well as cause resentment toward relatives who participated in his court commitments. The majority of sociopaths can benefit from help even if that help is confined to crisis outpatient therapy as the need arises, or treatment of the wife who provokes the homicidal threats she fears. Acting out, slight apparent motivation for treatment, and refusal to acknowledge illness are too often regarded as portents of therapeutic failure rather than as a therapeutic challenge.

RELEASE FROM JAIL ON BOND

Persons charged with serious crimes, other than murder, are entitled as a matter of law to be released on bond. The suspected offender cannot be kept in custody because he is likely to commit further crimes. The purpose of the bond is not to protect the public, but merely to assure appearance of the defendant in court at the time of the trial. It is illegal to set an excessive bond for the sole purpose of preventing a person to leave jail before trial. There are no available statistics to show how many murders are committed by suspects while free on bond.

Dangerous offenders should be tried without delay and not released on bond. Some criminals consider the cost of bail bonds a routine business expense, although not approved as tax deductions by the Internal Revenue Service. Many armed robbers while on bond commit further robberies. They feel they have nothing to lose by committing more armed robberies, they wish to continue the style of living to which they have been accustomed, or they want money to hire a private attorney. In the minds of these men PD stands for penitentiary deliverer rather than public defender.

Criminals free on bond have intimidated or even killed witnesses against them. Others have absconded. One of three suspects in the

holdup slaying of a world famous Columbia University law professor
had been arrested four times that year and warrants for his arrest had
been issued two months before the homicide for failure to appear in
court on charges of robbery and possession of narcotics. A New York
City police spokesman said that the police were unable to cope with the
volume of arrest warrants issued by the courts.

Andy Lopez age forty-five of Santa Fe, New Mexico in February
1985 was sentenced to seven years in prison for the second degree murder of Andy Hernandez. A psychologist testified that he had no criminal
record, the killing was an isolated incident in a long-standing family
feud, and he was unlikely to hurt anyone before reporting to prison. On
Wednesday the judge ordered Lopez to report to prison the follwing
Monday.

On Friday Lopez went to the home of the widow of his victim, and
killed her with a single shot in her face in the presence of her three young
children. She had opposed his request to be allowed to plead guilty to a
lesser charge of voluntary manslaughter in the killing of her husband.
After killing Regina Hernandez, Lopez seized nine persons in the court-
house as hostages. He asked to exchange the hostages for the district attorney and judge, who had sentenced him. He was fatally wounded
when he shot at a deputy sheriff while attempting to leave the court-
house.

LAW ENFORCEMENT

According to the **Uniform Crime Reports** of the FBI 92.3 percent of
murders in the United States in 1960 were cleared or solved by arrests,
86 percent in 1970, 72 percent in 1980 and 76 percent in 1983. Although
the clearance rate is higher for murder than for any other **Crime Index**
offense almost one in four homicides are not solved by the police.

It is, of course, impossible to estimate accurately the number of unsolved homicides. Death from homicide, which is falsely attributed to accidental or natural causes, will not appear in homicide statistics. It has been
suggested that if all coroners were required to have a medical degree, fewer
murders would be passed off as suicides or accidental deaths. However, the
laxity of some doctors in completing death certificates, without adequate
investigation encourages the poisoner to continue his trade.

More effective law enforcement increases the likelihood of the detection, conviction, and punishment of homicide offenders. The FBI

National Academy has done much to improve police standards throughout the United States as well as in other countries. The work of the Behavioral Science Unit of the FBI at Quantico, Virginia on profiling the various types of murderers and on devising police responses to trap the murderer have been the most exciting contributions in many years to the criminal investigation of homicide. Aggressive police patrol can do much to reduce the risk of homicide, especially robbery homicides. Random patrol is more effective than routine patrol in which businessmen and householders can set their watches by the appearance of the local precinct police cruiser.

The problem of the serial murderer who goes from state to state killing citizens, moving quickly from the scene of his crime to travel to another location hundreds or thousands of miles away, is being tackled by the Violent Criminal Apprehension Program (VI-CAP) of the FBI. A centralized data information center and crime analysis section have been designed to collect and analyze data on similar pattern multiple murderers within the United States.

Crimes that will be included are most murders by mutilation, dismemberment, torture or with violent sexual trauma; attacks on victims who survive criminal assaults that fit the VI-CAP crime pattern; missing children when there is reason to believe the child has been kidnapped or will be harmed; the mysterious disappearance of any person when there is substantial proof of foul play and unidentified bodies when death has resulted from homicide.

FAMILY VIOLENCE

Nearly 20 percent of all murders involve family relationships and almost a third of female homicide victims are killed by their husbands or boyfriends. These murders are often preceded by assaults that are reported to the police. In Kansas City, Missouri the police found that they had prior contact with 85 percent of the couples whose fights ended in homicide. Police responding to a report of domestic violence will usually attempt to restore peace at the scene or will order the offender to leave the house for the night. They are reluctant to make an arrest unless there is serious injury or continuing threats of violence, because victims either do not want the offender arrested or later fail to cooperate with the prosecutor.

A Justice Department Task Force has urged the nation's criminal justice system to treat physical and sexual abuse within the family as being no less serious than such acts when they occur outside the family unit. The legal response to family violence should be guided by the nature of the abusive act, not the relationship between the victim and abuser. The Task Force recommended that abusers should be arrested, and encouraged prosecutors to cease requiring victims to sign a formal complaint to initiate prosecution. When appropriate, weekend or evening incarceration was suggested to preserve the family's financial stability.

Some state laws do not permit police officers to make arrests for minor assaults they did not witness. In Minnesota such arrests are permitted and in Minneapolis a scientifically controlled study was made of the relative effectiveness in domestic violence of counselling both parties, sending the assailant away from the home and arresting the assailant. It was found that arresting the assailant was the most effective method of preventing further violence within a period of six months.

According to official records on 314 cases of domestic violence 10 percent of those arrested repeated violence compared with 19 percent of those advised and 24 percent of those suspects sent away from the home. Interviews with 161 victims showed that 19 percent of those arrested, 37 percent of those advised and 33 percent of those suspects sent away from the home repeated violence within six months (9). Only three of the 136 arrested offenders were punished by fines or a prison sentence. This suggests that arrest and a night in jail without formal punishment have a deterrent effect.

PRISON SENTENCES

Clarence Burns in 1982 was charged with first degree murder after shooting his wife five times in the head shortly after she had filed for divorce. To avoid a jury trial Burns pleaded guilty to second degree murder, which then carried a sentencing range of eight to twelve years. Denver District Court Judge Alvin Lichtenstein sentenced Burns to four years in prison but suspended the sentence on condition that Burns serve two years in a work-release program and two years on probation. This would have allowed him to keep his job as a butcher as he would spend only nights and weekends in the Denver County Jail.

At the sentencing hearing the prosecutor contended that Mrs. Burns was a battered wife whose beatings at her husband's hands resulted in bruises, black eyes and stitches. Burns was also a compulsive gambler who had left his family deeply in debt. Judge Lichtenstein said he believed Burns had been provoked by his wife who had deceived him by being extremely loving and caring up to the morning when she left him. At a rally of the National Organization for Women on the steps of the State Capitol protesting the sentence, one woman carried a sign "Lichtenstein has provoked me. Can I shoot him five times in the face?"

A woman discussed the case with a friend and told her "If that man can get off with such a short sentence, I know I can get away with it too." About a week later she shot and killed her husband. She was found guilty of first degree murder.

A week after the public outcry over the sentencing of Burns, Judge Lichtenstein, saying that he had just learned that the couple's fifteen year old son was to inherit $100,000 from his mother's estate, reversed himself and ordered Burns to spend four years in prison. The Colorado Supreme Court ruled that the sentence was illegal because it did not meet the standards of Colorado law. Another judge sentenced Burns to eight years in prison.

Murderers should be sent to prison for many years to deter others from committing this crime, to impress upon the murderer that his crime can have painful consequences for him for many years, and to protect law abiding citizens from being murdered by him so long as he is confined. Unfortunately prison guards do not have such protection. Short prison sentences for murder do not deter others inclined to kill. The murderer does not suffer the pain of prolonged confinement that after his release might cause him to think twice before pulling the trigger. He is free to kill again within a few years as in the following example.

In October 1966 Charles W. Yukl told police he found the nude body of Suzanne Reynolds, a model, in a vacant apartment in his building, an hour after she had finished a voice lesson and left his apartment. The police noticed semen stains on his trousers and he confessed to strangling, raping and mutilating the body of his victim. The District Attorney concerned that the confession might be thrown out by an appeal court accepted a plea of guilty to manslaughter which had a maximum penalty of twenty years.

The judge sentenced Yukl to seven to fifteen years but released him on bond while he appealed his conviction. After his appeal was rejected he was confined in prison from April 1969 to June 1973—less than five years. A state prison psychiatrist later stated, "We were sure he was rehabilitated and one of the best, brightest, most articulate prisoners I have ever seen." He committed an almost identical murder in 1974. The victim was an actress who replied to his advertisement seeking actresses to appear in a movie. Her body, nude, strangled, raped and battered was found on the roof of a building where Yukl lived. This time he got a life sentence.

Life sentences, however, are seldom life sentences. Nearly three-fifths of prisoners with life sentences released in the United States during 1982 had served seven years or less in prison. Almost a fourth of them served three years or less (10). There is seldom public outcry over quick release from prison because the public is seldom informed or the victim's relatives have no clout.

The quick release of a prisoner who has murdered a police officer is not likely to escape notice. In 1969 the police chief of Bellevue, Iowa was found lying face down in a pool of blood at the scene of a forced entry into an auto-dealer's garage. Apparently he surprised his murderers in the commission of the break-in and was bludgeoned to death with a shovel. William P. Sweeney know to have a history of assault and battery charges was arrested and charged with first-degree murder along with another man and an eighteen year old girl. Sweeney was convicted and sentenced to seventy-five years in prison.

Two years and eight months after entering prison he was freed on parole. An Iowa corrections official commenting on the case said, "He has received the maximum amount of treatment, his attitude and progress were excellent, and it was the staff opinion that now was the best time to release him if we expect complete rehabilitation... Our only excuse for keeping him incarcerated any longer would have been just to punish him. And to keep him only to punish him is not in keeping with the attitude of correcting."

PRISONS

"Prisons are not meant to be comfortable which is no doubt the consideration that reconciled Pontius Pilate to the practice of crucifixion."

Bernard Shaw, *The Crime of Imprisonment*

Many of our prisons give the appearance of having been expressly designed to reinforce the prisoner's grudge against society rather than to serve the purpose of rehabilitation. A study of life within a penitentiary often shows a combination of idleness, boredom and regimented useless-ness. Any other closed community, such as an army or a monastery, re-gards its discipline and discomfort as a means to an end, but penitentiary institutional life is sometimes an end in itself—a dead end.

Regimentation and removal of all responsibility have their dangers. Men can only learn to accept responsibility when they are given an op-portunity to exercise it. In the restrictive mental atmosphere of the con-ventional prison the inmate becomes progressively less well equipped to return to a useful life within society. Winston Churchill, while Home Secretary in charge of British prisons, made this statement in favor of improvements in the penal system:

> A desire and eagerness to rehabilitate in the world of industry all those who have paid their dues in the hard coinage of punishment, tireless efforts towards the discovery of curative and regenerating processes, and an un-faltering faith that there is a treasure if you can find it, in the heart of every man—these are the symbols which in the treatment of crime and criminals mark and measure the stored-up strengths of a nation, and are the sign and proof of living virture in it.

Reformers are seldom popular, and in this regard Churchill was no exception. When he was transferred from his position in charge of prisons to the Admiralty to take responsibility for the Royal Navy, an overjoyed prison governor, on hearing the news, at once instructed the chaplain that the two hymns to be sung in chapel the next morning should be "Now thank we all our God" and "For those in peril on the sea." Efforts to improve our prisons meet with slight public support. Even the longest penitentiary sentences come to an end. If prisoners emerge no better than when they went in, it will be the public which pays the price (6).

PREVENTION OF SELF-MURDER

Contrary to the general impression that a truly suicidal person "just goes ahead and does it," many patients reveal their plans beforehand. Days, weeks or even months before the suicide, reference may be made, quietly or melodramatically, to the intended event. Suicide may occur in the background of severe depression or schizophrenia, but only about one in five suicides are the result of psychosis. Alcoholics and impulsive persons with a low tolerance for frustration are a constant source of sui-cidal threats.

Unfortunately, relatives are reluctant to take threats of suicide seriously. "I didn't think he meant it." "He seemed to be improving." "He'd been saying it so long, I stopped worrying about it." Psychiatric evaluation should always be obtained promptly, especially when the suicidal person expresses no hope for the future, condemns himself for past transgressions, shows unreasonable concern over his financial position or complains of loss of appetite, lack of energy and insomnia, with early morning awakening. The death of a relative or an emotional crisis increases the danger. An unsuccessful attempt at suicide is another danger signal.

REFERENCES

1. Allen, Clifford: *A Textbook of Psychosexual Disorders.* London, Oxford University Press, 1969.
2. Greenwood, Colin: *Firearms Control.* London, Routledge and Kegan Paul, 1972.
3. Jones, Howard: *Crime and the Penal System.* London, University Tutorial Press, 1965.
4. Macdonald, J. M.: *Armed Robbery.* Springfield, Charles C Thomas, 1975.
5. Macdonald, J. M.: *Homicidal Threats.* Springfield, Charles C Thomas, 1968.
6. Macdonald, J. M.: *Psychiatry and the Criminal.* Springfield, Charles C Thomas, 1976.
7. Newman, Oscar: *Defensible Space: Crime Prevention Through Urban Design.* New York, Macmillan, 1972.
8. Radzinowicz, Leon and King, Joan: *The Growth of Crime.* New York, Basic Books, 1977.
9. Sherman, L. W. and Berk, R. A.: The specific deterrent effects of arrest for domestic assault. *Amer Sociol Rev 49:*261, 1984.
10. US Justice Department: *Time Served in Prison,* 1984.
11. Wolfgang, M. E.: *Patterns in Criminal Homicide.* Philadelphia, University of Pennsylvania Press, 1958.

CHAPTER 16

HOMICIDE IN FICTION

By

Stuart Boyd

"If wishes were horses they would pull the hearse
of our dearest friends and nearest relatives.
All men are murderers at heart."
"A thought-murder a day keeps the doctor away."

Theodore Reik

HOMICIDE only occurs in one kind of fiction — the detective story. In all other kinds of fiction it is murder, "murder most foul!" "Homicide" is a poltroon of a word, a Latin intruder, legalistic and pompous. Can anyone really hear the housemaid running from the gory corpse in the bedroom screaming "homicide!"? "Murder" is a gutty word, capable of expressing all subtle and sinister shades of meaning — it is a verb, a noun, and in various forms is able to encompass the fiend, his deed and the victim. So, "Murder" it will be.

It is surprising with what éclat one undertakes tasks that are impossible. The thought of covering the subject of "Murder in Fiction" appealed to this writer immediately. Eventually there came the realization that one could only hope to pen an entertaining essay on some aspects of murder in some works of fiction. The vasty compendium, the definitive statement, vanished like the clues before the gaze of the ponderous policeman.

Murder is the great, the ultimate crime. All else fades before its power to hold and repel at one and the same time. The act of murder, even the very thought of it, is the classic approach-avoidance situation where the goal both repels and attracts. I venture to suggest that all reasonably intelligent and imaginative men have thought of committing a murder. Many of us perhaps have felt the very impulse rising dangerously within us at one time or another. It is such a serious subject that, unless one is actually writing fiction, there is a natural defensive retreat to the light touch as in De Quincey and Ambrose Bierce. The writer is driven to this defense and the reader gratefully accepts it. Alfred Hitchcock has mastered this method in his television presentations. If this defense is recognized for what it is, I submit no great harm has been done to this most profound of all human acts.

When one first encounters the real murderer in professional work one is sadly aware that he is not vastly different from oneself. He does not have the look, the feel, the sense of murder about him. One's sadness may well turn to anger at having been taken in. I do not think one says "But this is me!" But I do think, if honest, one says "But this could be me." And if one had not misspent the youthful years reading "Penny Horribles" and instead had read Shakespeare or Dostoevsky one would not have been thus deceived. For if I have a central point to my essay it is this—The great writers did not and do not deceive, but an increasing sophistication is to be found today, even among the Spillane "Best Sellers," which reflects the general influence of Freud's mind.

Shakespeare and Dostoevsky did not need Freud. But we others did. It is somehow given to a few creative geniuses to know the stuff of life, and to be able to express it in subtle splendid writing. Too often we see the splendor and miss the subtlety. We others had to be taught the painful lessons of psychoanalysis to be able to see more to life than a series of exhortatory homilies couched in the language of "good" and "bad." By this I do not mean formal lessons in psychoanalysis but the informal teachings of an experience which today reflects Freud in art, literature, poetry and drama at high, middle and low levels of competence and taste, from Joyce to Spillane, from Picasso to the beatnik dauber, from T. S. Eliot to Ginsberg. Whether one chooses to disagree with what Freud said is irrelevant here, one cannot disagree as to the fact of influence, good or bad, on many important forms of artistic production to which one is inevitably exposed. The proponents of the good influence have on occasion proved themselves extremists and fanatics, while the recent **The Freudian Ethic** is an example of the fanaticism of the proponent of the bad.

Every great writer deals with murder because he knows it lies in the human heart. Many, considerably less than great, deal with murder (sometimes exclusively) because they know it sells books. In this second category I believe one must distinguish between the writer who ties up the murder in an ingenious knot, leaving the reader the cozy rationalization of an intellectual unravelling game to explain away his vicarious interest in the bloody deed itself; and the writer who makes no pretence in his appeal to hob-nailed emotions.

Arthur Conan Doyle is a good example of the first, with his irritating logical deductions (which only have the ring of logic after the reader has frustratedly wandered to the page where the Baker Street sleuth sneeringly confounds the dishonest human policemen, the only real people in his stories). How easy it is to disclaim interest in the murder itself when it is so skillfully tricked up in this intellectual puzzle. The English detective story writers are particularly adept at this trick of presenting the ultimate crime in the language of Lamb and the logic of the Jesuit. Michael Innes comes to mind as the master of the genre.

But the gentle ladies of murder, Dorothy Sayers and Agatha Christie, are no slouches when it comes to taking the guilt off the gingerbread by an appeal to style and reason. The professed interest of the reader is in the puzzle, with the blood and sex necessary but offensive, and to be skipped over with as much good taste and reserve as can be mustered.

Spillane, on the other hand, is more honest but uncivilized. His readers, avid millions according to the book-jackets, must find the puzzle a tedious link between the boot in face, death-by-scattering episodes, which abound, and which usually culminate in orgasmic crisis. There is no pretence here, but also no style, taste, rhyme nor reason. His books go for the groin, either with a caress or a knife — usually the latter. But even in these astounding monuments to cultural and educational deficiencies there is a glimmer or understanding that life cannot be arbitrarily divided into "the good" and "the bad."

Spillane is aware that badness is complex and dynamic. He is unaware that goodness is equally complex and dynamic. In fact he does not seem to be aware of goodness at all. Certainly his Neanderthal hero, Hammer, is no credit to the forces of justice and might — winning always by out-brutalizing, out-cunninging, and out-sexing his opponents. Hammer (and surely the name is subtle) is above the law, sometimes taking on the role of a mythological avenging Fury wearing brass knuckles — but always the tough realist, physically and psychologically.

The realism may well be a veneer for psychopathic expediency. If he has a super-ego it is whimsical and cynical. Mainly he is a walking compromise between the aggressive-sexual id and a cunning ego. One feels he is very much at home with the psychopaths he always manages to exterminate.

These then represent extremes—the urbane English stylist, Innes, and the very popular Spillane, the covert and the overt in murder. Innes is too defensive, Spillane too offensive about the necessary human fact of murder. Spillane almost reaches the level of "hardcore" violence, if I may use a term suggested by the Doctors Kronhauser in their recent **Pornography and the Law** in connection with sexual writings. Violence and murder are undeniable facts of human experience, no matter whether that experience be internal (in fantasy), or external (in action). When they are dealt with by the writer as an essential part of life, and shown in relation to tenderness and compassion, then we may talk of realism, or violent realism. When the theme of violence comes to dominate and overwhelm the life experience as presented, then this comes close to being "hard-core" sadism, in much the same way as erotic realism (as in **Ulysses**) gives place to hard-core pornography (as in **The Memoirs of Fanny Hill**).

One does not have to be a psychologist to understand why erotic realism and hard-core pornography attract the reader. They are intended to induce sexual excitement. Readers like to be sexually excited, and therefore **Lady Chatterley's Lover** and **Peyton Place** become best sellers. This applies to you and me, if we may call ourselves "normal," not just to the sexual pervert. But we, you and I, like a change of pace. We can face and enjoy sex in literature, but not as a steady diet. We cannot apply the same line of necessarily over-simplified reasoning to the attraction of murder and violence in literature. The physiological aspect of reaction to the sex theme is surely not present in the murder theme except in the case of the psychopathological sadist who reacts with definite sexual excitement.

There would seem to be no physiological involvement at all in the murder story. What then is the attraction? Theodore Reik seems to me to have exposed the dynamic relationship between the reader and his murderous material—"all men are murderers at heart." Now this statement does not simply mean that each of us, under sufficient stress and appropriate circumstance, could and would commit murder. It means also, and more meaningfully, that each of us **has** committed murder—in thought and emotion. Not "we are all **potential** murderers" but, "we have all murdered." Thus we are all guilty and concerned to be caught, but we prefer to shed our guilt and need for punishment on the murderer and perhaps also on to his victim.

We also like to play the policeman. In the typical murder theme someone kills; someone is killed; someone catches the killer; and, classically, the killer is in turn killed. In this simple theme the great tragedy of murder touches and compels the attention. "We have all murdered" means that we have wished for the death of someone, or have even acted it out in fantasy or perhaps even in a dream. We are all guilty. We all seek punishment. We all, according to the principle of repetition-compulsion, must repeat the deed. What better way to do, to be done to and to do it again than by vicarious identification through the pages of literature.

There seems to me to be two classes of addicted, compulsive readers, readers who only come to a peak of attention if their noses are plunged between the covers of their particular class of fiction. The obvious class is the reader addicted to sexual literature, who will go out of his way, pay exaggerated prices, even take risks in terms of his social and professional relationships, to obtain the printed intoxicant. The other, less obvious, is the reader addicted to crime or murder fiction.

Stereotypes are dangerous, I know, but who does not immediately recognize the quiet little old lady with her pile of violent thrillers or the kindly prelate or don with his eager anticipation of the new Christie or Ellery Queen? But then who are the millions who read everything Spillane writes? What do "they" look like? I have no facts of any kind to go on—"they" might be the same quiet little old ladies and kindly prelates or dons. If this is so then old age, religion and learning have even more hidden depths than I suspect.

However, I stray from the subject. Reik, in his **Myth and Guilt,** develops the idea of the first god-murder and sees this as the source of the sense of "original sin." He adds to this primal crime, murder, the ultimate abomination, cannibalism, but sees this as a symbolic act, not hunger. "We are what we eat," he says. In his **Compulsion to Confess** however, (written many years before his analysis of religious ritual and belief) he had not apparently seen this relationship between murder and cannibalism.

He does not revise or even mention his confession theory in **Myth and Guilt** and seems to me to have missed the opportunity to relate all three concepts—murder, cannibalism and confession. Confession may be the symbolic vomiting up of the symbolically ingested victim, a cleansing refection of the awful deed, a "spitting-out" of the act. Cannibalism has suddenly become mentionable, as in Tennessee Williams' **Suddenly Last Summer.** Note that this is not the cannibalism of the savage, nor the final indignity of the Donner Party, but a symbolic act among relatively civilized people. Cannibalism is usually dealt with historically, as in the Donner Party tragedy, or lightly as in Gilbert's **Bab Ballads** — sometimes horribly hinted at, as in Golding's masterly **Lord of the Flies.**

This last tale is of interest to the psychologist above and beyond its suspense and shock. The theme of a child murdering other children has been dealt with in terms of a widely disbelieved theory of constitutional psychopathy in March's **The Bad Seed** — a gripping drama, but based on a psychological improbability. In **Lord of the Flies** a more plausible theory and idea is presented. The marooned children begin their story as children, no better, no worse. By the end they are savage killers, lost in a mystery; and it is with a shock of surprise that the reader finally sees them through the eyes of the naval officer, come to rescue them, as little dirty frightened children once again, no better, no worse. It is possible to accept Golding's parable as a dramatic representation of Freud's battling Id, Ego and Superego, with reality, the adult world, stepping in dressed in its mature military uniform to take them off to the mature adult world of a battle cruiser.

Four main characters carry the symbolism to its mature but cynical conclusion. "Ralph," intelligent, administratively competent, "There aren't any grownups. We shall have to look after ourselves" speaks for the ego. "Piggy," fat, asthmatic, myopic, but above all concerned, "which is better, law and rescue, or hunting and breaking things up?" speaks for the superego. "Jack," the hunter, the power-seeker, "Who'll join my tribe and have fun?" is the id. "Simon," the mystic, who knows what is the beast of the island, terrorizing the dreams and night-thoughts of these little children, for he has talked with the Lord of the Flies.

The child-tribe is initially organized by Ralph; but Jack, the hunter, rebels against the attempt to control his need to kill. He breaks with Ralph and leads away the main body of the tribe. They hunt and kill pigs, but in the process a terrible savagery and fulfillment become obvious, and the reader waits for the first human child-victim to be butchered as the pigs are. Jack has left, as a sacrifice to the "Beast," a severed pig's head impaled on a stake in a jungle clearing. Simon finds it and in a moment of epileptic truth realizes the nature of the "Beast" — Beelzebub, the Lord of the Flies. The severed pig's head speaks to him,

"What are you doing out here all alone? Aren't you afraid of me?" Simon shook. "There isn't anyone to help you. Only me. And I'm the Beast." Simon's mouth laboured, brought forth audible words, "Pig's head on a stick."

"Fancy thinking the Beast was something you could hunt and kill!" said the head. For a moment or two the forest and all the other dimly appreciated places echoed with the parody of laughter. "You knew didn't you? I'm part of you? Close, close, close! I'm the reason why it's no go? Why things are what they are?"

Simon wakes and later finds the decayed body of a flyer which, still in its parachute harness, has moved with the wind and, seen dimly by Ralph and Jack, has terrified the children. He returns to tell the tribe that they need no longer be afraid. A terrible thunderstorm has broken over the island and the children seek comfort in a stamping ritualistic dance, chanting "Kill the Beast! Cut his throat! Spill his blood!" Simon stumbles into this nightmare scene only to have the now psychotic tribe fall on him, believing him to be the Beast. He is killed, with the awful hint of cannibalism.

"The sticks fell and the mouth of the new circle crunched and screamed. The beast was on its knees in the center, its arms folded over its face. It was crying out against the abominable noise something about a body on the hill. The beast struggled forward, broke the ring and fell over the steep edge of the rock to the sand by the water. At once the crowd surged after it, poured down the rock, leapt on to the beast, screamed, struck, bit, tore. There were no words, and no movements but the tearing of teeth and claws." Piggy is next destroyed, at the instigation of Jack, by having a boulder rolled onto him. "The rock struck Piggy a glancing blow from chin to knee . . . Piggy, saying nothing, with no time for even a grunt, travelled through the air sideways from the rock, turning over as he went. The rock bounded twice and was lost in the forest. Piggy fell forty feet and landed on his back across that square, red rock in the sea. His head opened and stuff came out and turned red." Finally the hunt is on for Ralph, a hunt by naked painted savages intent on his capture so that they may gut him like a pig, sever his head and impale it on a stake. He is saved, and the children are rescued by the naval officer—"And who will rescue the adult and his cruiser?"*

---

*From **Lord of the Flies** by William G. Golding. Copyright (c) 1954 by William Gerald Golding. Used by permission of Coward-McCann, Inc. (New York), and Faber and Faber Ltd. (London), publishers.

Golding's fable reaches the height of horror by his skillful use of the child characters. Nothing, in this reviewer's experience, matches this tale as a tour de force, as sheer psychological impact. Followers of Melanie Klein will find in this masterly story some very real food for thought. Golding's **Pincher Martin** takes the theme of oral aggressive symbolism to a final and full development.

Beelzebub, the Lord of the Flies, also appears as the friend of a little child in John Collier's short story **Thus I Refute Beelzy.** The young boy, who plays with some imaginary companion at the secluded end of the garden, is given a ham-fisted lesson in reality-testing by his psychologically indoctrinated father.

". . . But Small Simon is in the fantasy stage. Are you not, Small Simon. You just make things up."

"No, I don't," said the boy.

"You do," said his father. "And because you do, it is not too late to reason with you. There is no harm in fantasy, old chap. There is no harm in a bit of make-believe. Only you have to know the difference between day dreams and real things, or your brain will never grow. It will never be the brain of a Big Simon. So come on. Let us hear about this Beelzy of yours. Come on. What is he like?"

"He isn't like anything," said the boy.

"Like nothing on earth," said his father. "That's a terrible fellow."

"I'm not frightened of him," said the child, smiling. "Not a bit." . . . "I love him," said the small boy. "He loves me." Father, offended by his small son's refusal to give up the reality of Beelzy, sends the boy up to his room to prepare for a thrashing. Father follows, and the story ends with only one of his feet left in reality. "It was on the second-floor landing that they found the shoe, with the man's foot still in it, like that morsel of a mouse which sometimes falls unnoticed from the side of the jaws of the cat." Beelzebub has protected his own.

This is not a pleasant theme, but then murder never is. Children who kill are among us in reality. A few more examples from fiction will suffice, and then we can return to the safer murder of adults.

Saki, in **Sredni Vashtar,** uses the familiar fairytale defense of attacking the wicked aunt as a substitute for the hated parent. In this tale we find, as in Collier's story, the child in superb alliance with the powers of darkness. The boy is oppressed by the stern aunt who will not let him be free. His only friend in the restrictive atmosphere of his home is his giant ferret, Sredni Vashtar, who lives in a cage in the dark at the back of the garden shed. Sredni Vashtar is his God, who will bring death. He brings offerings to his ferret and prays to him for release from his oppressor. He chants to him,

> "Sredni Vashtar went forth,
> His thoughts were red thoughts and his teeth were white.
> His enemies called for peace, but he brought them death.
> Sredni Vashtar the Beautiful."

The aunt discovers Sredni Vashtar and goes to the shed to destroy him, while the boy waits in the house in the agony of his dark prayer. The minutes pass and lengthen as he gazes through the window toward the shed. "And presently his eyes were rewarded: out through that doorway came a long, low, yellow-and-brown beast, with eyes a-blink at the morning daylight and dark wet stains around the fur of jaws and throat." The boy happily makes hot buttered toast and listens to the loud foolish screams of the household as it discovers the tragedy.

Ray Bradbury, in **The Small Assassin,** tells of the tiniest murderer of them all, an infant of a few months who kills first his mother, then his father, and who is finally caught and killed by an injection from the kindly family physician. Bradbury is a science-fiction writer, praised by Harper's Magazine as "America's finest living fantasist." His tale does not ring true, but nevertheless is an example of this particular theme of the child who kills.

The stories and dictionary of Ambrose Bierce have long delighted the literate psychologist, and his **The Parenticide Club** is an example of the pathological attack on the parents which may be seen as the dynamic motivation of much of his bitterly sad writings. One cannot take much of Bierce seriously without becoming almost physically sick. We are living in an age when the word "sick" is used deliberately as a form of humor. There is the cult of the "sick joke" and the "sick comedian." **The Parenticide Club** is the most pathological "sick joke" of them all, and very much predates present attempts. Again it is to be noted that when a certain level of horror is reached the author can only retreat into the light touch. The reader can then psychologically handle the grisly material better by saying to himself, "It's really all a joke, and a little in bad taste at that, but I am not being asked to take any of this seriously." Perhaps the author also, in his inner need to spin these horrors, defends himself by savage irony.

The Parenticide Club is, perhaps fortunately, a collection of only four short stories. They deal, obviously, with the destruction ("killing" is far too mild a word to use here) of parents by their children. Although he writes with tongue in cheek, the Bierce tongue is flickering, loathsome, and poisoned. In **My Favorite Murder** Bierce begins with a Baconian economy of words "having murdered my mother under conditions of singular atrocity . . . " and goes on to relate how the murder of the mother was so trivial, in comparison with the earlier murder of the uncle, that the court acquitted him.

The uncle was murdered by the ingenious procedure of cutting his hamstrings, stuffing him in a sack, suspending the sack from a tree limb, and having a ferocious ram butt him to pulp. In **Oil of Dog** Bierce boils the mother and father. He begins, "I was born of honest parents in one of the humbler walks of life, my father being a manufacturer of dog-oil and my mother having a small studio in the shadow of the village church, where she disposed of unwelcome babies." The son helps his father by finding dogs to boil down into *Ol. can.*, which was then sold to the local physicians, who then dispensed it to their patients. He also helped his mother by dropping the baby corpses into the river.

One night he dropped a corpse into the bubbling dog-vat. This greatly improved the quality of the dog-oil, and the whole family scoured the village for bodies, child and adult. Soon they were killing, and soon the irate villagers banded together and demanded that they stop. Heartbroken over the loss of a lucrative business father decides to kill mother and use her to put the family economy back on its feet. Mother has the same idea, and the child watches as they surprise each other in their intentions, grapple, and finally fall together into the vat. In **An Imperfect Conflagration** the son kills the mother and father with an axe, then tries to burn the bodies by setting fire to the house — incidentally with intention of collecting the house insurance.

In **The Hypnotist,** the son, by the use of hypnosis, persuades his mother and father that they are wild broncos, then watches as they kick and batter each other to death — "At the end of it all two battered, tattered, bloody and fragmentary vestiges of mortality attested the solemn fact that the author of the strife was an orphan." He ends on a note of near-psychotic cynicism. "Such are a few of my principal experiments in the mysterious force or agency known as hypnotic suggestion. Whether or not it could be employed by a bad man for an unworthy purpose I am unable to say."

In defense of presenting these monstrosities of Bierce it may be said that all is grist to the mill of the psychologist, he must hide his eyes from nothing. Bierce is not an example of "hard-core violence"; he does not paint his scenes with blood and bruises as does Spillane. He is economical and precise in many instances, but the effect of his ideas is, by accumulation, decayed and psychotic. He lashes out indiscriminately, everything is a target. There is, in his writings, the sound of screaming rather than the cold tones of the cynic. However as studies in murder, they have a wild fascination unique in the English language.

Friedrich Duerrenmatt, in **The Pledge,** deals with the sombre theme of child murder. A little girl has been assaulted and murdered, and a Swiss policeman undertakes the tracking down of the murderer. He is unsuccessful within any reasonable time that the police organization can afford, so he devotes the rest of his life to the private, non-professional, solution of the wretched crime. His method is to live with a woman who has a small girl of about the same age as the murdered child. This weird obsession with the crime leads him deliberately to expose this other child to the same situations and circumstances which culminated in the murder of the first one. He does not inform the child or her mother what his terrible plan is. He follows the child around setting the stage for her attempted assault and murder. The culprit is finally revealed, but not before he himself has sunk into the degradation of his obsession. This is a disturbing story, where the focal point of interest is the overwhelming passion of the policeman in the search for his victim, who is a mental defective in a nearby community. The personality of the police officer is drawn with a skillful brevity which hints at the darker motivations involved in the pledge to see justice done.

Let us shift from these scenes of childhood to the world of the adult (and his battle cruiser). Lord Dunsany, in **Two Bottles of Relish,** deals with murder with the now familiar mechanism of the light touch. I do not believe his story could have been published were it not for the "punch line." One line of dialogue, seven spoken words, the last in the story, rescues us from the pit. Dunsany, despite the "punch line" comes close to the completely unacceptable. The story concerns a vegetarian who is suspected of killing a girl and disposing of her body. The cottage is under constant supervision, nothing has been smuggled out, no telltale smoke comes from the chimney, nothing has been buried in the garden. Some trees in the garden have been chopped down and sawn into logs by the suspect. It is discovered that he has bought two bottles of relish—a relish only used on meats or savories, a relish which if once used mistakenly by a vegetarian on his salad would not be used again.

But he has bought two bottles — six days apart. The story does not have to go into details. One loose end is left; the "punch line" clears it up, and provides the merciful release. Why the chopping and sawing of wood? "Solely," said Linley, "in order to get an appetite."

Cannibalism may be seen as ritual; as tragic necessity in the case of the Donner Party;* as a means to avoid conviction; but only has acceptability as seen through the eyes of W. G. Gilbert's sailor who survives because of cannibalism:

> "Oh, I am a cook and a captain bold,
> And the mate of the Nancy brig,
> And a bo'sun tight, and a midshipmite,
> And the crew of the captain's gig!"

An interesting variation on murder is seen in Romain Gary's **Lady L.** Usually murder is committed because of hate, or to achieve some personal goal or gain. In **Lady L** the motivation is love, deep, enduring, real. Annette, the heroine, has a bad start in life. Poor, the daughter of an anarchist, she is early exposed to both his wild theories and his incestuous advances. She successfully resists both and turns to prostitution as a business venture. She meets a wild-eyed, beautiful young man, who is to be the only true love of her life.

Unfortunately he is also an anarchist, so in love with abstract humanity that his whole life is dedicated to the destruction of authority. Most of the time he is blowing up kings and assassinating presidents; or plotting, or running from the police. A tiny corner only is left for Annette, who sees that her rival is humanity itself. By a series of fortunate incidents, marriages and deceptions she rises to the position of belle dame of European society, Lady "L." After many years of relative security her lover returns and she sadly plots with him the wholesale theft of jewels from the guests at a splendid fancy dress ball in her country house.

She bids farewell again to him after the theft, in his arms in her summer pavilion. Then she recognizes the hopelessness of her personal fight against his love of all the teeming unknown millions of the world. She hears sounds of pursuit and search, and urges him to hide in a huge trunk. He does. She sadly turns the key and locks it. Everyone wonders why she spends so much time thereafter in her summer pavilion, sometimes talking to herself apparently. Twenty years later she reveals her

---

*The Donner party set out for California from Illinois in 1846. Trapped by snow in the Sierra mountains the emigrant band spent the winter at Donner Lake under conditions of starvation and great hardship. In order to survive some members of the group resorted to cannibalism. Forty-two members of the party of ninety persons perished.

history to her old friend, the Poet Laureate of England, and opens the trunk to show the crouching skeleton of her lover, still bearing the shreds of his fancy dress costume of a French aristocrat.

Franz Kafka, the brilliant father-dominated neurotic, deals with murder as a solution to man's wandering, stumbling confusion. In **The Trial** Joseph K. finds the answer, the only real answer, in his murder by the two grotesque representatives of authority. Joseph K. is a reasonable, decent man, trying hard not to offend, living quietly and apparently decorously. He is man in this modern age, trying very hard to abide by rules which he can never define, in a game which he does not understand. One day there comes a knock at the door and he is told by police officers that he is accused. He clings to rationality and common sense in the nightmare that follows. He is charged, found guilty, sentenced. He never finds out what he is accused of, what charged with, what found guilty of, what sentenced to. He is led to a deserted part of town by two men, ridiculously polite and deferential in their manner and garb, who lay him down on the ground, place his head on a rock, and then press a knife through his heart. They seem to encourage him to grasp the knife and push it in by himself.

As he waits for the knife to press through into him he sees a figure waving from a window in a house on the edge of the deserted place. Perhaps help is on the way? But he dies. He never knew who? how? why? The murder of K. is dreadful; but, apart from the physical act, the reader feels that he himself is being murdered, that he himself has been exposed to the knife-like question, who? how? why? Kafka can be a shuddering experience to the sensitive reader, for there is no justice, no retribution, no purification, no tacit permission to sin again.

In **The Sentence** Kafka deals explicitly with the father domination which was to influence so much of his own life and writing. George Bendemann has succeeded in taking over his father's business when the father becomes too old to run it himself. George is growing to manhood, even planning marriage. He tells his father of his plans; but, to his consternation his father, increasingly resentful of the enforced dependence on his son, condemns him to death. His father says, "I am still much stronger. How long you hesitated before becoming mature . . . Now you know what was going on outside yourself. Before you only knew about yourself. You really were an innocent child, but in reality, diabolical! — Listen: I now condemn you to death by drowning."

The son, robot-like, promptly rushes to the river and flings himself from the bridge to his death. His last words are, "Dear parent! Yes, I have always loved you." It would seem that the only possible explanation as to why Kafka believed that such an ending would be believable is to be found in his own twisted relationship with his father. While it is sense in terms of present day concepts in psychology to understand all writing as in some degree autobiographical, Kafka goes farther than most in this kind of unwitting self-revelation.

Georges Simenon, the astonishingly productive source of the modern French detective story, has written in **The Murderer** an incisive study of the mind of a murderer. This is no intellectual puzzle, no patient unraveling of clues, but a straightforward analysis of a complex phenomenon. The compulsion to confess or reveal is strikingly presented in the thoughts and behavior of the physician who has murdered his faithless wife and her lover. The psychologist cannot but be impressed again by the insight of the artist in demonstrating the motivation of self-destruction in this tale. The guilty one is unable to retain his sanity at the thought of escape from punishment. Perhaps it is going too far to insist that all murders are committed because of the need, operating at the unconscious level, to be caught and punished, at least after the event, in the majority of cases.

The peculiar relationship between the murderer and his victim, the symbiosis of death, is becoming increasingly understood in criminal psychology. Macdonald has commented on this in his **Psychiatry and the Criminal.** It is as though in some cases the victim needs to be killed as much as the murderer needs to kill. This need to be killed may range all the way from the person who "asks for it," (the example comes to mind of the not uncommon case of the marital partner who goads or nags the other into murder) to the one who wanders off to a deserted place with a stranger who acts peculiarly. Hemingway touches on this idea in **The Killers,** his short story in which the victim waits for death at the hands of the fated killers, almost peacefully and expectantly. This may, in a sense, be compared to the symbiosis between the murderer and the instruments of fate, the police. The murderer often experiences a similar sense of release once he has consciously or unconsciously delivered himself up to their hands.

A point of departure in this essay was the popularity of the novels of Mickey Spillane. He unfortunately has his imitators, even in the land of Dorothy L. Sayers, Agatha Christie, and Michael Innes. He even has his source in the writings of the English author, James Hadley Chase. In 1939, Chase wrote **No Orchids for Miss Blandish,** a work which has been widely read in England, and perhaps justifiably criticized as an attack on morality, law, and "the rules of the game" in general. George Orwell in an essay entitled **Raffles and Miss Blandish** contrasts the cricketing burglar, Raffles, with his own relatively inviolable role, with the lurching psychotics and sadistic psychopaths who infest the world of Miss Blandish. Raffles is a gentleman, moving in and stealing from the upper circles, accepted for his charm, intelligence and skill as a cricketer. Raffles operates, within his own set of taboos, as a decent sort of chap going the wrong way with the wrong taboos. He is an educated picaresque hero.

There are no heroes of any kind in **No Orchids for Miss Blandish.** She, the daughter of a rich businessman, is kidnapped by a group of small time gangsters, who are in turn wiped out by bigger time gangsters. The brains of this second gang is a woman whose son is sexually impotent. She sees Miss Blandish as a solution to her son's sexual problem and, under her motherly tuition, he finally succeeds in raping the kidnapped victim. The private eye rescues her and prepares to return her to her father. She seems to have become addicted to the slobbering brutality of the rapist, however, and leaps from a high window, preferring death to the mundane life of the daughter of a rich businessman.

Within the confines of this simple story murder stumbles around on defective, psychotic, brutally sadistic feet. This is "hard-core" realism of the worst type — meaningless, tasteless, serving no purpose, compensated for in no way. It is to be noted that the rescuer of Miss Blandish is barely distinguishable from the gangsters. Like Spillane's Mike Hammer he happens to be on one side rather than the other more by luck than choice. It should be noted also that "No Orchids" was a fantastic success in an England hungering apparently for action (its great sales success was in 1940).

England has a successful, new, educated version of Mickey Spillane. Ian Fleming has written a series of very popular novels (**Dr. No, From Russia with Love, Casino Royale, Live and Let Die**) in which a Mike Hammer type secret agent, James Bond, smashes everything in sight to the accompaniment of good music, superb wine and a touch of the old school tie. Fingers are broken, faces smashed in and bullets sent ripping through vainly protesting bellies, with all the gory insanity that pervades Spillane at his best worst. In **Dr. No,** James Bond triumphs finally over the evil doctor by burying him in a huge mound of guano.

In **Casino Royale** Bond is tortured by the Russian agent in a fashion calculated to upset the book's anxious male readers. Bond is stripped, tied into a bottomless chair, then whacked on the genitals with an old-fashioned carpet-beater by the bad Russian. In his books victims are shredded by fish, blown up by explosives, burned, usually just plain smashed. The "hero," like Hammer, is a psychopathic thug operating on the side of justice. Unlike Hammer he talks, perhaps even thinks, polysyllabically. Fleming, unlike Spillane, does not attempt to moralize about the activities of his avenging fury.

One of the strangest styles in modern fiction, and one of the most compelling from the standpoint of the reader, is seen in the work of the French author Alain Robbe-Grillet. Two of his novels, **The Voyeur** and **Jealousy,** have received considerable attention both in America and Britain. Robbe-Grillet places you, the reader, right into the action of the story. **Jealousy** involves murder, and is therefore, of the two novels, more appropriate for discussion here. The story of **Jealousy** is supremely simple, an adulterous relationship ends in murder. The novel introduces the unfaithful wife and her lover, also married.

The lover comes to her house every evening, for a drink, and usually to have dinner. The scene is set in Africa and those involved are obviously colonial planters. The behaviour of the adulterous couple is minutely analyzed in a series of vivid descriptive passages. They plan (openly, for who would suspect them?) to drive into town so that she may shop, he may attend to business. They will have time for dinner in town before they leave. They do not get back that night, but of course anything may have happened — car trouble, a fellow motorist in trouble, a chance meeting with an old friend that delayed them until it was too late to start back.

He comes for dinner in the evening again, she sits by him, pours him his drink, they plan (openly, for who would suspect them?) to drive into town so that she may shop, he may attend to business. At dinner she sees a huge centipede on the wall, he gets up, squashes it under his balled-up napkin, then crushes it under his foot. After dinner she asks how his wife and child are, and they are much the same, unable to stand the heat and the colonial way of life. He comes for dinner again, she sits by him, pours his drink; and they discuss a novel they both are reading about French colonial life in Africa. They eat, and she sees a huge centipede on the wall. He gets up, squashes it under his balled-up napkin, then crushes it under his feet.

After dinner he goes home, and she goes to her room, and combs her hair stroke by stroke by stroke. During the day she writes on her blue stationery, and at night the pocket of his colonial shirt does not quite cover a letter on blue stationery. They drink, they eat, the centipede is killed, the town-trip is planned, the questions are asked about the wife and child, eyes meet, fingertips touch, goodnights are said, the hair is brushed, the stationery written on.

This terrible round of commonplaces begins to grip you, the reader, by the throat. The third member of this triangular relationship, the cuckolded husband, is never mentioned, described, talked to, or seen. He is you, the reader. Yours are the eyes that prey, the ears that hear, the mind that builds up the repetitive scenes of adultery until the mind explodes in murder and violence. But does it happen? Here he comes again for a drink before dinner, there is the centipede, there they are planning again. In this novel Robbe-Grillet has developed a superb fictional approach to the "projective hypothesis" of the psychologist.

It is quite clear to the reader that he is dealing with two very real people in a very real situation — the brilliant economy of style makes them come to sinister life in the mere description of how he eats, or she walks. But what is happening has no meaning unless there is a third person. The action is seen through his eyes, he is the narrator, but beyond this he is blank. You are given the eyes and the ears, and before long you are the third person. You are the jealous one, you are the killer. This is a subtle refinement of the literary technique of inducing identification with a particular character (usually the hero) by sympathy, empathy, depth of understanding, or because of deeper unconscious factors and motivations. The reader has no one to identify with (no hero that is) and yet he is so involved in the story that he himself becomes the third member of the party.

The series of images draw the reader even deeper and deeper into the story — he becomes inevitably the participant-observer. The explanation of the behavior of the couple can only come from the reader, which means of course that a variety of explanations is possible. What is important, however, is not the story as a projective test, but the experience of personal involvement. The interpretation I found may, or may not, reveal something of myself. The interpretation found by another reader may, or may not, reveal something of himself. This is rather beside the point of finding oneself, literally, swept along and into the story, and finding one's own personal reaction becoming central to the story. These following lines indicate the photographic clarity of Robbe-Grillet's writing:

"The lamp is set on the dressing table. A. . . . is putting on the last of her discreet makeup: the lipstick which merely accentuates the natural

colour of her lips, but which seems darker in this glaring light. . . .
Dawn has not yet broken. Frank will come soon to call for A. . . . and
take her down to the port.

"She is sitting in front of the oval mirror where her full face is reflected, lit from only one side, at a short distance from her own face seen
in profile.

"A. . . . bends toward the mirror. The two faces come closer. They are
no more than four inches from each other, but they keep their forms and
their respective positions; a profile and a full face, parallel to each other.

"The right hand and the hand in the mirror trace on the lips and on
their reflection the exact image of the lips, somewhat brighter, clearer,
slightly darker.

"Two light knocks sound at the hallway door.

"Two bright lips and the lips in profile move in perfect synchroniza-
tion: 'Yes, what is it?'

"The voice is restrained, as in a sickroom, or like the voice of a thief
talking to his accomplice.

" 'The gentleman, he is here,' the boy's voice answers on the other side
of the door.

"No sound of a motor, however, has broken the silence (which was no
silence, but the continuous hissing of the kerosene lamp.)

"A. . . . says: 'I'm coming.'

"She calmly finishes the curving rim above her chin with an assured
gesture.

"She stands up, crosses the room, walks around the big bed, picks up
her handbag on the chest and the white wide-brimmed straw hat.

"She opens the door without making any noise (though without excessive precautions), goes out, closes the door behind her.

"The sound of her steps fades down the hallway.

"The entrance door opens and closes.

"It is six-thirty."

Six-thirty in the morning and you, dear reader, are left with your
own jealous, murderous thoughts—for she has walked out on you.

Actor-director Robert Montgomery used this technique in a movie
made just after World War II, entitled **The Lady in the Lake,** based
on the murder-mystery of that name written by Raymond Chandler.
Montgomery filmed this with a camera strapped to his own shoulder,
so that you in the audience, became the actor, seeing through the images of the camera. However, in the movie there was little ambiguity or
uncertainty of motivation, and reality was completely present. In

Robbe-Grillet's novel things are a little hazy and indefinite. It is by no means sure that violence and death occur, or do they only happen in your imagination?

One of the most fascinating books ever written about the immediate field of abnormality and psychopathology is **Auto Da Fe** by Elias Cannetti (also published in the United States under the title of **Tower of Babel**). There is an interesting murder, and also a powerful suicide scene. One of the most intriguing features of the book is that every main character is recognizably psychotic, with the exception perhaps of the psychiatrist, and he is insufferably dull by comparison. The story concerns the world's greatest Sinologist, Professor Kien, who has almost decided to forsake the world of reality for the world of his books.

He contracts an unfortunate marriage with his housekeeper, and faces up to the impending loss of his virginity and consummation of his marriage in what he feels is the most tasteful way possible. He decides that the consummation will take place on the couch in his study. He lovingly lines the couch with his most beautiful, prized and rarest books. She storms into the study, sweeps the books to the floor, spreadeagles herself on the couch and shamelessly shouts encouragement to him. In total defeat he runs to the bathroom and cries, like a little lost child, as he sits on the toilet.

To avoid any further contact with his wife he practices turning himself into stone for hours at a time. This overly deliberate catatonic defense breaks down, however, when his wife boxes his ears. His final defense is retreat into schizophrenic madness, and he wanders the city with the delusion that he has stuffed his entire library into his head. A deluded Don Quixote, he sets out to save books from the cannibalism of bookstore owners. His Sancho Panza is a dwarf, Fischerle, who believes himself to be the greatest, but as yet unrecognized, chess player in the world.

Fischerle lives with a prostitute, and he hides under her bed while she entertains her customers. However, as he crouches beneath the bed with his grandiose chess fantasies he often wonders if the man just over his head might be a chess player too. So he crawls out, taps the busy stranger on the shoulder and says "Do you play chess?" The answers differ in expression, but the content is usually the same. One day the answer is a knife in the hand of a customer-acquaintance who dismembers his wretched little body. Kien locks himself in his beloved library and sets fire to it. He climbs the small library ladder, and sits on top, reading, as the flames reach for his life.

This extraordinary novel has all the tumultuous vigour of Céline, and the classic descriptive simplicity of Kraepelin. The madmen who run and tumble through its pages are sympathetically and skillfully drawn; and with the kind of technical excellence so miserably lacking in Tennessee Williams' **Suddenly Last Summer.** It is difficult for the reader to maintain perspective and reality in this brilliant psychotic kaleidoscope, where the only recognizably "normal" person is Kien's brother, the stuffy psychiatrist. The sensitive reader may well find himself drifting away with these weird and wonderful characters in more than the usual and appropriate suspension of judgment—in a dangerously seductive "imaginary puissance."

Suicide, in one of the forms suggested by Menninger, insidiously wanders the pages of Goncharov's masterly novel, **Oblomov.** Oblomov is unable to commit himself to any course of action and he ultimately dies of this inaction—he dies in fact of "Oblomovism" (a condition which has been discussed by British psychiatrists). Oblomov suffers from a weariness of life which is recognizable as Menninger's concept of slow, lifetime suicide. Oblomov is a type, in the sense that Pecksniff and Babbit are types, but he is an undeniable suicide, and one of the most pitiful in the pages of literature.

> "Lying down was not for Ilya Ilyitch either a necessity as it is for a sick or a sleepy man, or an occasional need as it is for a person who is tired, or a pleasure as it is for a sluggard: it was his normal state. When he was at home—and he was always at home—he was lying down, and invariably in the same room, the one in which we have found him and which served him as bedroom, study and reception room. He had three more rooms, but he seldom looked into them, only, perhaps, in the morning when his servant swept his study—which did not happen every day. In those other rooms the furniture was covered and the curtains were drawn."

This house is not the meaningful morgue of Miss Haversham in **Great Expectations**—this house is almost meaningless.

> "If it had not been for this plate and for a freshly smoked pipe by the bed, and for the owner himself lying in it, one might have thought that the room was uninhabited—everything was so dusty and faded and devoid of all traces of human presence. It is true there were two or three open books and a newspaper on the chiffoniers, an inkstand and pens on the bureau; but the open pages were covered with dust, evidently they had been left so for weeks; the newspaper dated from last year, and if one dipped a pen into the inkstand a startled fly might perhaps come buzzing out of it.
> "As soon as he woke he made up his mind to get up and wash; and, after drinking tea, to think matters over, taking various things into consideration

and writing them down, and altogether to go into the subject thoroughly. He lay for half an hour tormented by his decision; but afterwards he reflected that he would have time to think after breakfast, which he could have in bed as usual, especially since one can think just as well lying down."

Oblomov drifts toward his inevitable death, his every thought and relationship dying just ahead of his physical dissolution. At the end there is no reason, no meaning.

"And who is this Ilya Ilyitch he mentioned?" the writer asked.

"Oblomov: I have often spoken to you about him."

"Yes, I remember the name: he was your friend and school-fellow. What became of him?"

"He is dead, and how he was wasted!"

Stolz sighed and sank into thought.

"And he was as intelligent as other people, his soul was pure and clear as crystal; he was noble and affectionate — and yet he did nothing!"

"But why? What was the reason?"

"The reason . . . what reason was there? Oblomovism!"

Very few writers have succeeded in making a farce (intentionally, that is) out of murder. Nabokov almost succeeds in **Lolita,** but his intention is not altogether clear, and the reader is left to gag on his chuckles. Humbert-Humbert has finally tracked down the dispoiler of his nymphet, and kills him in the following fantastic scene:

"My next bullet caught him somewhere in the side, and he rose from his chair higher and higher, like old, gray, mad Nijinski, like Old Faithful, like some old nightmare of mine, to a phenomenal altitude, or so it seemed, as he rent the air — still shaking with the rich black music — head thrown back in a howl, hand pressed to his brow, and with his other hand clutching his armpit as if stung by a hornet, down he came on his heels and, again a normal robed man, scurried out into the hall. . . .

"Suddenly dignified, and somewhat morose, he started to walk up the broad stairs; and shifting my position, but not actually following him up the steps, I fired three or four times in quick succession, wounding him at every blaze; and every time I did it to him, that horrible thing to him, his face would twitch in an absurd clownish manner, as if he were exaggerating the pain; he slowed down, rolled his eyes half closing them and made a feminine 'ah!' and he shivered every time a bullet hit him as if I were tickling him, and every time I got him with those slow, clumsy, blind bullets of mine, he would say under his breath, with a phony British accent — all the while twitching, shivering, smirking, but withal talking in a curiously detached and even amiable manner: 'Ah, that hurts, sir, enough! Ah, that hurts atrociously, my dear fellow. I pray you, desist. Ah — very painful, very painful indeed . . . God! Hah! This is abominable, you should really not — !' His voice trailed off as he reached the landing, but he steadily walked on despite all the lead I had lodged in his bloated body; and in distress, in dismay, I understood that far from killing him I was injecting spurts of energy into the poor fellow, as if the bullets had been capsules wherein a heady elixir danced.

"I reloaded the thing with hands that were black and bloody—I had touched something he had anointed with his thick gore. Then I rejoined him upstairs, the keys jangling in my pockets like gold.

"He was trudging from room to room, bleeding majestically, trying to find an open window, shaking his head, and still trying to talk me out of murder. I took aim at his head, and he retired to the master bedroom with a burst of royal purple where his ear had been.

" 'Get out, get out of here,' he said, coughing and spitting; and in a night-mare of wonder, I saw this blood spattered, but still buoyant person get into his bed and wrap himself up in the chaotic bed clothes. I hit him at very close range through the blankets; and then he lay back, and a big pink bubble with juvenile connotations formed on his lips, grew to the size of a toy balloon, and vanished.

"I may have lost contact with reality for a second or two—oh, nothing of the I-just-blacked-out sort that your common criminal enacts; on the contrary I want to stress the fact that I was responsible for every shed drop of his bubblehood; . . .

"Quilty was a very sick man. I held one of his slippers instead of the pistol—I was sitting on the pistol. Then I made myself a little more comfort-able in the chair near the bed, and consulted my wrist watch. The crystal was gone, but it ticked. The whole sad business had taken more than an hour. He was quiet at last. Far from feeling any relief, a burden even weightier than the one I had hoped to get rid of was with me, upon me, over me. I could not bring myself to touch him in order to make sure he was really dead. He looked it: a quarter of his face gone, and two flies beside themselves with a dawning sense of unbelievable luck."*

Mine Own Executioner by Nigel Balchin, stands out as a fine piece of psychological writing, perhaps because Balchin was trained as a psy-chologist. The novel pictures the psychologist trying to help a paranoid schizophrenic, trying to save his own marriage, and fighting a status battle with professional colleagues. The schizophrenic murders his wife then commits suicide. The psychologist wins the other two rounds with his wife and his colleagues. The story is convincingly told without the usual excesses in portraying the psychotherapist—either as sicker than his patients, or as a Freudian Socrates.

The political murder is well handled in Koestler's **Darkness at Noon.** The old brigade communist is subjected to the powerful subtleties of in-terrogation, and then is destroyed in the inevitable climax. Political murder is also disturbingly presented in Orwell's **1984.** The hero

---

*From **Lolita** by Vladimir Nabokov. Copyright (c) 1955 by Vladimir Nabokov. Used by permission of G. P. Putnam's Sons, publishers.

and heroine have committed the terrible crime of loving each other.
They are caught and condemned to a living death. What is murdered is
the conviction, the integrity, the total being of the victims. Winston, the
hero, breaks under the threat of having a mask containing ferociously
hungry sewer rats strapped over his face. The following passages outline, in a philosophy of violence, the murder of his soul. The inquisitor,
O'Brien, speaks,

" 'How does one man assert his power over another, Winston?' Winston thought, 'by making him suffer,' he said.

" 'Exactly. By making him suffer. Obedience is not enough. Unless he
is suffering, how can you be sure that he is obeying your will and not his
own? Power is in inflicting pain and humiliation. Power is in tearing human minds to pieces and putting them together again in new shapes of
your own choosing. Do you begin to see, then, what kind of world we
are creating? It is the exact opposite of the stupid hedonistic utopias that
the old reformers imagined. A world of fear and treachery and torment,
a world of trampling and being trampled upon, a world which will grow
not less but *more* merciless as it refines itself. Progress in our world will
be progress toward more pain. The old civilizations claimed that they
were founded on love and justice. Ours is founded upon hatred. In our
world there will be no emotions except fear, rage, triumph, and self-
abasement. Everything else we shall destroy—everything. Already we
are breaking down the habits of thought which have survived from before the Revolution. We have cut the links between child and parent,
and between man and man, and between man and woman. No one
dares trust a wife or child or a friend any longer. But in the future there
will be no wives and no friends. Children will be taken from their
mothers at birth, as one takes eggs from a hen. The sex instinct will be
eradicated. Procreation will be an annual formality like the renewal of a
ration card. We shall abolish the orgasm. Our neurologists are at work
upon it now. There will be no loyalty, except loyalty to the Party. There
will be no love except the love of Big Brother. There will be no laughter,
except the laugh of triumph over a defeated enemy. There will be no art,
no literature, no science. When we are omnipotent we shall have no
more need of science. There will be no distinction between beauty and
ugliness. There will be no curiosity, no enjoyment of the process of life.
All competing pleasures will be destroyed. But always—do not forget
this, Winston, always there will be the intoxication of power, constantly
increasing and constantly growing subtler. Always, at every moment,
there will be the thrill of victory, the sensation of trampling on an enemy

who is helpless. If you want a picture of the future, imagine a boot stamping on a human face—forever!"

Winston tries to protest that humanity will never tolerate this philosophy, that life itself will defeat the Party. O'Brien replies,

"Do you see any evidence that that is happening? Or any reason why it should?"

"No, I believe it. I *know* that you will fail. There is something in the universe—I don't know, some spirit, some principle—that you will never overcome."

"Do you believe in God, Winston?"

"No."

"Then what is it, this principle that will defeat us?"

"I don't know. The spirit of Man."

"And do you consider yourself a man?"

"Yes."

"If you are a man, Winston, you are the last man."

Winston is forced to look at himself in a mirror, and collapses in tears at the sight of his filthy, ruined body. All he has left is his knowledge that he has not betrayed his love for Julia, by ceasing to love her. He has by this time, however, betrayed her in every other way. The rat mask is presented to him and he screams for them to do it to Julia, not to him. The end has come nothing is left—not even love. One day they will shoot him. He is released to await his execution. He hears a speech proclaiming another victory for the Party and he looks up at the face of Big Brother on the telescreen.

> "He gazed up at the enormous face. Forty years it had taken him to learn what kind of smile was hidden beneath the dark moustache. O cruel, needless misunderstanding! O stubborn, self-willed exile from the loving breast! Two gin-scented tears trickled down the side of his nose. But it was all right, the struggle was finished. He had won the victory over himself. He loved Big Brother."*

Winston will go through the formality of dying later, but humanity, the spirit of man, is dead, in the most heartbreaking murder of all. Orwell's shocking climax must emerge as a possible epitaph for this desperate age.

There are countless examples of the theme of murder in the literature of the world. Some, perhaps not so well known (with the exception of the

---

*From **Nineteen Eighty Four** by George Orwell. Copyright 1949 by Harcourt, Brace and Company, Inc. and Secker and Warburg.

"hard-core" sadistic writers who are usually only too well-known) have been presented here. Theodore Reik, I believe, has seen most clearly into this dark region. There is a necessity for murder in fiction. Reik is not joking when he says "A thought-murder a day keeps the doctor away." To accept the idea of murder, without anxiety, may well be therapeutic. To accept the presentation of murder in fiction, without anxiety, may be similarly useful. To become addicted to murder and violence in literature, however, may reflect a continuing struggle to master such impulses within the psychological system of the reader. An interesting hypothesis to the experimental psychopathologist was the Freudian suggestion that the person showing a decided preference for various kinds of infantile humour (anal, genital, oral, etc.) was the person who was unable to master anxiety in connection with these areas of psychosexual development. It may well be that a similar set of factors is operating in the area of violence preference.

It is also obvious that murder is a necessity in fiction because it is a fact of experience — however unpleasant this may be, and however much we may be unwilling to accept this. Does this then place murder and violence at the level of experience lovingly described by those writers who have been caught up in the mystique de la merde? I think not. The "put-everything-in" school suffers from an enormous imbalance. They are so busy with sexual, anatomical, excretory details that no recognition is made of other experience details. I am not for one moment saying that these sexual, anatomical, excretory details are less important or less valuable. To be unaware of them leads to the crass literature of moral uplift (which is crass precisely because there is nothing else in them, they are unbalanced). However, to present these earthy details in isolation, or even in dominant emphasis, is to wrench them out of their human gestalt. In this sense the hostile, murderous impulses of men are a fact of experience and should be dealt with as they have meaning in the development of story and character.

The "put-everything-in" school in fact does not put everything in. The essential ambivalence of man is lost. Of course man defecates — he also prays. Of course man kills — he also has been know to lay down his life for his friend. Whether one interprets prayer and altruism as neurotic is beside the point. They are facts of experience. The great killers of literature and drama (Macbeth, Othello, Oedipus) are timeless and fascinating precisely because of their ambivalence. The Mike Hammers and James Bonds are tedious not only in terms of literary depicture, but also because they do violence to their adversaries and the

facts of experience at the same time. Iago has a meaning and a place in
Othello, but to place him as the central character of unrelieved villany
would be to reduce Shakespeare almost to the level of Grand Guignol.

The murderer in fiction is almost always a comprehensible person for
perhaps two main reasons. First the reader demands comprehensibility,
second the murderer is a creation of the writer; and as such, reflects his
logic, insight and demand for order. The motive, once revealed, is
clearly sufficient and reasonable. The killer is presented often as someone whose behavior is rational (although often stupid) once the dominant motive is revealed — greed, lust, revenge, power. When the central
motive is lacking in fiction, the attempt is made to paddle in the dangerous waters of symbolism and psychopathology. A murder in real life
rarely show the comprehensibility of fiction.

There is a logic and a central motive in fiction which are hard to find
with any exactness in the John Gilbert Grahams of experience. The fiction writer is prone to deal in a kind of predictive typology which would
delight a Sheldon and appall the experimentalist. Shifty eyes, square
jaws, honest expressions, menacing glances, consistent traits for good or
ill, have meaning only in fiction; but, once grant that meaning, and
comprehensibility is only a description away. Perhaps one of the great
attractions of literature as a form of escape is this world of order, reason,
predictability, comprehensibility, which is in such open contrast to the
real world, often meaningless, inconsistent and incomprehensible.

The psychologist may break his heart and mind in trying to comprehend the behaviour of John Gilbert Graham; he has no such problem in
comprehending the behaviour of the murderer in **A Study in Scarlet**.
He may wrestle in agony with the problem of Leopold and Loeb; he will
not do so with the killers in **Compulsion**. Even Dostoevsky's complex
characters, Raskolnikov and Stavrogin, have this air of comprehensibility which is not found in even a simple petty thief in reality. The author
is infinitely more skilled in presenting comprehensibility than is the psychologist, because he is creating rather than describing. He is dealing in
abstractions which have no essential counterpart in life; and ultimately
the rationality of his characters bears the stamp of his own rationalizing.
If he were to deal with reality he would be writing case histories rather
than fiction.

Very few writers attempt to portray the witchdoctors of modern society, the psychiatrist and psychologist, and those who do fail ludicrously
(with the notable exceptions of T. S. Eliot and Nigel Balchin). Tennessee
Williams is the latest to convince a gullible public (and an equally

gullible critic) that he is peering wisely into the depths of humanity. In **Suddenly Last Summer** Williams transforms the incredible complexities of homosexuality, incest and cannibalism into a one-act play (made worse by Hollywood's expansion of it into a full-length movie) described by one influential critic as ". . . A triumphant piece of dramatic literature." The Rogerian neuro-surgeon, Dr. "Sugar," nondirectively "theraps" his way through a plot as thick and steamy as the weird garden-jungle which is the cutely symbolic backdrop to the action, and finally catalyses the abreaction of villainous memories before the rest of the suspects in a manner more reminiscent of the Thin Man conducting the last scene dénouement than a professional psychiatrist at work. The **Manchester Guardian** critic did not see this work as a triumphant piece of dramatic literature, in the film version at least.

"The trouble with this kind of entertainment, if that is the word for it, is that it is so very subject to the law of diminishing returns. In his other contributions to dramatic literature, Mr. Williams has treated us to such rich feasts of human degradation, of sexual complication, and what not, that now, when he serves up a little piece in which we find that a young man (dead before the story starts) was a rabid homosexual, that he had been murdered in sunny Spain by a crowd of his young victims (who, being poor and hungry, had also eaten him), that his mother (Katherine Hepburn) and his beautiful cousin (Elizabeth Taylor) had been used by him to procure young men, that the beautiful cousin has now gone mad and that the mother is even madder, the effect is not so much one of horror as of hilarious incredulity. Poor Mr. Williams, we feel, has tried so hard to shock us that now he can do so no longer, and in his zeal to do so he has had to go beyond realism into a world of laughable monstrosity."

The point which seems to have been missed by Brooks Atkinson and by the anonymous critic of the Guardian is that such events could happen in reality, and would shock us into silence. When they are contrived to happen in literature they produce, not the shock, but the "hilarious incredulity"—no matter how skillfully or artistically they are contrived. The mechanism of denial is a very powerful defensive operation for many of us. We do not deny the plane bomber, Graham, *after* he has acted; we do not deny Gein, the necrophiliac, *after* he has acted; but we would strenuously deny the probability of such behavior, by human beings, before they take place—and the novel essentially enters the realm of probability and credibility, the realm of "this could be."

Here, I am not talking of the psychiatrist and psychologist, to whom anything in possible human behaviour is probable, but of the reading public at its several levels of intelligence and sophistication. What happens in reality, particularly with respect to violence, murder and cannibalism, is often incredible and incomprehensible; to represent such reality within the demanded credible, comprehensible, framework of literature is a contradiction in terms. It is possible to achieve this goal, however, in poetry where these tight demands are not made (although, of course, other even stricter demands are made).

Dylan Thomas can write, in **The Burning Baby** of a preacher who incestuously seduces his daughter, then, in a wild hilltop scene, burns their bodies, watched from cover by his demented son. But I feel he can only escape "hilarious incredulity" because he is writing in a poetic form stemming from the unconscious and appealing to the unconscious. The novelist as a sensitive creator of human character is usually far superior to the psychologist. The novelist as psychologist, and most unfortunately in his portrayal of the psychologist, often operates at a level analogous to the physics of a Buck Rogers cartoon strip.

The technique of appeal, if the unscrupulous author wishes to use it, is becoming apparent. We are, perhaps, becoming increasingly tolerant to the portrayal of sexual details in literature, and this is healthy as long as they are presented in context and in balance. It would seem to be tasteless when such portrayal becomes the selling point of a book, rather than an idea. **Peyton Place** tends to evoke "hilarious incredulity," and **Return to Peyton Place** reminds this reader, at least, of the wartime British poster "Is this journey really necessary"? In **Peyton Place**, Metalious hits her enthralled (this was a best seller?) audience right in the groin, with the pornography of life and the pornography of death. Violence and sadism, attention to the act and details of killing rather than the meaning of murder, have become a selling point which may well exceed the drawing power of sex.

The literature of murder is enormous, and little more can be done in this chapter than to scan the great highlights and the unfortunately numerous lowlights. The selection may, to some small extent, interest the psychiatrist and the psychologist immersed in his technical battles and the unending struggle to understand and help the mentally ill, the unbalanced, the criminal. It is better in the long run if we psychiatrists and psychologists settle back to poetry and philosophy in our leisure reading. Too often this leisure time becomes technical browsing. The literature of murder often combines technical interest with compelling art, and may be a reasonable compromise between the text and the texture of life.

The selections presented here, although in some cases a trifle gruesome, do not in any sense compare with the horror of reality. It is my belief that no creative artist can ever match the insanity and savagery of certain aspects of human existence. There is no war novel to equal the fury and tragedy and misery of war — nor ever will be. Farmer Gein belongs to life, not literature — not because our sensitivities must be spared, but because the creative writer cannot, in these areas, match the darkness of human motivation and behaviour. The writer fails if his characters, good or evil, sick or well, are not believable, and here one faces a paradox. Many of the murderers of life, the Petiots, the Haarmans, the Kurtens, are not believable — they just exist; and by no stretch of the Freudian imagination does their behaviour become essentially understandable. Similarly, Jean-Paul Sartre, in **The Wall** and Leo Andreyev, in **The Seven Who Were Hanged** do not chill the blood as do the factual official statements on execution methods given in this book. The creative imagination of the great writer is pale in comparison with the febrile imagination and behaviour of Neville Heath — or our official executioners. If the novelist were to go that far, it would be too far.

REFERENCES

1. Bierce, Ambrose: *The Collected Writings of Ambrose Bierce.* New York, The Citadel Press, 1946.
2. Collier, J.: Thus I refute Beelzy. In Davenport, Basil (Ed.): *Tales to be Told in the Dark.* New York, Ballentine Books, 1953.
3. Dunsany, Lord: The two bottles of relish. In Davenport, Basil (Ed.): *Tales to be Told in the Dark.* New York, Ballentine Books, 1953.
4. Goncharov, Ivan: *Oblomov.* New York, Macmillian Company, 1929.
5. Munro, H. H.: *The Short Stories of Saki.* New York, The Viking Press Inc., 1930.
6. Reik, Theodor: *Myth and Guilt.* New York, George Braziller Inc., 1957.
7. Reik, Theodor: *The Compulsion to Confess.* New York, Farrar, Straus and Cudahy, 1959.
8. Robbe-Grillet, Alain: *Jealousy.* New York, Grove Press Inc., 1959.

INDEX